STEM CELL BIOLOGY: FUNDAMENTALS

Edited by
Dr Ashwani Kumar

ArclerPress

Stem Cell Biology: Fundamentals

Edited by Dr Ashwani Kumar

Edition 2018

Published by
Arcler Press LLC
708 3rd Avenue, 6th Floor
New York
NY 10017
United States of America
www.arclerpress.com

ISBN: 978-1-68094-538-6 (Hardback)

Printed in United States of America

Library of Congress Control Number: 2017933111

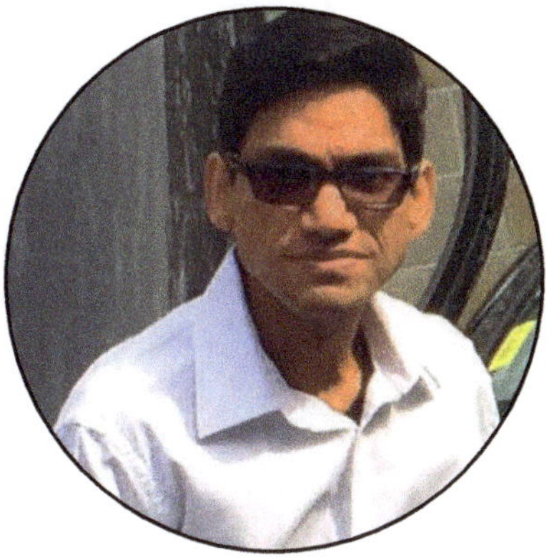

About the Editor

Dr Ashwani Kumar

Ashwani obtained his Master's degree in Clinical Pharmacology from Delhi University, India in 2007. Over the years, he has handled roles of increasing responsibilities including developing, reviewing, and approving medical and scientific literature and communications, e.g. manuscripts, and abstracts for the high indexed peer-reviewed journals; research proposal, posters, blogs, and articles. His major interest's areas include pharmacogenomics, onco-pharmacogenomics, and neuroscience. He is currently working as freelance healthcare consultant at Sydney, Australia.

Table of Contents

2 INDUCED STEM CELLS

3 STEM-CELL THERAPY

4 CELL POTENCY

5 STEM CELL LAWS AND POLICY

6 CANCER AND STEM CELL

7 STEM CELL CONTROVERSY

8 SPINAL CORD: STRUCTURE AND FUNCTION

9 EPIGENETICS IN STEM-CELL DIFFERENTIATION

List of Abbreviations

BPAI	Board of Patent Appeals and Interferences
BMP	Bone morphogenetic protein
CMC	Cambial Meristematic Cells
CSC	Cancer stem cell
CNS	Central nervous system
CAFC	Cobblestone area-forming cell
CMP	Common myeloid progenitor
CRC	Conditionally Reprogrammed Cells
CAFC	Court of Appeals for the Federal Circuit
DC	Dendritic cells
ES	Embryonic stem
ESC	Embryonic stem cell
EPC	Endothelial progenitor cells
EGF	Epidermal growth factor
EMT	Epithelial-mesenchymal transition
ECM	Extracellular matrices
FACS	Fluorescence-activated cell sorting
GFAP	Glial fibrillary acidic protein
GMP	Granulocyte-macrophage progenitor
HSC	Hematopoietic stem cells
IVF	In vitro fertilization
iPSC	Induced pluripotent stem cells
ICM	Inner cell mass

IVF	Intervertebral foramen
LIF	Leukemia inhibitory factor
LRPs	Lineage-restricted progenitor cells
MEP	Megakaryocyte-erythroid progenitor
MSCs	Mesenchymal stem cells
MSCs	Mesenchymal Stromal Cells
MSC	Migrating cancer stem cells
MEFs	Mouse embryonic fibroblasts
MDR	Multidrug resistance
MPPs	Multipotent progenitor cells
NSPCs	Neural stem cells and progenitors
OEC's	Olfactory ensheathing cells
OIS	oncogene-induced senescence
PGD	Prenatal genetic diagnosis
RGCs	Radial glial cells
RS	Replicative senescence
RBPs	RNA binding proteins
RAM	Root apical meristem
STT	Schirmer tear tests
SAM	Shoot apical meristem
SCNT	Somatic-cell nuclear transfer
SCOTS	Stem Cell Ophthalmology Treatment Study
SVZ	Subventricular zone
USPTO	US Patent and Trademark Office
VPL	Ventral posterolateral nucleus
VM	Ventromedial
YAP	Yes-associated protein

Preface

Stem cells are mother cells that have the potential to become any type of cell in the body. One of the main characteristics of stem cells is their ability to self-renew or multiply while maintaining the potential to develop into other types of cells. Stem cells can become cells of the blood, heart, bones, skin, muscles, brain etc. There are different sources of stem cells but all types of stem cells have the same capacity to develop into multiple types of cells. Stem cells are the foundation for every organ and tissue in your body. There are many different types of stem cells that come from different places in the body or are formed at different times in our lives. These include embryonic stem cells that exist only at the earliest stages of development and various types of tissue-specific (or adult) stem cells that appear during fetal development and remain in our bodies throughout life. All stem cells can self-renew and differentiate. Beyond these two critical abilities, though, stem cells vary widely in what they can and cannot do and in the circumstances under which they can and cannot do certain things. Stem cells have the remarkable potential to develop into many different cell types in the body during early life and growth. In addition, in many tissues they serve as a sort of internal repair system, dividing essentially without limit to replenish other cells as long as the person or animal is still alive. When a stem cell divides, each new cell has the potential either to remain a stem cell or become another type of cell with a more specialized function, such as a muscle cell, a red blood cell, or a brain cell. Stem cells are distinguished from other cell types by two important characteristics. First, they are unspecialized cells capable of renewing themselves through cell division, sometimes after long periods of inactivity. Second, under certain physiologic or experimental conditions, they can be induced to become tissue- or organ-specific cells with special functions. In some organs, such as the gut and bone marrow, stem cells regularly divide to repair and replace worn out or damaged tissues. In other organs, however, such as the pancreas and the heart, stem cells only divide under special conditions. Stem cell research is improving by leaps and bounds. These may soon become the basis for treating diseases such as Parkinson's disease, diabetes, heart failure, cerebral palsy, heart disease and host of other chronic ailments. Stem cells may also be used for screening new drugs and toxins and understanding birth defects without subjecting human volunteers to the toxins and drugs.

Content Coverage

Chapters One and *Two* present an introduction of stem cells and induced stem cells, correspondingly.

Chapters Three and *Four* present a coverage of stem cell therapy and cell potency, respectively. Stem-cell therapy is the use of stem cells to treat or prevent a disease or condition. Bone marrow transplant is the most widely used stem-cell therapy, but some therapies derived from umbilical cord blood are also in use.

Chapter Five is intended to focus on stem cell laws and policy in different countries.

Stem cells have been used to repair tissue damaged by disease or age. Cloning also might be done with stem cells. Pluripotent stem cells can also be derived from Somatic cell nuclear transfer which is a laboratory technique where a clone embryo is created from a donor nucleus. Somatic cell nuclear transfer is also tightly regulated amongst various countries.

Chapter Six presents an overview of cancer stem cells that possess characteristics associated with normal stem cells, specifically the ability to give rise to all cell types found in a particular cancer sample.

Chapter Seven focuses on stem cell controversy which is the consideration of the ethics of research involving the development, use, and destruction of human embryos.

Chapters Eight and Nine present about spinal cord and epigenetics in stem cell differentiation. The spinal cord has three major functions: as a conduit for motor information, which travels down the spinal cord, as a conduit for sensory information in the reverse direction, and finally as a center for coordinating certain reflexes. Epigenetics, however, has been used to refer to changes in gene expression, which are heritable through modifications not affecting the DNA sequence.

CHAPTER 1

Stem Cells: An Overview

Chapter Contents

Stem cells are special cells in multicellular organisms that are capable of differentiating into a wide range of other cells as needed. In other words, the cells themselves are not specialized, like blood cells, nerve cells, and so forth, but they can make specialized cells to form an embryo or repair damage to an adult organism. This property has suggested that they could be extremely useful in medical treatment, and many nations have established stem cell funding to explore the possibility of research and development.

All multicellular organisms actually start out as a cluster of stem cells. As they divide and multiply, they differentiate themselves to make organs, muscle, bone, and so forth until a complete embryo is formed. Adults also have stem cells, although their precise origin is not fully understood. These adult cells trigger in response to serious injury to replace damaged tissues.

INTRODUCTION

Stem cells are undifferentiated biological cells that can differentiate into specialized cells and can divide (through mitosis) to produce more stem cells. They are found in multicellular organisms. In mammals, there are two broad types of stem cells: embryonic stem cells, which are isolated from the inner cell mass of blastocysts, and adult stem cells, which are found in various tissues. In adult organisms, stem cells and progenitor cells act as a repair system for the body, replenishing adult tissues. In a developing embryo, stem cells can differentiate into all the specialized cells—ectoderm, endoderm and mesoderm (see induced pluripotent stem cells)—but also maintain the normal turnover of regenerative organs, such as blood, skin, or intestinal tissues.

There are three known accessible sources of autologous adult stem cells in humans:

- Bone marrow, which requires extraction by *harvesting*, that is, drilling into bone (typically the femur or iliac crest).
- Adipose tissue (lipid cells), which requires extraction by liposuction.
- Blood, which requires extraction through apheresis, wherein blood is drawn from the donor (similar to a blood donation), and passed through a machine that extracts the stem cells and returns other portions of the blood to the donor.

Stem cells can also be taken from umbilical cord blood just after birth. Of all stem cell types, autologous harvesting involves the least risk. By definition, autologous cells are obtained from one's own body, just as one may bank his or her own blood for elective surgical procedures.

Adult stem cells are frequently used in various medical therapies (e.g., bone marrow transplantation). Stem cells can now be artificially grown and transformed (differentiated) into specialized cell types with characteristics consistent with cells of various tissues such as muscles or nerves. Embryonic cell lines and autologous embryonic stem cells generated through somatic cell nuclear transfer or dedifferentiation have also been proposed as promising candidates for future therapies. Research into stem cells grew out of findings by Ernest A. McCulloch and James E. Till at the University of Toronto in the 1960s.

PROPERTIES

The classical definition of a stem cell requires that it possess two properties:

- *Self-renewal*: the ability to go through numerous cycles of cell division while maintaining the undifferentiated state.
- *Potency*: the capacity to differentiate into specialized cell types. In the strictest sense, this requires stem cells to be either totipotent or pluripotent—to be able to give rise to any mature cell type, although multipotent or unipotent progenitor cells are sometimes referred to as stem cells. Apart from this it is said that stem cell function is regulated in a feedback mechanism.

Self-Renewal

Two mechanisms exist to ensure that a stem cell population is maintained:

- Obligatory asymmetric replication: a stem cell divides into one mother cell that is identical to the original stem cell, and another daughter cell that is differentiated.
- Stochastic differentiation: when one stem cell develops into two differentiated daughter cells, another stem cell undergoes mitosis and produces two stem cells identical to the original.

Potency Definition

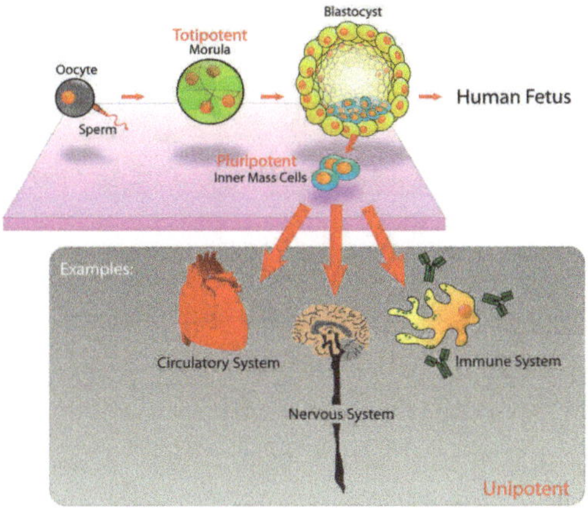

Pluripotent, embryonic stem cells originate as inner cell mass (ICM) cells within a blastocyst. These stem cells can become any tissue in the body, excluding a placenta. Only cells from an earlier stage of the embryo, known as the morula, are totipotent, able to become all tissues in the body and the extraembryonic placenta.

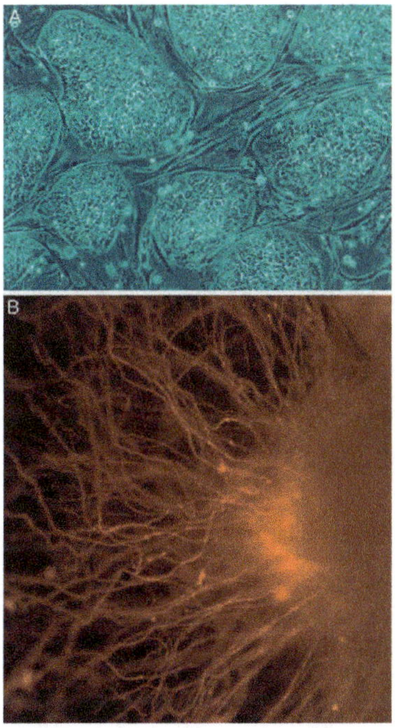

Human embryonic stem cells

A: Stem cell colonies that are not yet differentiated.

B: Nerve cells, an example of a cell type after differentiation.

Potency specifies the differentiation potential (the potential to differentiate into different cell types) of the stem cell.

- Totipotent (a.k.a. omnipotent) stem cells can differentiate into embryonic and extraembryonic cell types. Such cells can construct a complete, viable organism. These cells are produced from the fusion of an egg and sperm cell. Cells produced by the first few divisions of the fertilized egg are also totipotent.
- Pluripotent stem cells are the descendants of totipotent cells and can differentiate into nearly all cells, i.e. cells derived from any of the three germ layers.
- Multipotent stem cells can differentiate into a number of cell types, but only those of a closely related family of cells.
- Oligopotent stem cells can differentiate into only a few cell types, such as lymphoid or myeloid stem cells.
- Unipotent cells can produce only one cell type, their own, but have the property of self-renewal, which distinguishes them from non-stem cells (e.g. progenitor cells, which cannot self-renew).

Identification

In practice, stem cells are identified by whether they can regenerate tissue. For example, the defining test for bone marrow or hematopoietic stem cells (HSCs) is the ability to transplant the cells and save an individual without HSCs. This demonstrates that the cells can produce new blood cells over a long term. It should also be possible to isolate stem cells from the transplanted individual, which can themselves be transplanted into another individual without HSCs, demonstrating that the stem cell was able to self-renew.

Properties of stem cells can be illustrated *in vitro*, using methods such as clonogenic assays, in which single cells are assessed for their ability to differentiate and self-renew. Stem cells can also be isolated by their possession of a distinctive set of cell surface markers. However, *in vitro* culture conditions can alter the behavior of cells, making it unclear whether the cells shall behave in a similar manner *in vivo*. There is considerable debate as to whether some proposed adult cell populations are truly stem cells.

EMBRYONIC

Embryonic stem (ES) cells are the cells of the inner cell mass of a blastocyst, an early-stage embryo.Human embryos reach the blastocyst stage 4–5 days post fertilization, at which time they consist of 50–150 cells. ES cells are pluripotent and give rise during development to all derivatives of the three primary germ layers: ectoderm, endoderm and mesoderm. In other words, they can develop into each of the more than 200 cell types of the adult body when given sufficient and necessary stimulation for a specific cell type. They do not contribute to the extra-embryonic membranes or the placenta.

During embryonic development these inner cell mass cells continuously divide and become more specialized. For example, a portion of the ectoderm in the dorsal part of the embryo specializes as ‹neurectoderm›, which will become the future central nervous system. Later in development, neurulation causes the neurectoderm to form the neural tube. At the neural tube stage, the anterior portion undergoes encephalization to generate or 'pattern' the basic form of the brain. At this stage of development, the principal cell type of the CNS is considered a neural stem cell. These neural stem cells are pluripotent, as they can generate a large diversity of many different neuron types, each with unique gene expression, morphological, and functional characteristics. The process of generating neurons from stem cells is called neurogenesis. One prominent example of a neural stem cell is the radial glial cell, so named because it has a distinctive bipolar morphology with highly elongated processes spanning the thickness of the neural tube wall, and because historically it shared some glial characteristics, most notably the expression of glial fibrillary acidic protein (GFAP). The radial glial cell is the primary neural stem cell of the developing vertebrate CNS, and its cell body resides in the ventricular zone, adjacent to the developing ventricular system. Neural stem cells are committed to the neuronal lineages (neurons, astrocytes, and oligodendrocytes), and thus their potency is restricted.

Nearly all research to date has made use of mouse embryonic stem cells (mES) or human embryonic stem cells (hES) derived from the early inner cell mass. Both have the essential stem cell characteristics, yet they require very different environments in order to maintain an undifferentiated state. Mouse ES cells are grown on a layer of gelatin as an extracellular matrix (for support) and require the presence of leukemia inhibitory factor (LIF) in serum media. A drug cocktail containing inhibitors to GSK3B and the MAPK/ERK pathway, called 2i, has also been shown to maintain pluripotency in stem cell culture. Human ES cells are grown on a feeder layer of mouse embryonic fibroblasts (MEFs) and require the presence of basic fibroblast growth factor (bFGF or FGF-2). Without optimal culture conditions or genetic manipulation, embryonic stem cells will rapidly differentiate.

A human embryonic stem cell is also defined by the expression of several transcription factors and cell surface proteins. The transcription factors Oct-4, Nanog, and Sox2 form the core regulatory network that ensures the suppression of genes that lead to differentiation and the maintenance of pluripotency. The cell surface antigens most commonly used to identify hES cells are the glycolipids stage specific embryonic antigen 3 and 4 and the keratan sulfate antigens Tra-1-60 and Tra-1-81. By using human embryonic stem cells to produce specialized cells like nerve cells or heart cells in the lab, scientists can gain access to adult human cells without taking tissue from patients. They can then study these specialized adult cells in detail to try and catch complications of diseases, or to study cells reactions to potentially new drugs. The molecular definition of a stem cell includes many more proteins and continues to be a topic of research.

There are currently no approved treatments using embryonic stem cells. The first human trial was approved by the US Food and Drug Administration in January 2009. However, the human trial was not initiated until October 13, 2010 in Atlanta for spinal cord injury research. On November 14, 2011 the company conducting the trial (Geron Corporation) announced that it will discontinue further development of its stem cell programs. ES cells, being pluripotent cells, require specific signals for correct differentiation—if injected directly into another body, ES cells will differentiate into many different types of cells, causing a teratoma. Differentiating ES cells into usable cells while avoiding transplant rejection are just a few of the hurdles that embryonic stem cell researchers still face. Due to ethical considerations, many nations currently have moratoria or limitations on either human ES cell research or the production of new human ES cell lines. Because of their combined abilities of unlimited expansion and pluripotency, embryonic stem cells remain a theoretically potential source for regenerative medicine and tissue replacement after injury or disease.

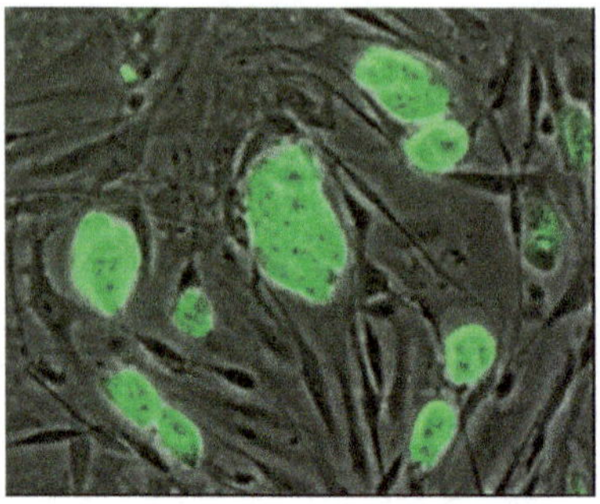

Mouse embryonic stem cells with fluorescent marker

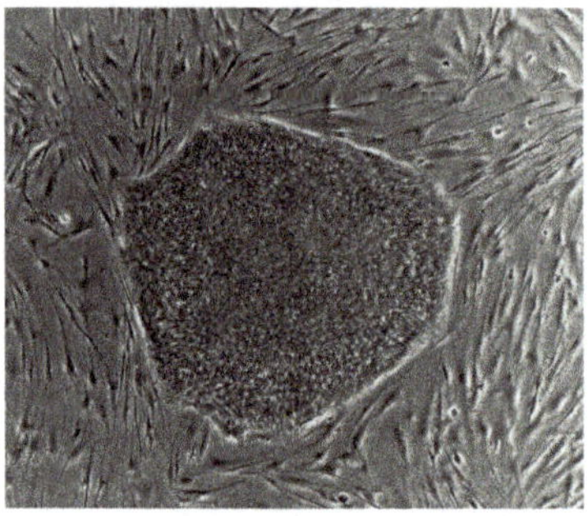

Human embryonic stem cell colony on mouse embryonic fibroblast feeder layer

FETAL

The primitive stem cells located in the organs of fetuses are referred to as fetal stem cells. There are two types of fetal stem cells:

- Fetal proper stem cells come from the tissue of the fetus proper, and are generally obtained after an abortion. These stem cells are not immortal but have a high level of division and are multipotent.
- Extraembryonic fetal stem cells come from extraembryonic membranes, and are generally not distinguished from adult stem cells. These stem cells are acquired after birth, they are not immortal but have a high level of cell division, and are pluripotent.

ADULT

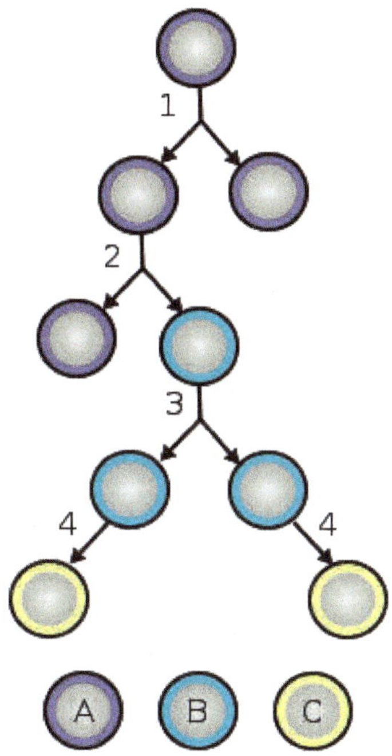

Stem cell division and differentiation. A: stem cell; B: progenitor cell; C: differentiated cell; 1: symmetric stem cell division; 2: asymmetric stem cell division; 3: progenitor division; 4: terminal differentiation.

Adult stem cells, also called somatic (from Greek σωματικός, "of the body") stem cells, are stem cells which maintain and repair the tissue in which they are found. They can be found in children, as well as adults.

Pluripotent adult stem cells are rare and generally small in number, but they can be found in umbilical cord blood and other tissues. Bone marrow is a rich source of adult stem cells, which have been used in treating several conditions including liver cirrhosis, chronic limb ischemia and endstage heart failure. The quantity of bone marrow stem cells declines with age and is greater in males than females during reproductive years. Much adult stem cell research to date has aimed to characterize their potency and self-renewal capabilities. DNA damage accumulates with age in both stem cells and the cells that comprise the stem cell environment. This accumulation is considered to be responsible, at least in part, for increasing stem cell dysfunction with aging (see DNA damage theory of aging).

Most adult stem cells are lineage-restricted (multipotent) and are generally referred to by their tissue origin (mesenchymal stem cell, adipose-derived stem cell, endothelial stem cell, dental pulp stem cell, etc.).Muse cells (multi-lineage differentiating stress enduring cells) are a recently discovered pluripotent stem cell type found in multiple adult tissues, including adipose, dermal fibroblasts, and bone marrow. While rare, muse cells are identifiable by their expression of SSEA-3, a marker for undifferentiated stem cells, and general mesenchymal stem cells markers such as CD105. When subjected to single cell suspension culture, the cells will generate clusters that are similar to embryoid bodies in morphology as well as gene expression, including canonical pluripotency markers Oct4, Sox2, and Nanog.

Adult stem cell treatments have been successfully used for many years to treat leukemia and related bone/blood cancers through bone marrow transplants. Adult stem cells are also used in veterinary medicine to treat tendon and ligament injuries in horses.

The use of adult stem cells in research and therapy is not as controversial as the use of embryonic stem cells, because the production of adult stem cells does not require the destruction of an embryo. Additionally, in instances where adult stem cells are obtained from the intended recipient (an autograft), the risk of rejection is essentially non-existent. Consequently, more US government funding is being provided for adult stem cell research.

AMNIOTIC

Multipotent stem cells are also found in amniotic fluid. These stem cells are very active, expand extensively without feeders and are not tumorigenic. Amniotic stem cells are multipotent and can differentiate in cells of adipogenic, osteogenic, myogenic, endothelial, hepatic and also neuronal lines. Amniotic stem cells are a topic of active research.

Use of stem cells from amniotic fluid overcomes the ethical objections to using human embryos as a source of cells. Roman Catholic teaching forbids the use of embryonic stem cells in experimentation; accordingly, the Vatican newspaper “Osservatore Romano called amniotic stem cells the future of medicine.

It is possible to collect amniotic stem cells for donors or for autologuous use: the first US amniotic stem cells bank was opened in 2009 in Medford, MA, by Biocell Center Corporation and collaborates with various hospitals and universities all over the world.

INDUCED PLURIPOTENT

Adult stem cells have limitations with their potency; unlike ESCs, they are not able to differentiate into cells from all three germ layers. As such, they are deemed multipotent.

However, reprogramming allows for the creation of pluripotent cells, induced pluripotent stem cells, from adult cells. It is important to note that these are not adult stem cells, but adult cells (e.g. epithelial cells) reprogrammed to give rise to cells with pluripotent capabilities. Using genetic reprogramming with protein transcription factors, pluripotent stem cells with ESC-like capabilities have been derived. The first demonstration of Induced Pluripotent Stem Cells was conducted by Shinya Yamanaka and his colleagues at Kyoto University. They used the transcription factors Oct3/4, Sox2, c-Myc, and Klf4 to reprogram mouse fibroblast cells into pluripotent cells. Subsequent work was able to induce pluripotency in human derived cells. Yamanaka›s research group was able to induce pluripotency in human fibroblast cells using the four Yamanaka Factors. Junying Yu, James Thomson, and their colleagues at the University of Wisconsin–Madison used a different set of factors, Oct4, Sox2, Nanog and Lin28, and carried out their experiments using cells from human foreskin. However, they were able to replicate Yamanaka›s finding that inducing pluripotency in human cells was possible. It is important to note that iPSCs and ESCs are not equivalent. They have many similar properties, such as pluripotency and differentiation potential, the expression of pluripotency genes, epigenetic patterns, embryoid body and teratoma formation, and viable chimera formation.However, similar does not mean they are the same. In fact, there are many differences within these properties. Importantly, the chromatin of iPSCs appears to be more closed or methylated than that of ESCs. Similarly, the gene expression pattern between ESCs and iPSCs, or even iPSCs sourced from different origins. There are thus questions about the completeness of reprogramming and the somatic memory of induced pluripotent stem cells. Despite this, inducing adult cells to be pluripotent appears to be viable.

As a result of the success of these experiments, Ian Wilmut, who helped create the first cloned animal Dolly the Sheep, has announced that he will abandon somatic cell nuclear transfer as an avenue of research.

Furthermore, induced pluripotent stem cells provide several therapeutic advantages. Like ESCs, they are pluripotent. They thus have great differentiation potential; theoretically, they could produce any cell within the human body (if reprogramming to pluripotency was "complete").Moreover, unlike ESCs, they potentially could allow doctors to create a pluripotent stem cell line for each individual patient. In fact, frozen blood samples can be used as a source of induced pluripotent stem cells, opening a new avenue for obtaining the valued cells. Patient specific stem cells allow for the screening for side affects before drug treatment, as well as the reduced risk of transplantation rejection. Despite their current limited use therapeutically, iPSCs hold create potential for future use in medical treatment and research.

LINEAGE

To ensure self-renewal, stem cells undergo two types of cell division (see *Stem cell division and differentiation* diagram). Symmetric division gives rise to two identical daughter cells both endowed with stem cell properties. Asymmetric division, on the other hand, produces only one stem cell and a progenitor cell with limited self-renewal potential. Progenitors can go through several rounds of cell division before terminally differentiating into a mature cell. It is possible that the molecular distinction between symmetric and asymmetric divisions lies in differential segregation of cell membrane proteins (such as receptors) between the daughter cells.

An alternative theory is that stem cells remain undifferentiated due to environmental cues in their particular niche. Stem cells differentiate when they leave that niche or no longer receive those signals. Studies in *Drosophila* germarium have identified the signals decapentaplegic and adherens junctions that prevent germarium stem cells from differentiating.

TREATMENTS

Stem cell therapy is the use of stem cells to treat or prevent a disease or condition. Bone marrow transplant is a form of stem cell therapy that has been used for many years without controversy. No stem cell therapies other than bone marrow transplant are widely used.

Disadvantages

Stem cell treatments may require immunosuppression because of a requirement for radiation before the transplant to remove the person's previous cells, or because the patient's immune system may target the stem cells. One approach to avoid the second possibility is to use stem cells from the same patient who is being treated.

Pluripotency in certain stem cells could also make it difficult to obtain a specific cell type. It is also difficult to obtain the exact cell type needed, because not all cells in a population differentiate uniformly. Undifferentiated cells can create tissues other than desired types.

Some stem cells form tumors after transplantation; pluripotency is linked to tumor formation especially in embryonic stem cells, fetal proper stem cells, induced pluripotent stem cells. Fetal proper stem cells form tumors despite multipotency.

RESEARCH

Some of the fundamental patents covering human embryonic stem cells are owned by the Wisconsin Alumni Research Foundation (WARF) – they are patents 5,843,780, 6,200,806, and 7,029,913 invented by James A. Thomson. WARF does not enforce these patents against academic scientists, but does enforce them against companies.

In 2006, a request for the US Patent and Trademark Office (USPTO) to re-examine the three patents was filed by the Public Patent Foundation on behalf of its client, the non-profit patent-watchdog group Consumer Watchdog (formerly the Foundation for Taxpayer and Consumer Rights). In the re-examination process, which involves several rounds of discussion between the USTPO and the parties, the USPTO initially agreed with Consumer Watchdog and rejected all the claims in all three patents, however in response, WARF amended the claims of all three patents to make them more narrow, and in 2008 the USPTO found the amended claims in all three patents to be patentable. The decision on one of the patents (7,029,913) was appealable, while the decisions on the other two were not. Consumer Watchdog appealed the granting of the '913 patent to the USTPO's Board of Patent Appeals and Interferences (BPAI) which granted the appeal, and in 2010 the BPAI decided that the amended claims of the ‹913 patent were not patentable. However, WARF was able to re-open prosecution of the case and did so, amending the claims of the ‹913 patent again to make them more narrow, and in January 2013 the amended claims were allowed.

In July 2013, Consumer Watchdog announced that it would appeal the decision to allow the claims of the ‹913 patent to the US Court of Appeals for the Federal Circuit (CAFC), the federal appeals court that hears patent cases. At a hearing in December 2013, the CAFC raised the question of whether Consumer Watchdog had legal standing to appeal; the case could not proceed until that issue was resolved.

Treatment

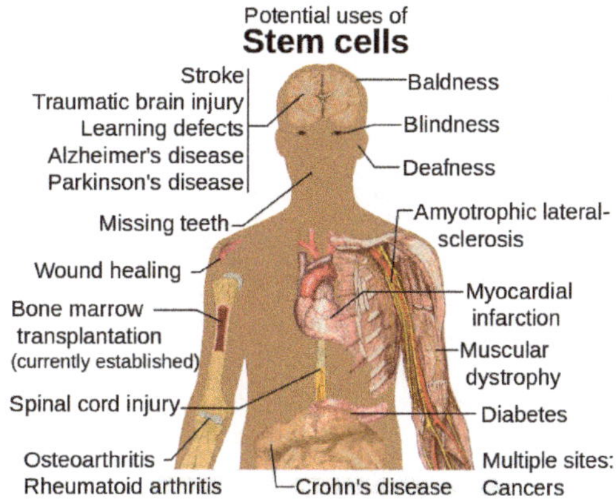

Diseases and conditions where stem cell treatment is being investigated.

Diseases and conditions where stem cell treatment is being investigated include:

- Diabetes
- Rheumatoid arthritis
- Parkinson's disease
- Alzheimer's disease
- Osteoarthritis
- Stroke and traumatic brain injury repair
- Learning disability due to congenital disorder
- Spinal cord injury repair
- Heart infarction
- Anti-cancer treatments
- Baldness reversal
- Replace missing teeth
- Repair hearing
- Restore vision and repair damage to the cornea
- Amyotrophic lateral sclerosis
- Crohn›s disease
- Wound healing
- Male infertility due to absence of spermatogonial stem cells

Research is underway to develop various sources for stem cells, and to apply stem cell treatments for neurodegenerative diseases and conditions, diabetes, heart disease, and other conditions. Research is also underway in generating organoids using stem cells, which would allow for further understanding of human development, organogenesis, and modeling of human diseases.

In more recent years, with the ability of scientists to isolate and culture embryonic stem cells, and with scientists› growing ability to create stem cells using somatic cell nuclear transfer and techniques to create induced pluripotent stem cells, controversy has crept in, both related to abortion politics and to human cloning.

Hepatotoxicity and drug-induced liver injury account for a substantial number of failures of new drugs in development and market withdrawal, highlighting the need for screening assays such as stem cell-derived hepatocyte-like cells, that are capable of detecting toxicity early in the drug development process.

PLANT STEM CELL

Plant stem cells are innately undifferentiated cells located in the meristems of plants. Plant stem cells serve as the origin of plant vitality, as they maintain themselves while providing a steady supply of precursor cells to form differentiated tissues and organs in plants. Two distinct areas of stem cells are recognised: the apical meristem and the lateral meristem.

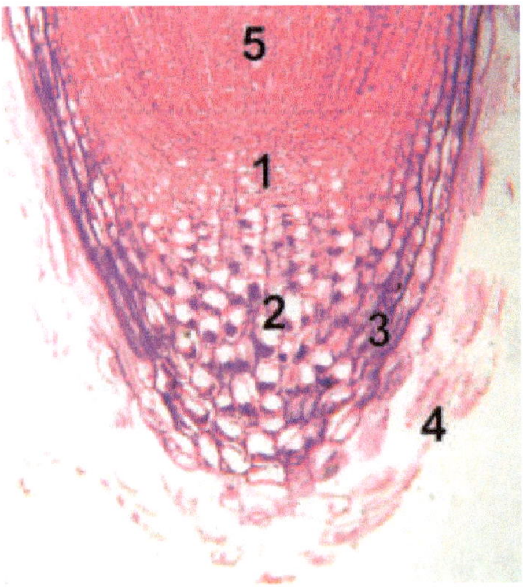

Root tip (10X) 1) Meristem; 2)Columelle 3)Lateral part of the tip; 4)Dead Cells; 5)Elongation zone.

Plant stem cells are characterized by two distinctive properties, which are: the ability to create all differentiated cell types and the ability to self-renew such that the number of stem cells is maintained.Plant stem cells never undergo aging process but immortally give rise to new specialized and unspecialized cells, and they have the potential to grow into any organ, tissue, or cell in the body. Thus they are totipotent cells equipped with regenerative powers that facilitate plant growth and production of new organs throughout lifetime.

Unlike animals, plants are immobile. As plants cannot escape from danger by taking motion, they need a special mechanism to withstand various and sometimes unforeseen environmental stress. Here, what empowers them to withstand harsh external influence and preserve life is stem cell. In fact, plants comprise the oldest and the largest living organisms on earth, including Bristlecone Pines in California, U.S. (4,842 years old), and the Giant Sequoia in mountainous regions of California, U.S. (87 meters in height and 2,000 tons in weight). This is possible because they have a modular body plan that enables them to survive substantial damage by initiating continuous and repetitive formation of new structures and organs such as leaves and flowers.

Plant stem cells are also characterized by their location in specialized structures called meristematic tissues, which are located in root apical meristem (RAM), shoot apical meristem (SAM), and vascular system ((pro)cambium or vascular meristem.)

Research and Development

Traditionally, plant stem cells were thought to only exist in SAM and RAM and studies were conducted based on this assumption. However, recent studies have indicated that (pro)cambium also serves as a niche for plant stem cells: "Procambium cells fulfill the criteria for being stem cells since they have the capacity for long-term self renewal and being able to differentiate into one or more specialized cell types."

- **Cambium** is a type of meristem with thin walls which minutely exist in small populations within a plant. Due to this structural characteristic, once physical force is applied to it, it is easily damaged in the very process of isolation, losing its stem cell characteristics. Despite 160 years of biological effort to isolate and retrieve plant stem cells, none succeeded in the isolation due to the distinct structural characteristics of plant stem cell: "[t]he cambium consists of a few layers of narrow elongated, thin-walled cells, easily damaged during sampling." This highly vulnerable feature has made studies on cambial structure and ultrastructure difficult to achieve with conventional methods. Thus failure to isolate plant stem cells from meristematic tissues prompted scientists to administer plant cell culture by using callus (dedifferentiated cells) as an alternative to plant stem cells.
- **Callus**, or dedifferentiated cells, are somatic cells that undergo dedifferentiation to give rise to totipotent embryogenic cells, which temporarily gains the ability to proliferate and/or regenerate an embryo. Since embryogenic cells were considered totipotent cells based on their ability to regenerate or develop into an embryo under given conditions, dedifferentiated cells were generally regarded as stem cells of plant: ...we propose to extend the concept of stem cells to include embryogenic stem cells that arise from plant somatic cells. We examine the cellular, physiological and molecular similarities and differences between plant meristematic stem cells and embryogenic stem cells originating directly from single somatic cells.

Plant stem cell vs. Callus

Despite that callus exhibits a number of stem cell-like properties for a temporary period and that it has been cultured for useful plant compounds as an alternative source of plant stem cell, callus and plant stem cell are fundamentally different from each other. Callus is similar to plant stem cell in its ability to differentiate, but the two are different in their origin. While plant stem cell exists in the meristematic tissues of plant, callus is obtained as a temporary response to cure wounds in somatic cell.

Moreover, callus undergoes dedifferentiation as differentiated cells acquire ability to differentiate; but genetic variation is inevitable in the process because the cells consist of somatic undifferentiated cells from an adult subject plant. Unlike true stem cells, callus is heterogeneous. Due to this reason, continuous and stable cell division of callus is difficult. Hence plant stem cell originated from cambium is an immortal cell while callus is a temporary dediffertiated cell obtained from stimulating the somatic cell.

Furthermore, the ability to differentiate and proliferate is different that differences between plant stem cell and callus are prevalent in culture and research. Only plant stem cells embedded in meristems can divide and give rise to cells that differentiate while giving rise to new stem cells. These immortal cells divide infinitely.

Bioprocess Innovation

Plant cells are cultured to acquire plant useful compounds. However cell cultures are often hindered by various factors especially if cell culture continues long-term. However, strong vitality and structural characteristics of plant stem cell overcome previous drawbacks to plant cell culture. Thus plant stem cell culture is the most ideal and productive method of cell culture and phytochemical production as cells are successfully mass cultured while maintaining quality.

Further Applications

Numerous medicines, perfumes, pigments, antimicrobials, and insecticides are derived from plant natural products. Cultured **C**ambial **M**eristematic **C**ells (CMC) may provide a cost-effective, environmentally friendly, and sustainable source of important natural products, including paclitaxel. Unlike plant cultivation, this approach is not subject to the unpredictability caused by variation in climatic conditions or political instability in certain part of the world. Also, CMCs from reference specifies may also provide an important biological tool to explore plant stem cell function.

In 2010, researchers from the Plant Stem Cell Institute (formerly Unhwa Institute of Science and Technology) presented their data to the world via Nature Biotechnology. Their research demonstrated the world's first cambial meristematic cell isolation. Due to the valuable and beneficial compounds for human health (i.e. paclitaxel) which are secreted by the CMC's, this technology is considered a serious breakthrough in plant biotechnology.

STEM CELL CONTROVERSY

The **stem cell controversy** is the consideration of the ethics of research involving the development, use, and destruction of human embryos. Most commonly, this controversy focuses on embryonic stem cells. Not all stem cell research involves the human embryos. For example, adult stem cells, amniotic stem cells, and induced pluripotent stem cells do not involve creating, using, or destroying human embryos, thus are minimally, if at all, controversial. Many less controversial sources of acquiring stem cells include using cells from the umbilical cord, breast milk, and bone marrow, which are not pluripotent.

For many decades, stem cells have played an important role in medical research, beginning in 1868 when Ernst Haeckel first used the phrase to describe the fertilized egg which eventually gestates into an organism. The term was later used in 1886 by William Sedgwick to describe the parts of a plant that grow and regenerate. Further work by Alexander Maximow and Leroy Stevens introduced the concept that stem cells are pluripotent, i.e. able to become many types of different cell. This significant discovery led to the first human bone marrow transplant by E. Donnal Thomas in 1968, which although successful in saving lives, has generated much controversy since. This has included the many complications inherent in stem cell transplantation (almost 200 allogeneic marrow transplants were performed in humans, with no long-term successes before the first successful treatment was made), through to more modern problems, such as how many cells are sufficient for engraftment of various types of hematopoietic stem cell transplants, whether older patients should undergo transplant therapy, and the role of irradiation-based therapies in preparation for transplantation.

The discovery of adult stem cells led scientists to develop an interest in the role of embroynic stem cells, and in separate studies in 1981 Gail Martin and Martin Evans derived pluripotent stem cells from the embryos of mice for the first time. This paved the way for Mario Capecchi, Martin Evans, and Oliver Smithies to create the first knockout mouse, ushering in a whole new era of research on human disease.

In 1998, James Thomson and Jeffrey Jones derived the first human embryonic stem cells, with even greater potential for drug discovery and therapeutic transplantation. However, the use of the technique on human embryos led to more widespread controversy as criticism of the technique now began from the wider non-scientific public who debated the moral ethics of questions concerning research involving human embryonic cells.

Potential use in Therapy

Since pluripotent stem cells have the ability to differentiate into any type of cell, they are used in the development of medical treatments for a wide range of conditions. Treatments that have been proposed include treatment for physical trauma, degenerative conditions, and genetic diseases (in combination with gene therapy). Yet further treatments using stem cells could potentially be developed due to their ability to repair extensive tissue damage.

Great levels of success and potential have been realized from research using adult stem cells. In early 2009, the FDA approved the first human clinical trials using embryonic stem cells. These can become any cell type of the body, excluding placental cells. This ability is called pluripotency. Only cells from an embryo at the morula stage or earlier are truly totipotent, meaning that they are able to form all cell types including placental cells. Adult stem cells are generally limited to differentiating into different cell types of their tissue of origin. However, some evidence suggests that adult stem cell plasticity may exist, increasing the number of cell types a given adult stem cell can become.

Points of Controversy

Many of the debates surrounding human embryonic stem cells concern issues such as what restrictions should be made on studies using these types of cells. At what point does one consider life to begin? Is it just to destroy an embryo cell if it has the potential to cure countless numbers of patients? Political leaders are debating how to regulate and fund research studies that involve the techniques used to remove the embryo cells. No clear consensus has emerged. Other recent discoveries may extinguish the need for embryonic stem cells.

Much of the criticism has been a result of religious beliefs, and in the most high-profile case, Christian US President George W Bush signed an executive order banning the use of federal funding for any cell lines other than those already in existence, stating at the time, "My position on these issues is shaped by deeply held beliefs," and "I also believe human life is a sacred gift from our creator." This ban was in part revoked by his successor Barack Obama, who stated As a person of faith, I believe we are called to care for each other and work to ease human suffering. I believe we have been given the capacity and will to pursue this research and the humanity and conscience to do so responsibly.

Potential Solutions

Some stem cell researchers are working to develop techniques of isolating stem cells that are as potent as embryonic stem cells, but do not require a human embryo.

Foremost among these was the discovery in August 2006 that adult cells can be reprogrammed into a pluripotent state by the introduction of four specific transcription factors, resulting in induced pluripotent stem cells. This major breakthrough won a Nobel Prize for the discoverers, Shinya Yamanaka and John Gurdon.

In an alternative technique, researchers at Harvard University, led by Kevin Eggan and Savitri Marajh, have transferred the nucleus of a somatic cell into an existing embryonic stem cell, thus creating a new stem cell line.

Researchers at Advanced Cell Technology, led by Robert Lanza and Travis Wahl, reported the successful derivation of a stem cell line using a process similar to preimplantation genetic diagnosis, in which a single blastomere is extracted from a blastocyst. At the 2007 meeting of the International Society for Stem Cell Research (ISSCR), Lanza announced that his team had succeeded in producing three new stem cell lines without destroying the parent embryos. These are the first human embryonic cell lines in existence that didn›t result from the destruction of an embryo. Lanza is currently in discussions with the National Institutes of Health to determine whether the new technique sidesteps U.S. restrictions on federal funding for ES cell research.

Anthony Atala of Wake Forest University says that the fluid surrounding the fetus has been found to contain stem cells that, when used correctly, "can be differentiated towards cell types such as fat, bone, muscle, blood vessel, nerve and liver cells". The extraction of this fluid is not thought to harm the fetus in any way. He hopes "that these cells will provide a valuable resource for tissue repair and for engineered organs, as well".

Viewpoints

The status of the human embryo and human embryonic stem cell research is a controversial issue, as with the present state of technology, the creation of a human embryonic stem cell line requires the destruction of a human embryo. Most of these embryos are discarded. Stem cell debates have motivated and reinvigorated the pro-life movement, whose members are concerned with the rights and status of the embryo as an early-aged human life. They believe that embryonic stem cell research instrumentalizes and violates the sanctity of life and is tantamount to murder. The fundamental assertion of those who oppose embryonic stem cell research is the belief that human life is inviolable, combined with the belief that human life begins when a sperm cell fertilizes an egg cell to form a single cell. The view of those in favor is that these embryos would otherwise be discarded, and if used as stem cells, they can survive as a part of a living human being.

A portion of stem cell researchers use embryos that were created but not used in *in vitro* fertility treatments to derive new stem cell lines. Most of these embryos are to be destroyed, or stored for long periods of time, long past their viable storage life. In the United States alone, an estimated at least 400,000 such embryos exist. This has led some opponents of abortion, such as Senator Orrin Hatch, to support human embryonic stem cell research. See also embryo donation.

Medical researchers widely report that stem cell research has the potential to dramatically alter approaches to understanding and treating diseases, and to alleviate suffering. In the future, most medical researchers anticipate being able to use technologies derived from stem cell research to treat a variety of diseases and impairments. Spinal cord injuries and Parkinson›s disease are two examples that have been championed by high-profile media personalities (for instance, Christopher Reeve and Michael J. Fox, who have lived with these conditions, respectively). The anticipated medical benefits of stem cell research add urgency to the debates, which has been appealed to by proponents of embryonic stem cell research.

In August 2000, The U.S. National Institutes of Health›s Guidelines stated:

...research involving human pluripotent stem cells...promises new treatments and possible cures for many debilitating diseases and injuries, including Parkinson›s disease, diabetes, heart disease, multiple sclerosis, burns and spinal cord injuries. The NIH believes the potential medical benefits of human pluripotent stem cell technology are compelling and worthy of pursuit in accordance with appropriate ethical standards.

In 2006, researchers at Advanced Cell Technology of Worcester, Massachusetts, succeeded in obtaining stem cells from mouse embryos without destroying the embryos. If this technique and its reliability are improved, it would alleviate some of the ethical concerns related to embryonic stem cell research.

Another technique announced in 2007 may also defuse the longstanding debate and controversy. Research teams in the United States and Japan have developed a simple and cost-effective method of reprogramming human skin cells to function much like embryonic stem cells by introducing artificial viruses. While extracting and cloning stem cells is complex and extremely expensive, the newly discovered method of reprogramming cells is much cheaper. However, the technique may disrupt the DNA in the new stem cells, resulting in damaged and cancerous tissue. More research will be required before noncancerous stem cells can be created.

Update article to include 2009/2010 current stem cell usages in clinical trials. The planned treatment trials will focus on the effects of oral lithium on neurological function in people with chronic spinal cord injury and those who have received umbilical cord blood mononuclear cell transplants to the spinal cord. The interest in these two treatments derives from recent reports indicating that umbilical cord blood stem cells may be beneficial for spinal cord injury and that lithium may promote regeneration and recovery of function after spinal cord injury. Both lithium and umbilical cord blood are widely available therapies that have long been used to treat diseases in humans.

Endorsement

- Embryonic stem cells have the potential to grow indefinitely in a laboratory environment and can differentiate into almost all types of bodily tissue. This makes embryonic stem cells a prospect for cellular therapies to treat a wide range of diseases.

Human potential and humanity

This argument often goes hand-in-hand with the utilitarian argument, and can be presented in several forms:

- Embryos are not equivalent to human life while they are still incapable of surviving outside the womb (i.e. they only have the potential for life).
- More than a third of zygotes do not implant after conception. Thus, far more embryos are lost due to chance than are proposed to be used for embryonic stem cell research or treatments.
- Blastocysts are a cluster of human cells that have not differentiated into distinct organ tissue, making cells of the inner cell mass no more human than a skin cell.
- Some parties contend that embryos are not humans, believing that the life of *Homo sapiens* only begins when the heartbeat develops, which is during the fifth week of pregnancy, or when the brain begins developing activity, which has been detected at 54 days after conception.

Efficiency

- *In vitro* fertilization (IVF) generates large numbers of unused embryos (e.g. 70,000 in Australia alone). Many of these thousands of IVF embryos are slated for destruction. Using them for scientific research uses a resource that would otherwise be wasted.
- While the destruction of human embryos is required to establish a stem cell line, no new embryos have to be destroyed to work with existing stem cell lines. It would be wasteful not to continue to make use of these cell lines as a resource.

Superiority

This is usually presented as a counter-argument to using adult stem cells as an alternative that does not involve embryonic destruction.

- Embryonic stem cells make up a significant proportion of a developing embryo, while adult stem cells exist as minor populations within a mature individual (e.g. in every 1,000 cells of the bone marrow, only one will be a usable stem cell). Thus, embryonic stem cells are likely to be easier to isolate and grow *ex vivo* than adult stem cells.
- Embryonic stem cells divide more rapidly than adult stem cells, potentially making it easier to generate large numbers of cells for therapeutic means. In contrast, adult stem cell might not divide fast enough to offer immediate treatment.
- Embryonic stem cells have greater plasticity, potentially allowing them to treat a wider range of diseases.
- Adult stem cells from the patient›s own body might not be effective in treatment of genetic disorders. Allogeneic embryonic stem cell transplantation (i.e. from a healthy donor) may be more practical in these cases than gene therapy of a patient's own cell.
- DNA abnormalities found in adult stem cells that are caused by toxins and sunlight may make them poorly suited for treatment.
- Embryonic stem cells have been shown to be effective in treating heart damage in mice.
- Embryonic stem cells have the potential to cure chronic and degenerative diseases which current medicine has been unable to effectively treat.

Individuality

- Before the primitive streak is formed when the embryo attaches to the uterus around 14 days after fertilization, two fertilized eggs can combine by fusing together and develop into one person (a tetragametic chimera). Since a fertilized egg has the potential to be two individuals or half of one, some believe it can only be considered a ‹potential› person, not an actual one. Those who subscribe to this belief then hold that destroying a blastocyst for embryonic stem cells is ethical.

Viability

- Viability is another standard under which embryos and fetuses have been regarded as human lives. In the United States, the 1973 Supreme Court case of *Roe v. Wade* concluded that viability determined the permissibility of abortions performed for reasons other than the protection of the woman's health, defining viability as the point at which a fetus is "potentially able to live outside the mother's womb, albeit with artificial aid." The point of viability was 24 to 28 weeks when the case was decided and has since moved to about 22 weeks due to advancement in medical technology. Embryos used in medical research for stem cells are well below development that would enable viability.

Objection

Alternatives

This argument is used by opponents of embryonic destruction, as well as researchers specializing in adult stem cell research.

Pro-life supporters often claim that the use of adult stem cells from sources such as umbilical cord blood has consistently produced more promising results than the use of embryonic stem cells. Furthermore, adult stem cell research may be able to make greater advances if less money and resources were channeled into embryonic stem cell research.

In the past, it has been a necessity to research embryonic stem cells and in doing so destroy them for research to progress. As a result of the research done with both embryonic and adult stem cells, new techniques may make the necessity for embryonic cell research obsolete. Because many of the restrictions placed on stem cell research have been based on moral dilemmas surrounding the use of embryonic cells, there will likely be rapid advancement in the field as the techniques that created those issues are becoming less of a necessity. Many funding and research restrictions on embryonic cell research will not impact research on IPSCs (induced pluripotent stem cells) allowing for a promising portion of the field of research to continue relatively unhindered by the ethical issues of embryonic research.

Adult stem cells have provided many different therapies for illnesses such as Parkinson's disease, leukemia, multiple sclerosis, lupus, sickle-cell anemia, and heart damage (to date, embryonic stem cells have also been used in treatment), Moreover, there have been many advances in adult stem cell research, including a recent study where pluripotent adult stem cells were manufactured from differentiated fibroblast by the addition of specific transcription factors. Newly created stem cells were developed into an embryo and were integrated into newborn mouse tissues, analogous to the properties of embryonic stem cells.

Stated views of Groups

Government Policy Stances

Europe

Austria, Denmark, France, Germany, and Ireland do not allow the production of embryonic stem cell lines, but the creation of embryonic stem cell lines is permitted in Finland, Greece, the Netherlands, Sweden, and the United Kingdom.

United States

Origins

In 1973, *Roe v. Wade* legalized abortion in the United States. Five years later, the first successful human *in vitro* fertilization resulted in the birth of Louise Brown in England. These developments prompted the federal government to create regulations barring the use of federal funds for research that experimented on human embryos. In 1995, the NIH Human Embryo Research Panel advised the administration of President Bill Clinton to permit federal funding for research on embryos left over from *in vitro* fertility treatments and also recommended federal funding of research on embryos specifically created for experimentation. In response to the panel's recommendations, the Clinton administration, citing moral and ethical concerns, declined to fund research on embryos created solely for research purposes, but did agree to fund research on leftover embryos created by *in vitro* fertility treatments. At this point, the Congress intervened and passed the Dickey Amendment in 1995 (the final bill, which included the Dickey Amendment, was signed into law by Bill Clinton) which prohibited any federal funding for the Department of Health and Human Services be used for research that resulted in the destruction of an embryo regardless of the source of that embryo.

In 1998, privately funded research led to the breakthrough discovery of human embryonic stem cells (hESC). This prompted the Clinton administration to re-examine guidelines for federal funding of embryonic research. In 1999, the president›s National Bioethics Advisory Commission recommended that hESC harvested from embryos discarded after *in vitro* fertility treatments, but not from embryos created expressly for experimentation, be eligible for federal funding. Though embryo destruction had been inevitable in the process of harvesting hESC in the past (this is no longer the case), the Clinton administration had decided that it would be permissible under the Dickey Amendment to fund hESC research as long as such research did not itself directly cause the destruction of an embryo. Therefore, HHS issued its proposed regulation concerning hESC funding in 2001. Enactment of the new guidelines was delayed by the incoming George W. Bush administration which decided to reconsider the issue.

President Bush announced, on August 9, 2001, that federal funds, for the first time, would be made available for hESC research on currently existing embryonic stem cell lines. President Bush authorized research on existing human embryonic stem cell lines, not on human embryos under a specific, unrealistic timeline in which the stem cell lines must have been developed. However, the Bush Administration chose not to permit taxpayer funding for research on hESC cell lines not currently in existence, thus limiting federal funding to research in which the life-and-death decision has already been made. The Bush Administration›s guidelines differ from the Clinton Administration guidelines which did not distinguish between currently existing and not-yet-existing hESC. Both the Bush and Clinton guidelines agree that the federal government should not fund hESC research that directly destroys embryos.

Neither Congress nor any administration has ever prohibited private funding of embryonic research. Public and private funding of research on adult and cord blood stem cells is unrestricted.

U.S. Congressional Response

In April 2004, 206 members of Congress signed a letter urging President Bush to expand federal funding of embryonic stem cell research beyond what Bush had already supported.

In May 2005, the House of Representatives voted 238–194 to loosen the limitations on federally funded embryonic stem-cell research—by allowing government-funded research on surplus frozen embryos from in vitro fertilization clinics to be used for stem cell research with the permission of donors—despite Bush's promise to veto the bill if passed. On July 29, 2005, Senate Majority Leader William H. Frist. announced that he too favored loosening restrictions on federal funding of embryonic stem cell research. On July 18, 2006, the Senate passed three different bills concerning stem cell research. The Senate passed the first bill (the Stem Cell Research Enhancement Act) 63–37, which would have made it legal for the federal government to spend federal money on embryonic stem cell research that uses embryos left over from *in vitro* fertilization procedures. On July 19, 2006 President Bush vetoed this bill. The second bill makes it illegal to create, grow, and abort fetuses for research purposes. The third bill would encourage research that would isolate pluripotent, i.e., embryonic-like, stem cells without the destruction of human embryos.

In 2005 and 2007, Congressman Ron Paul introduced the Cures Can Be Found Act, with 10 cosponsors. With an income tax credit, the bill favors research upon non–embryonic stem cells obtained from placentas, umbilical cord blood, amniotic fluid, humans after birth, or unborn human offspring who died of natural causes; the bill was referred to committee. Paul argued that hESC research is outside of federal jurisdiction either to ban or to subsidize.

Bush vetoed another bill, the Stem Cell Research Enhancement Act of 2007, which would have amended the Public Health Service Act to provide for human embryonic stem cell research. The bill passed the Senate on April 11 by a vote of 63-34, then passed the House on June 7 by a vote of 247–176. President Bush vetoed the bill on July 19, 2007.

On March 9, 2009, President Obama removed the restriction on federal funding for newer stem cell lines. Two days after Obama removed the restriction, the president then signed the Omnibus Appropriations Act of 2009, which still contained the long-standing Dickey-Wicker provision which bans federal funding of "research in which a human embryo or embryos are destroyed, discarded, or knowingly subjected to risk of injury or death;" the Congressional provision effectively prevents federal funding being used to create new stem cell lines by many of the known methods. So, while scientists might not be free to create new lines with federal funding, President Obama's policy allows the potential of applying for such funding into research involving the hundreds of existing stem cell lines as well as any further lines created using private funds or state-level funding. The ability to apply for federal funding for stem cell lines created in the private sector is a significant expansion of options over the limits imposed by President Bush, who restricted funding to the 21 viable stem cell lines that were created before he announced his decision in 2001. The ethical concerns raised during Clinton's time in office continue to restrict hESC research and dozens of stem cell lines have been excluded from funding, now by judgment of an administrative office rather than presidential or legislative discretion.

Funding

In 2005, the NIH funded $607 million worth of stem cell research, of which $39 million was specifically used for hESC. Sigrid Fry-Revere has argued that private organizations, not the federal government, should provide funding for stem-cell research, so that shifts in public opinion and government policy would not bring valuable scientific research to a grinding halt.

In 2005, the State of California took out $3 billion in bond loans to fund embryonic stem cell research in that state.

Asia

China has one of the most permissive human embryonic stem cell policies in the world. In the absence of a public controversy, human embryo stem cell research is supported by policies that allow the use of human embryos and therapeutic cloning.

Catholicism

The Catholic Church opposes human embryonic stem cell research calling it "an absolutely unacceptable act." The Church supports research that involves stem cells from adult tissues and the umbilical cord, as it "involves no harm to human beings at any state of development."

Baptists

The Southern Baptist Convention opposes human embryonic stem cell research on the grounds that "Bible teaches that human beings are made in the image and likeness of God (Gen. 1:27; 9:6) and protectable human life begins at fertilization." However, it supports adult stem cell research as it does "not require the destruction of embryos."

Methodism

The United Methodist Church opposes human embryonic stem cell research, saying, "a human embryo, even at its earliest stages, commands our reverence. However, it supports adult stem cell research, stating that there are few moral questions raised by this issue.

Pentecostalism

The Assemblies of God opposes human embryonic stem cell research, saying, it "perpetuates the evil of abortion and should be prohibited."

Islam

The religion of Islam favors the stance that scientific research and development in terms of stem cell research is allowed as long as it benefits society while using the least amount of harm to the subjects. "Stem cell research is one of the most controversial topics of our time period and has raised many religious and ethical questions regarding the research being done. With there being no true guidelines set forth in the Qur'an against the study of biomedical testing, Muslims have adopted any new studies as long as the studies do not contradict another teaching in the Quran. One of the teachings of the Qur'an states that "Whosoever saves the life of one, it shall be if he saves the life of humankind" (5:32), it is this teaching that makes stem cell research acceptable in the Muslim faith because of its promise of potential medical breakthrough."

The Church of Jesus Christ of Latter-day Saints

The First Presidency of The Church of Jesus Christ of Latter-day Saints "has not taken a position regarding the use of embryonic stem cells for research purposes. The absence of a position should not be interpreted as support for or opposition to any other statement made by Church members, whether they are for or against embryonic stem cell research."

REFERENCES

1. Appendix E: Stem Cell Markers. Stem Cell Information. Bethesda, Maryland: National Institutes of Health. 17 June 2001. Retrieved 23 July 2009.
2. Petrenko O, Beavis A, Klaine M, Kittappa R, Godin I, Lemischka IR (June 1999). The molecular characterization of the fetal stem cell marker AA4. Immunity. **10** *(6): 691–700.* doi:10.1016/S1074-7613(00)80068-0. PMID 10403644.
3. Taoudi S, Morrison AM, Inoue H, Gribi R, Ure J, Medvinsky A (September 2005). Progressive divergence of definitive haematopoietic stem cells from the endothelial compartment does not depend on contact with the foetal liver. Development. **132** *(18): 4179–91. doi:10.1242/dev.01974. PMID 16107475.*
4. Islam MO, Kanemura Y, Tajria J, et al. (July 2005). Characterization of ABC transporter ABCB1 expressed in human neural stem/progenitor cells. FEBS Letters. **579** *(17): 3473–80. doi:10.1016/j.febslet.2005.05.019. PMID 15950972.*

5. Frank NY, Margaryan A, Huang Y, et al. (May 2005). ABCB5-mediated doxorubicin transport and chemoresistance in human malignant melanoma. Cancer Research. **65** *(10): 4320–33. doi:10.1158/0008-5472.CAN-04-3327. PMID 15899824.*

6. Bernardo AS, Barrow J, Hay CW, et al. (July 2006). Presence of endocrine and exocrine markers in EGFP-positive cells from the developing pancreas of a nestin/EGFP mouse. Molecular and Cellular Endocrinology. **253** *(1–2): 14–21. doi:10.1016/j.mce.2006.03.003. PMID 16698177.*

7. Chute JP, Muramoto GG, Whitesides J, et al. (August 2006). Inhibition of aldehyde dehydrogenase and retinoid signaling induces the expansion of human hematopoietic stem cells. Proceedings of the National Academy of Sciences of the United States of America. **103** *(31): 11707–12. doi:10.1073/pnas.0603806103. PMC 1544234. PMID 16857736.*

8. Nagafuchi S, Katsuta H, Kogawa K, et al. (July 1999). Establishment of an embryonic stem (ES) cell line derived from a non-obese diabetic (NOD) mouse: in vivo differentiation into lymphocytes and potential for germ line transmission. FEBS Letters. **455** *(1–2): 101–4.* doi:10.1016/S0014-5793(99)00801-7. PMID 10428481.

9. Shinohara T, Avarbock MR, Brinster RL (May 1999). *1*- and α6-integrin are surface markers on mouse spermatogonial stem cells. Proceedings of the National Academy of Sciences of the United States of America. **96** *(10): 5504–9. doi:10.1073/pnas.96.10.5504. PMC 21889. PMID 10318913.*

10. Katoh M (December 2005). WNT2B: comparative integromics and clinical applications (Review). International Journal of Molecular Medicine. **16** *(6): 1103–8. doi:10.3892/ijmm.16.6.1103. PMID 16273293.*

11. Gordon B, Haire W, Ruby E, et al. (March 1997). Factors predicting morbidity following hematopoietic stem cell transplantation. Bone Marrow Transplantation. **19** *(5): 497–501. doi:10.1038/sj.bmt.1700684. PMID 9052918.*

12. Harris MT, Schwarting GA, Stout RD (September 1981). Selective expression of asialo GM1 on maturational subsets of lymphocytes in normal and athymic mice. Thymus. **3** *(3): 153–67. PMID 6171918.*

13. Polakowska RR, Piacentini M, Bartlett R, Goldsmith LA, Haake AR (March 1994). Apoptosis in human skin development: morphogenesis, periderm, and stem cells. Developmental Dynamics. **199** *(3): 176–88. doi:10.1002/aja.1001990303. PMID 7517223.*

14. Asari S, Okada S, Ohkubo Y, et al. (August 2004). Beta-galactosidase of ROSA26 mice is a useful marker for detecting the definitive erythropoiesis after stem cell transplantation. Transplantation. **78** *(4): 516–23. doi:10.1097/01.TP.0000128854.20831.6F. PMID 15446309.*

15. Valente T, Junyent F, Auladell C (June 2005). Zac1 is expressed in progenitor/stem cells of the neuroectoderm and mesoderm during embryogenesis: differential phenotype of the Zac1-expressing cells during development. Developmental Dynamics. **233** *(2): 667–79. doi:10.1002/dvdy.20373. PMID 15844099.*

16. Raisky O, Nykänen AI, Krebs R, et al. (April 2007). VEGFR-1 and -2 regulate inflammation, myocardial angiogenesis, and arteriosclerosis in chronically rejecting cardiac allografts. Arteriosclerosis, Thrombosis, and Vascular Biology. **27** *(4): 819–25. doi:10.1161/01.ATV.0000260001.55955.6c. PMID 17290032.*

17. Suzuki A, Zheng YW, Fukao K, Nakauchi H, Taniguchi H (2004). Liver repopulation by c-Met-positive stem/progenitor cells isolated from the developing rat liver. Hepato-gastroenterology. **51** *(56): 423–6. PMID 15086173.*

18. Danet GH, Luongo JL, Butler G, et al. (August 2002). C1qRp defines a new human stem cell population with hematopoietic and hepatic potential. Proceedings of the National Academy of Sciences of the United States of America. **99** *(16): 10441–5. doi:10.1073/pnas.162104799. PMC 124933.* PMID 12140365.

19. Nagatomo K, Komaki M, Sekiya I, et al. (August 2006). "Stem cell properties of human periodontal ligament cells". Journal of Periodontal Research. **41** *(4): 303–10. doi:10.1111/j.1600-0765.2006.00870.x. PMID 16827724.*

20. Peichev M, Naiyer AJ, Pereira D, et al. (1 February 2000). Expression of VEGFR-2 and AC133 by circulating human CD34(+) cells identifies a population of functional endothelial precursors. Blood. **95** *(3): 952–8. PMID 10648408.*

21. Zhou L, Wei X, Cheng L, Tian J, Jiang JJ (March 2007). CD133, one of the markers of cancer stem cells in Hep-2 cell line. The Laryngoscope. **117** *(3): 455–60. doi:10.1097/01.mlg.0000251586.15299.35. PMID 17334305.*

22. Kania G, Corbeil D, Fuchs J, et al. (2005). Somatic stem cell marker prominin-1/CD133 is expressed in embryonic stem cell-derived progenitors. Stem Cells. **23** *(6): 791–804. doi:10.1634/stemcells.2004-0232. PMID 15917475.*

23. Herrera MB, Bruno S, Buttiglieri S, et al. (December 2006). Isolation and characterization of a stem cell population from adult human liver. Stem Cells. **24** *(12): 2840–50. doi:10.1634/stemcells.2006-0114. PMID 16945998.*

24. Pera MF, Herszfeld D (1998). Differentiation of human pluripotent teratocarcinoma stem cells induced by bone morphogenetic protein-2. Reproduction, Fertility, and Development. **10** *(7–8): 551–5.* doi:10.1071/RD98097. PMID 10612460.

25. Miranville A, Heeschen C, Sengenès C, Curat CA, Busse R, Bouloumié A (July 2004). Improvement of postnatal neovascularization by human adipose tissue-derived stem cells. Circulation. **110** *(3): 349–55. doi:10.1161/01.CIR.0000135466.16823.D0. PMID 15238461.*

26. Blakolmer K, Jaskiewicz K, Dunsford HA, Robson SC (June 1995). Hematopoietic stem cell markers are expressed by ductal plate and bile duct cells in developing human liver. Hepatology. **21** *(6): 1510–6. doi:10.1002/hep.1840210606. PMID 7539394.*

27. Ning H, Lin G, Lue TF, Lin CS (December 2006). Neuron-like differentiation of adipose tissue-derived stromal cells and vascular smooth muscle cells. Differentiation. **74** *(9–10): 510–8. doi:10.1111/j.1432-0436.2006.00081.x. PMID 17177848.*

28. Van Den Heuvel MC, Slooff MJ, Visser L, et al. (June 2001). Expression of anti-OV6 antibody and anti-N-CAM antibody along the biliary line of

normal and diseased human livers. Hepatology. **33** *(6): 1387–93. doi:10.1053/jhep.2001.24453. PMID 11391527.*

29. Kanatsu-Shinohara M, Toyokuni S, Shinohara T (January 2004). CD9 is a surface marker on mouse and rat male germline stem cells. Biology of Reproduction. **70** *(1): 70–5. doi:10.1095/biolreprod.103.020867. PMID 12954725.*
30. Okumoto K, Saito T, Hattori E, et al. (May 2003). Differentiation of bone marrow cells into cells that express liver-specific genes in vitro: implication of the Notch signals in differentiation. Biochemical and Biophysical Research Communications. **304** *(4): 691–5.* doi:10.1016/S0006-291X(03)00637-5. PMID 12727209.
31. Kimura H, Morii E, Ikeda JI, et al. (September 2006). Role of DNA methylation for expression of novel stem cell marker CDCP1 in hematopoietic cells. Leukemia. **20** *(9): 1551–6. doi:10.1038/sj.leu.2404312. PMID 16926850.*
32. Regauer S (May 2006). Extramammary Paget›s disease--a proliferation of adnexal origin?. *Histopathology.* **48** *(6): 723–9. doi:10.1111/j.1365-2559.2006.02405.x. PMID 16681689.*
33. Schoof H, Lenhard M, Haecker A, Mayer KF, Jürgens G, Laux T (March 2000). The stem cell population of Arabidopsis shoot meristems in maintained by a regulatory loop between the CLAVATA and WUSCHEL genes. Cell. **100** *(6): 635–44.* doi:10.1016/S0092-8674(00)80700-X. PMID 10761929.
34. Scavennec J, Carcassonne Y, Gastaut JA, Blanc A, Cailla HL (1 August 1981). Relationship between the levels of cyclic cytidine 3›:5›-monophosphate, cyclic guanosine 3›:5›-monophosphate, and cyclic adenosine 3›:5›-monophosphate in urines and leukocytes and the type of human leukemias. Cancer Research. **41** *(8): 3222–7. PMID 6265079.*
35. Boulter CA, Wagner EF (March 1988). The effects of v-src expression on the differentiation of embryonal carcinoma cells. Oncogene. **2** *(3): 207–14. PMID 3127777.*
36. Giuliano CJ, Kerley-Hamilton JS, Bee T, et al. (October 2005). Retinoic acid represses a cassette of candidate pluripotency chromosome 12p genes during induced loss of human embryonal carcinoma tumorigenicity. Biochimica et Biophysica Acta. **1731** *(1): 48–56. doi:10.1016/j.bbaexp.2005.08.006. PMID 16168501.*
37. Reid CD (June 1987). The significance of endogenous erythroid colonies (EEC) in haematological disorders. Blood Reviews. **1** *(2): 133–40.* doi:10.1016/0268-960X(87)90008-7. PMID 3332094.
38. Lane MA, Chen AC, Roman SD, Derguini F, Gudas LJ (November 1999). Removal of LIF (leukemia inhibitory factor) results in increased vitamin A (retinol) metabolism to 4-oxoretinol in embryonic stem cells. Proceedings of the National Academy of Sciences of the United States of America. **96** *(23): 13524–9. doi:10.1073/pnas.96.23.13524. PMC 23981. PMID 10557354.*
39. Christensen JL, Weissman IL (December 2001). Flk-2 is a marker in hematopoietic stem cell differentiation: A simple method to isolate long-term stem cells.

Proceedings of the National Academy of Sciences of the United States of America. **98** *(25): 14541–6. doi:10.1073/pnas.261562798. PMC 64718*. PMID 11724967.

40. Hu Y, Zhang Z, Torsney E, et al. (May 2004). Abundant progenitor cells in the adventitia contribute to atherosclerosis of vein grafts in ApoE-deficient mice. The Journal of Clinical Investigation. **113** *(9): 1258–65*. doi:10.1172/JCI19628. PMC 398426. PMID 15124016.

41. Anzai H, Nagayoshi M, Obata M, Ikawa Y, Atsumi T (February 1999). Self-renewal and differentiation of a basic fibroblast growth factor-dependent multipotent hematopoietic cell line derived from embryonic stem cells. Development, Growth & Differentiation. **41** *(1): 51–8. doi:10.1046/j.1440-169x.1999.00412.x. PMID 10445502.*

42. Rappold I, Ziegler BL, Köhler I, et al. (15 July 1997). Functional and phenotypic characterization of cord blood and bone marrow subsets expressing FLT3 (CD135) receptor tyrosine kinase. Blood. **90** *(1): 111–25. PMID 9207445.*

43. Pfeilstöcker M, Karlic H, Paukovits J, et al. (April 1999). In vivo and in vitro effects of cytokines and the hemoregulatory peptide dimer (pEEDCK)2 (pyroGlu-Glu-Asp-Cys-Lys)2 on G alpha16-positive hematopoiesis. Leukemia. **13** *(4): 590–4. doi:10.1038/*sj/leu/2401377. PMID 10214866.

44. Kume A, Hashiyama M, Suda T, Ozawa K (1999). Green fluorescent protein as a selectable marker of retrovirally transduced hematopoietic progenitors. Stem Cells. **17** *(4): 226–32. doi:10.1002/stem.170226. PMID 10437986.*

45. Sonoda T, Hayashi C, Seike H, et al. (February 1985). Extensive proliferation of subsequently injected marrow cells in parental-to-F1 hematopoietic chimeras that restored normal stem cell concentration after initial transplantation. Experimental Hematology. **13** *(2): 143–50. PMID 2857651.*

46. Perron M, Boy S, Amato MA, et al. (April 2003). A novel function for Hedgehog signalling in retinal pigment epithelium differentiation. Development. **130** *(8): 1565–77. doi:10.1242/dev.00391. PMID 12620982.*

47. Tschöpe D, Langer E, Schauseil S, Rösen P, Kaufmann L, Gries FA (February 1989). Increased platelet volume--sign of impaired thrombopoiesis in diabetes mellitus. Klinische Wochenschrift. **67** *(4): 253–9.* doi:10.1007/BF01717328. PMID 2927060.

48. Czerwinski M, Kiem HP, Slattery JT (March 1997). Human CD34+ cells do not express glutathione S-transferases alpha. Gene Therapy. **4** *(3): 268–70. doi:10.1038/sj.gt.3300381. PMID 9135742.*

49. Grskovic B, Pollaschek C, Mueller MM, Stuhlmeier KM (June 2006). Expression of hyaluronan synthase genes in umbilical cord blood stem/progenitor cells. Biochimica et Biophysica Acta. **1760** *(6): 890–5. doi:10.1016/j.bbagen.2006.02.002. PMID 16564133.*

50. Chapouton P, Adolf B, Leucht C, et al. (November 2006). her5 expression reveals a pool of neural stem cells in the adult zebrafish midbrain. Development. **133** *(21): 4293–303. doi:10.1242/dev.02573. PMID 17038515.*

51. Wang Q, Li N, Wang X, et al. (January 2007). Membrane protein hMYADM preferentially expressed in myeloid cells is up-regulated during differentiation of stem cells and myeloid leukemia cells. Life Sciences. **80** *(5): 420–9. doi:10.1016/j.lfs.2006.09.043. PMID 17097684.*

52. Stahl J, Wobus AM, Ihrig S, Lutsch G, Bielka H (September 1992). The small heat shock protein hsp25 is accumulated in P19 embryonal carcinoma cells and embryonic stem cells of line BLC6 during differentiation. Differentiation. **51** *(1): 33–7. doi:10.1111/j.1432-0436.1992.tb00677.x. PMID 1451960.*

53. Gultice AD, Selesniemi KL, Brown TL (June 2006). Hypoxia inhibits differentiation of lineage-specific Rcho-1 trophoblast giant cells. Biology of Reproduction. **74** *(6): 1041–50. doi:10.1095/biolreprod.105.047845. PMID 16481593.*

54. Testa U, Riccioni R, Diverio D, Rossini A, Lo Coco F, Peschle C (February 2004). Interleukin-3 receptor in acute leukemia. Leukemia. **18** *(2): 219–26. doi:10.1038/sj.leu.2403224. PMID 14671644.*

55. Hall PE, Lathia JD, Miller NG, Caldwell MA, ffrench-Constant C (September 2006). Integrins are markers of human neural stem cells. Stem Cells. **24** *(9): 2078–84. doi:10.1634/stemcells.2005-0595. PMID 16690778.*

56. Jordan CT, Upchurch D, Szilvassy SJ, et al. (October 2000). The interleukin-3 receptor alpha chain is a unique marker for human acute myelogenous leukemia stem cells. Leukemia. **14** *(10): 1777–84. doi:10.1038/sj.leu.2401903. PMID 11021753.*

57. Jendelová P, Herynek V, Urdzíková L, et al. (April 2004). Magnetic resonance tracking of transplanted bone marrow and embryonic stem cells labeled by iron oxide nanoparticles in rat brain and spinal cord. Journal of Neuroscience Research. **76** *(2): 232–43. doi:10.1002/jnr.20041. PMID 15048921.*

58. Ziegler BL, Valtieri M, Porada GA, et al. (September 1999). KDR receptor: a key marker defining hematopoietic stem cells. Science. **285** *(5433): 1553–8. doi:10.1126/science.285.5433.1553. PMID 10477517.*

59. Misago N, Narisawa Y (September 2006). Cytokeratin 15 expression in neoplasms with sebaceous differentiation. Journal of Cutaneous Pathology. **33** *(9): 634–41. doi:10.1111/j.1600-0560.2006.00500.x. PMID 16965339.*

60. Tiede S, Koop N, Kloepper JE, Fässler R, Paus R (November 2009). Nonviral in situ green fluorescent protein labeling and culture of primary, adult human hair follicle epithelial progenitor cells. Stem Cells. **27** *(11): 2793–803. doi:10.1002/stem.213. PMID 19750535.*

61. Nijhof JG, Braun KM, Giangreco A, et al. (August 2006). The cell-surface marker MTS24 identifies a novel population of follicular keratinocytes with characteristics of progenitor cells. Development. **133** *(15): 3027–37. doi:10.1242/dev.02443. PMID 16818453.*

62. Youn SW, Kim DS, Cho HJ, et al. (August 2004). Cellular senescence induced loss of stem cell proportion in the skin in vitro. Journal of Dermatological Science. **35** *(2): 113–23. doi:10.1016/j.jdermsci.2004.04.002. PMID 15265523.*

63. Fu XB, Sun TZ, Li XK, Sheng ZY (February 2005). Morphological and distribution characteristics of sweat glands in hypertrophic scar and their possible effects on sweat gland regeneration. Chinese Medical Journal. **118** *(3): 186–91. PMID 15740645.*

64. Clarke RB (December 2005). Isolation and characterization of human mammary stem cells. Cell Proliferation. **38** *(6): 375–86. doi:10.1111/j.1365-2184.2005.00357.x. PMID 16300651.*

65. Perry SS, Wang H, Pierce LJ, Yang AM, Tsai S, Spangrude GJ (April 2004). L-selectin defines a bone marrow analog to the thymic early T-lineage progenitor. Blood. **103** *(8): 2990–6.* doi:10.1182/blood-2003-09-3030. PMID 15070675.

66. Constantinescu D, Gray HL, Sammak PJ, Schatten GP, Csoka AB (January 2006). Lamin A/C expression is a marker of mouse and human embryonic stem cell differentiation. Stem Cells. **24** *(1): 177–85. doi:10.1634/stemcells.2004-0159. PMID 16179429.*

67. Muramatsu T, Muramatsu H (2004). Carbohydrate antigens expressed on stem cells and early embryonic cells. Glycoconjugate Journal. **21** *(1–2): 41–5. doi:10.1023/B:GLYC.0000043746.77504.28. PMID 15467397.*

68. Ganat YM, Silbereis J, Cave C, et al. (August 2006). Early postnatal astroglial cells produce multilineage precursors and neural stem cells in vivo. The Journal of Neuroscience. **26** *(33): 8609–21. doi:10.1523/JNEUROSCI.2532-06.2006. PMID 16914687.*

69. van Es JH, Kuipers J, Kujala P, van den Born M, Cozijnsen M, Haegebarth A, Korving J, Begthel H, Peters PJ, Clevers H (2007). Identification of stem cells in small intestine and colon by marker gene Lgr5. Nature. **449** *(7165): 1003–1007.* doi:10.1038/nature06196. PMID 17934449.

70. Yamaguchi YL, Tanaka SS, Kasa M, Yasuda K, Tam PP, Matsui Y (August 2006). Expression of low density lipoprotein receptor-related protein 4 (Lrp4) gene in the mouse germ cells. Gene Expression Patterns. **6** *(6): 607–12. doi:10.1016/j.modgep.2005.11.013. PMID 16434236.*

71. Mohan A, Kandalam M, Ramkumar HL, Gopal L, Krishnakumar S (July 2006). Stem cell markers: ABCG2 and MCM2 expression in retinoblastoma. The British Journal of Ophthalmology. **90** *(7): 889–93. doi:10.1136/bjo.2005.089219. PMC 1857132. PMID 16556617.*

72. Legg J, Jensen UB, Broad S, Leigh I, Watt FM (December 2003). Role of melanoma chondroitin sulphate proteoglycan in patterning stem cells in human interfollicular epidermis. Development. **130** *(24): 6049–63. doi:10.1242/dev.00837. PMID 14573520.*

73. Donnelly ET, Bardwell H, Thomas GA, et al. (June 2005). Metallothionein crypt-restricted immunopositivity indices (MTCRII) correlate with aberrant crypt foci (ACF) in mouse colon. British Journal of Cancer. **92** *(12): 2160–5. doi:10.1038/sj.bjc.6602633. PMC 2361830 PMID 15928667.*

74. Hutter JJ, Hecht F, Kaiser-McCaw B, et al. (1984). Bone marrow monosomy 7: hematologic and clinical manifestations in childhood and adolescence.

Hematological Oncology. **2** *(1): 5–12. doi:10.1002/hon.2900020103. PMID 6588021.*

75. Colombo E, Galli R, Cossu G, Gécz J, Broccoli V (November 2004). Mouse orthologue of ARX, a gene mutated in several X-linked forms of mental retardation and epilepsy, is a marker of adult neural stem cells and forebrain GABAergic neurons. Developmental Dynamics. **231** *(3): 631–9. doi:10.1002/dvdy.20164. PMID 15376319.*
76. Steinbach D, Wittig S, Cario G, et al. (December 2003). The multidrug resistance-associated protein 3 (MRP3) is associated with a poor outcome in childhood ALL and may account for the worse prognosis in male patients and T-cell immunophenotype. Blood. **102** *(13): 4493–8.* doi:10.1182/blood-2002-11-3461. PMID 12816874.
77. Clarke RB, Spence K, Anderson E, Howell A, Okano H, Potten CS (January 2005). A putative human breast stem cell population is enriched for steroid receptor-positive cells. Developmental Biology. **277** *(2): 443–56. doi:10.1016/j.ydbio.2004.07.044. PMID 15617686.*
78. Yoshida S, Shimmura S, Nagoshi N, et al. (December 2006). Isolation of multipotent neural crest-derived stem cells from the adult mouse cornea. Stem Cells. **24** *(12): 2714–22. doi:10.1634/stemcells.2006-0156. PMID 16888282.*
79. Staud F, Pavek P (April 2005). Breast cancer resistance protein (BCRP/ABCG2). The International Journal of Biochemistry & Cell Biology. **37** *(4): 720–5. doi:10.1016/j.biocel.2004.11.004. PMID 15694832.*
80. Loo DT, Althoen MC, Cotman CW (October 1995). Differentiation of serum-free mouse embryo cells into astrocytes is accompanied by induction of glutamine synthetase activity. Journal of Neuroscience Research. **42** *(2): 184–91. doi:10.1002/jnr.490420205. PMID 8568918.*
81. Okawa H, Okuda O, Arai H, Sakuragawa N, Sato K (December 2001). Amniotic epithelial cells transform into neuron-like cells in the ischemic brain. NeuroReport. **12** *(18): 4003–7.* doi:10.1097/00001756-200112210-00030. PMID 11742228.
82. Neudenberger J, Hotfilder M, Rosemann A, et al. (May 2006). Lack of expression of the chondroitin sulphate proteoglycan neuron-glial antigen 2 on candidate stem cell populations in paediatric acute myeloid leukaemia/abn(11q23) and acute lymphoblastic leukaemia/t(4;11). British Journal of Haematology. **133** *(3): 337–44. doi:10.1111/j.1365-2141.2006.06013.x. PMID 16643437.*
83. Umemoto T, Yamato M, Nishida K, et al. (December 2005). Rat limbal epithelial side population cells exhibit a distinct expression of stem cell markers that are lacking in side population cells from the central cornea. FEBS Letters. **579** *(29): 6569–74. doi:10.1016/j.febslet.2005.10.047. PMID 16297384.*
84. Imaoka S, Mori T, Kinoshita T (February 2007). Bisphenol A causes malformation of the head region in embryos of Xenopus laevis and decreases the expression of the ESR-1 gene mediated by Notch signaling. Biological & Pharmaceutical Bulletin. **30** *(2): 371–4. doi:10.1248/bpb.30.371. PMID 17268083.*

85. Kafienah W, Mistry S, Williams C, Hollander AP (April 2006). Nucleostemin is a marker of proliferating stromal stem cells in adult human bone marrow. Stem Cells. **24** *(4): 1113–20. doi:10.1634/stemcells.2005-0416. PMID 16282439.*

86. Sigal SH, Brill S, Reid LM, et al. (April 1994). Characterization and enrichment of fetal rat hepatoblasts by immunoadsorption (panning) and fluorescence-activated cell sorting. Hepatology. **19** *(4): 999–1006. doi:10.1002/hep.1840190427. PMID 7511129.*

87. Raman JD, Mongan NP, Liu L, et al. (March 2006). Decreased expression of the human stem cell marker, Rex-1 (zfp-42), in renal cell carcinoma. Carcinogenesis. **27** *(3): 499–507. doi:10.1093/*carcin/bgi299. PMID 16344273.

88. Maduro MR, Davis E, Davis A, Lamb DJ (May 2002). Osteotesticular protein tyrosine phosphatase expression in rodent testis. The Journal of Urology. **167** *(5): 2282–3.* doi:10.1016/S0022-5347(05)65143-9. PMID 11956493.

89. Tokura Y, Shikami M, Miwa H, et al. (January 2002). Augmented expression of P-gp/multi-drug resistance gene by all-trans retinoic acid in monocytic leukemic cells. Leukemia Research. **26** *(1): 29–36.* doi:10.1016/S0145-2126(01)00094-7. PMID 11734301.

90. Ramirez RD, Sheridan S, Girard L, et al. (December 2004). Immortalization of human bronchial epithelial cells in the absence of viral oncoproteins. Cancer Research. **64** *(24): 9027–34. doi:10.1158/0008-5472.CAN-04-3703. PMID 15604268.*

91. Wong CE, Paratore C, Dours-Zimmermann MT, et al. (December 2006). Neural crest–derived cells with stem cell features can be traced back to multiple lineages in the adult skin. The Journal of Cell Biology. **175** *(6): 1005–15. doi:10.1083/jcb.200606062. PMC 2064709. PMID 17158956.*

92. Kerosuo L, Juvonen E, Alitalo R, Gylling M, Kerjaschki D, Miettinen A (March 2004). Podocalyxin in human haematopoietic cells. British Journal of Haematology. **124** *(6): 809–18. doi:10.1111/j.1365-2141.2004.04840.x. PMID 15009070.*

93. Fu XB, Xing F, Yang YH, Sun TZ, Guo BC (September 2003). Activation of phosphorylating-p38 mitogen-activated protein kinase and its relationship with localization of intestinal stem cells in rats after ischemia-reperfusion injury. World Journal of Gastroenterology. **9** *(9): 2036–9. PMID 12970901.*

94. Doyonnas R, Nielsen JS, Chelliah S, et al. (June 2005). Podocalyxin is a CD34-related marker of murine hematopoietic stem cells and embryonic erythroid cells. Blood. **105** *(11): 4170–8.* doi:10.1182/blood-2004-10-4077. PMID 15701716.

95. Ortega M, Rovira M, Filella X, et al. (March 2006). Prospective evaluation of procalcitonin in adults with non-neutropenic fever after allogeneic hematopoietic stem cell transplantation. Bone Marrow Transplantation. **37** *(5): 499–502. doi:10.1038/sj.bmt.1705262. PMID 16415895.*

96. Suzuki A, Nakauchi H, Taniguchi H (August 2004). Prospective isolation of multipotent pancreatic progenitors using flow-cytometric cell sorting. Diabetes. **53** *(8): 2143–52. doi:10.2337/diabetes.53.8.2143. PMID 15277399.*

97. Bucchini D, Lasserre C, Kunst F, Lovell-Badge R, Pictet R, Jami J (1983). Stable transformation of mouse teratocarcinoma stem cells with the dominant selective marker Eco.gpt and retention of their developmental potentialities. The EMBO Journal. **2** *(2): 229–32. PMC 555118.* PMID 11894931.

98. Braun KM, Watt FM (September 2004). Epidermal label-retaining cells: background and recent applications. The Journal of Investigative Dermatology. **9** *(3): 196–201. doi:10.1111/j.1087-0024.2004.09313.x. PMID 15369213.*

99. Rubin DC, Swietlicki E, Roth KA, Gordon JI (25 July 1992). Use of fetal intestinal isografts from normal and transgenic mice to study the programming of positional information along the duodenal-to-colonic axis. The Journal of Biological Chemistry. **267** *(21): 15122–33. PMID 1634547.*

100. Nakafuku M, Nakamura S (June 1995). Establishment and characterization of a multipotential neural cell line that can conditionally generate neurons, astrocytes, and oligodendrocytes in vitro. Journal of Neuroscience Research. **41** *(2): 153–68. doi:10.1002/jnr.490410203. PMID 7650751.*

101. Lamoury FM, Croitoru-Lamoury J, Brew BJ (2006). Undifferentiated mouse mesenchymal stem cells spontaneously express neural and stem cell markers Oct-4 and Rex-1. Cytotherapy. **8** *(3): 228–42.* doi:10.1080/14653240600735875. PMID 16793732.

102. Asakura A, Seale P, Girgis-Gabardo A, Rudnicki MA (October 2002). Myogenic specification of side population cells in skeletal muscle. The Journal of Cell Biology. **159** *(1): 123–34. doi:10.1083/jcb.200202092. PMC 2173497. PMID 12379804.*

103. Timper K, Seboek D, Eberhardt M, et al. (March 2006). Human adipose tissue-derived mesenchymal stem cells differentiate into insulin, somatostatin, and glucagon expressing cells. Biochemical and Biophysical Research Communications. **341** *(4): 1135–40. doi:10.1016/j.bbrc.2006.01.072. PMID 16460677.*

104. Barone, Angela; Säljö, Karin; Benktander, John; Blomqvist, Maria; Månsson, Jan-Eric; Johansson, Bengt R.; Mölne, Johan; Aspegren, Anders; Björquist, Petter (2014-07-04). Sialyl-lactotetra, a novel cell surface marker of undifferentiated human pluripotent stem cells. The Journal of Biological Chemistry. **289** *(27): 18846–18859. doi:10.1074/jbc.M114.568832. ISSN 1083-351X. PMC 4081926. PMID 24841197.*

105. Hirao A, Arai F, Suda T (December 2004). Regulation of cell cycle in hematopoietic stem cells by the niche. Cell Cycle. **3** *(12): 1481–3. doi:10.4161/cc.3.12.1281. PMID 15539950.*

106. Munoz JR, Stoutenger BR, Robinson AP, Spees JL, Prockop DJ (December 2005). Human stem/progenitor cells from bone marrow promote neurogenesis of endogenous neural stem cells in the hippocampus of mice. Proceedings of the National Academy of Sciences of the United States of America. **102** *(50): 18171–6. doi:10.1073/pnas.0508945102. PMC 1312406. PMID 16330757.*

107. Sottile V, Li M, Scotting PJ (July 2006). Stem cell marker expression in the Bergmann glia population of the adult mouse brain. Brain Research. **1099** *(1): 8–17. doi:10.1016/j.brainres.2006.04.127. PMID 16797497.*

108. Smalley MJ, Clarke RB (January 2005). The mammary gland side population: a putative stem/progenitor cell marker?. *Journal of Mammary Gland Biology and Neoplasia.* **10** *(1): 37–47.* doi:10.1007/s10911-005-2539-0. PMID 15886885.

109. Furue M, Okamoto T, Hayashi Y, et al. (2005). Leukemia inhibitory factor as an anti-apoptotic mitogen for pluripotent mouse embryonic stem cells in a serum-free medium without feeder cells. In Vitro Cellular & Developmental Biology. Animal. **41** *(1–2): 19–28. doi:10.1290/0502010.1. PMID 15926856.*

110. Przyborski SA (2001). Isolation of human embryonal carcinoma stem cells by immunomagnetic sorting. Stem Cells. **19** *(6): 500–4. doi:10.1634/stemcells.19-6-500. PMID 11713341.*

111. D›Ippolito G, Howard GA, Roos BA, Schiller PC (2006). Sustained stromal stem cell self-renewal and osteoblastic differentiation during aging. Rejuvenation Research. **9** *(1): 10–9. doi:10.1089/rej.2006.9.10. PMID 16608390.*

112. Kues WA, Petersen B, Mysegades W, Carnwath JW, Niemann H (April 2005). Isolation of murine and porcine fetal stem cells from somatic tissue. Biology of Reproduction. **72** *(4): 1020–8. doi:10.1095/biolreprod.104.031229. PMID 15616223.*

113. Nemetz C, Hocke GM (March 1998). Transcription factor Stat5 is an early marker of differentiation of murine embryonic stem cells. Differentiation. **62** *(5): 213–20. doi:10.1046/j.1432-0436.1998.6250213.x. PMID 9566306.*

114. Falender AE, Freiman RN, Geles KG, et al. (April 2005). Maintenance of spermatogenesis requires TAF4b, a gonad-specific subunit of TFIID. Genes & Development. **19** *(7): 794–803. doi:10.1101/gad.1290105. PMC 1074317. PMID 15774719.*

115. Caddick J, Kingham PJ, Gardiner NJ, Wiberg M, Terenghi G (December 2006). Phenotypic and functional characteristics of mesenchymal stem cells differentiated along a Schwann cell lineage. Glia. **54** *(8): 840–9. doi:10.1002/glia.20421. PMID 16977603.*

116. Snipes RG, Lam KW, Dodd RC, Gray TK, Cohen MS (1 March 1986). Acid phosphatase activity in mononuclear phagocytes and the U937 cell line: monocyte-derived macrophages express tartrate-resistant acid phosphatase. Blood. **67** *(3): 729–34. PMID 3511985.*

117. Krause JR, Brody JP, Kaplan SS, Penchansky L (June 1986). Terminal deoxynucleotidyl transferase activity in acute leukemia: a study of 100 cases comparing an immunoperoxidase (PAP) vs immunofluorescent method. American Journal of Hematology. **22** *(2): 179–84. doi:10.1002/ajh.2830220208. PMID 3518417.*

118. Nakano T, Waki N, Asai H, Kitamura Y (1 December 1987). Long-term monoclonal reconstitution of erythropoiesis in genetically anemic W/Wv mice

by injection of 5-fluorouracil-treated bone marrow cells of Pgk-1b/Pgk-1a mice. Blood. **70** *(6): 1758–63. PMID 2890388.*

119. McNagny KM, Pettersson I, Rossi F, et al. (September 1997). Thrombomucin, a Novel Cell Surface Protein that Defines Thrombocytes and Multipotent Hematopoietic Progenitors. The Journal of Cell Biology. **138** *(6): 1395–407. doi:10.1083/jcb.138.6.1395. PMC 2132552. PMID 9298993.*

120. Masson NM, Currie IS, Terrace JD, Garden OJ, Parks RW, Ross JA (July 2006). Hepatic progenitor cells in human fetal liver express the oval cell marker Thy-1. American Journal of Physiology. **291** *(1): G45–54. doi:10.1152/ajpgi.00465.2005. PMID 16769813.*

121. Inniss K, Moore H (December 2006). Mediation of apoptosis and proliferation of human embryonic stem cells by sphingosine-1-phosphate. Stem Cells and Development. **15** *(6): 789–96. doi:10.1089/scd.2006.15.789. PMID 17253942.*

122. Miller SJ, Rangwala F, Williams J, et al. (March 2006). Large-scale molecular comparison of human schwann cells to malignant peripheral nerve sheath tumor cell lines and tissues. Cancer Research. **66** *(5): 2584–91. doi:10.1158/0008-5472.CAN-05-3330. PMID 16510576.*

123. Pyakurel P, Pak F, Mwakigonja AR, Kaaya E, Heiden T, Biberfeld P (September 2006). Lymphatic and vascular origin of Kaposi›s sarcoma spindle cells during tumor development. International Journal of Cancer. **119** *(6): 1262–7. doi:10.1002/ijc.21969. PMID 16615115.*

124. Walder S, Zhang F, Ferretti P (December 2003). Up-regulation of neural stem cell markers suggests the occurrence of dedifferentiation in regenerating spinal cord. Development Genes and Evolution. **213** *(12): 625–30.* doi:10.1007/s00427-003-0364-2. PMID 14608505.

125. Baker CV, Sharpe CR, Torpey NP, Heasman J, Wylie CC (April 1995). A Xenopus c-kit-related receptor tyrosine kinase expressed in migrating stem cells of the lateral line system. Mechanisms of Development. **50** *(2–3): 217–28.* doi:10.1016/0925-4773(94)00338-N. PMID 7619732.

CHAPTER 2

Induced Stem Cells

Chapter Contents

INTRODUCTION

Induced stem cells (**iSC**) are stem cells derived from somatic, reproductive, pluripotent or other cell types by deliberate epigenetic reprogramming. They are classified as either totipotent (iTC), pluripotent (iPSC) or progenitor (multipotent—iMSC, also called an induced multipotent progenitor cell—iMPC) or unipotent—(iUSC) according to their developmental potential and degree of dedifferentiation. Progenitors are obtained by so-called direct reprogramming or directed differentiation and are also called induced somatic stem cells.

Three techniques are widely recognized:

- Transplantation of nuclei taken from somatic cells into an oocyte (egg cell) lacking its own nucleus (removed in lab)
- Fusion of somatic cells with pluripotent stem cells and
- Transformation of somatic cells into stem cells, using the genetic material encoding reprogramming protein factors, recombinant proteins; microRNA, a synthetic, self-replicating polycistronic RNA and low-molecular weight biologically active substances.

Natural Processes

In 1895 Thomas Morgan removed one of a frog›s two blastomeres and found that amphibians are able to form whole embryos from the remaining part. This meant that the cells can change their differentiation pathway. In 1924 Spemann and Mangold demonstrated the key importance of cell–cell inductions during animal development. The reversible transformation of cells of one differentiated cell type to another is called metaplasia. This transition can be a part of the normal maturation process, or caused by an inducement.

One example is the transformation of iris cells to lens cells in the process of maturation and transformation of retinal pigment epithelium cells into the neural retina during regeneration in adult newt eyes. This process allows the body to replace cells not suitable to new conditions with more suitable new cells. In Drosophila imaginal discs, cells have to choose from a limited number of standard discrete differentiation states. The fact that transdetermination (change of the path of differentiation) often occurs for a group of cells rather than single cells shows that it is induced rather than part of maturation.

The researchers were able to identify the minimal conditions and factors that would be sufficient for starting the cascade of molecular and cellular processes to instruct pluripotent cells to organize the embryo. They showed that opposing gradients of bone morphogenetic protein (BMP) and Nodal, two transforming growth factor family members that act as morphogens, are sufficient to induce molecular and cellular mechanisms required to organize, *in vivo* or *in vitro*, uncommitted cells of the zebrafishblastula animal pole into a well-developed embryo.

Some types of mature, specialized adult cells can naturally revert to stem cells. For example, chief cells express the stem cell marker Troy. While they normally produce digestive fluids for the stomach, they can revert into stem cells to make temporary repairs to stomach injuries, such as a cut or damage from infection. Moreover, they can make this transition even in the absence of noticeable injuries and are capable of replenishing entire gastric units, in essence serving as quiescent reserve stem cells.Differentiated airway epithelial cells can revert into stable and functional stem cells in vivo.

After injury, mature terminally differentiated kidney cells dedifferentiate into more primordial versions of themselves and then differentiate into the cell types needing replacement in the damaged tissue Macrophages can self-renew by local proliferation of mature differentiated cells. In newts, muscle tissue is regenerated from specialized muscle cells that dedifferentiate and forget the type of cell they had been. This capacity to regenerate does not decline with age and may be linked to their ability to make new stem cells from muscle cells on demand.

A variety of nontumorigenic stem cells display the ability to generate multiple cell types. For instance, multilineage-differentiating stress-enduring (MUSE) cells are stress-tolerant adult human stem cells that can self-renew. They form characteristic cell clusters in suspension culture that express a set of genes associated with pluripotency and can differentiate into endodermal, ectodermal and mesodermal cells both in vitro and in vivo.

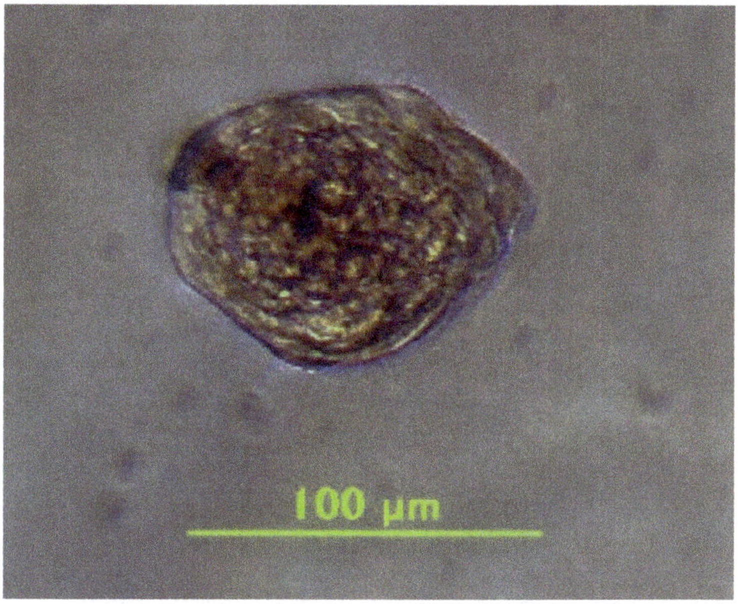

Cluster forming of pluripotent Muse/Stem cell.

Other well-documented examples of transdifferentiation and their significance in development and regeneration were described in detail.

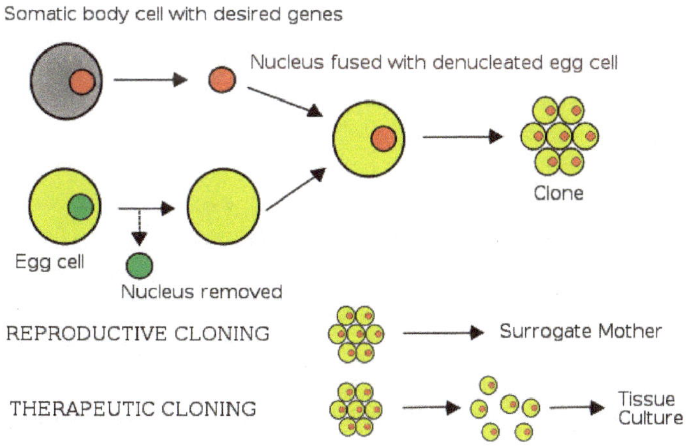

Induced totipotent cells usually can be obtained by reprogramming somatic cells by somatic-cell nuclear transfer (SCNT).

Induced Totipotent Cells

SCNT-mediated

Induced totipotent cells can be obtained by reprogramming somatic cells with somatic-cell nuclear transfer (SCNT). The process involves sucking out the nucleus of a somatic (body) cell and injecting it into an oocyte that has had its nucleus removed

Using an approach based on the protocol outlined by Tachibana et al., hESCs can be generated by SCNT using dermal fibroblasts nuclei from both a middle-aged 35-year-old male and an elderly, 75-year-old male, suggesting that age-associated changes are not necessarily an impediment to SCNT-based nuclear reprogramming of human cells. Such reprogramming of somatic cells to a pluripotent state holds huge potentials for regenerative medicine. Unfortunately, the cells generated by this technology, potentially are not completely protected from the immune system of the patient (donor of nuclei), because they have the same mitochondrial DNA, as a donor of oocytes, instead of the patients mitochondrial DNA. This reduces their value as a source for autologous stem cell transplantation therapy, as for the present, it is not clear whether it can induce an immune response of the patient upon treatment.

Induced androgenetic haploid embryonic stem cells can be used instead of sperm for cloning. These cells, synchronized in M phase and injected into the oocyte can produce viable offspring.

These developments, together with data on the possibility of unlimited oocytes from mitotically active reproductive stem cells, offer the possibility of industrial production of transgenic farm animals. Repeated recloning of viable mice through a SCNT method that includes a histone deacetylase inhibitor, trichostatin, added to the cell culture medium, show that it may be possible to reclone animals indefinitely with no visible accumulation of reprogramming or genomic errors However, research into technologies to develop sperm and egg cells from stem cells raises bioethical issues.

Such technologies may also have far-reaching clinical applications for overcoming cytoplasmic defects in human oocytes. For example, the technology could prevent inherited mitochondrial disease from passing to future generations. Mitochondrial genetic material is passed from mother to child. Mutations can cause diabetes, deafness, eye disorders, gastrointestinal disorders, heart disease, dementia and other neurological diseases. The nucleus from one human egg has been transferred to another, including its mitochondria, creating a cell that could be regarded as having two mothers. The eggs were then fertilised and the resulting embryonic stem cells carried the swapped mitochondrial DNA. As evidence that the technique is safe author of this method points to the existence of the healthy monkeys that are now more than four years old — and are the product of mitochondrial transplants across different genetic backgrounds.

In late-generation telomerase-deficient (Terc−/−) mice, SCNT-mediated reprogramming mitigates telomere dysfunction and mitochondrial defects to a greater extent than iPSC-based reprogramming.

Other cloning and totipotent transformation achievements have been described.

Obtained without SCNT

Recently some researchers succeeded to get the totipotent cells without the aid of SCNT. Totipotent cells were obtained using the epigenetic factors such as oocyte germinal isoform of histone.Reprogramming in vivo, by transitory induction of the four factors Oct4, Sox2, Klf4 and c-Myc in mice, confers totipotency features. Intraperitoneal injection of such in vivo iPS cells generates embryo-like structures that express embryonic and extraembryonic (trophectodermal) markers.

Rejuvenation to iPSc

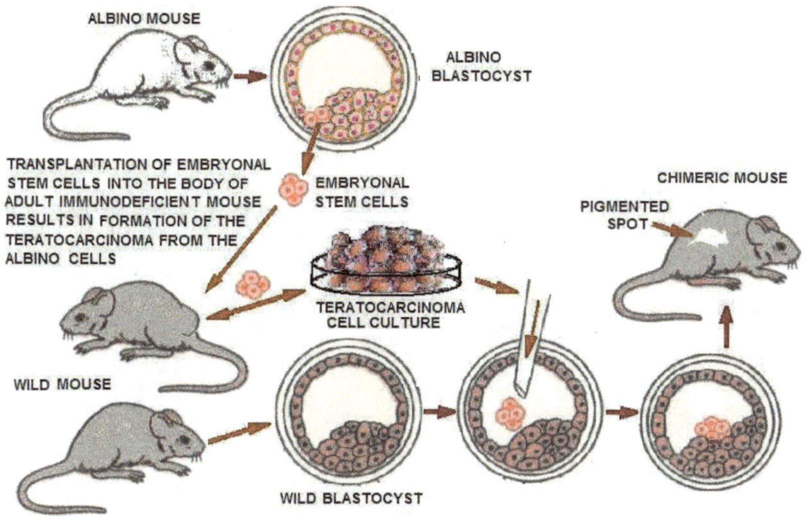

Transplantation of pluripotent/embryonic stem cells into the body of adult mammals, usually leads to the formation of teratomas, which can then turn into a malignant tumor teratocarcinoma. However, putting teratocarcinoma cells into the embryo at the blastocyst stage, caused them to become incorporated in the cell mass and often produced a normal healthy chimeric (i.e. composed of cells from different organisms) animal.

iPSc were first obtained in the form of transplantable teratocarcinoma induced by grafts taken from mouse embryos. Teratocarcinoma formed from somatic cells.Genetically mosaic mice were obtained from malignant teratocarcinoma cells, confirming the cells' pluripotency. It turned out that teratocarcinoma cells are able to maintain a culture of pluripotent embryonic stem cell in an undifferentiated state, by supplying the culture medium with various factors. In the 1980s, it became clear that transplanting pluripotent/embryonic stem cells into the body of adult mammals, usually leads to the formation of teratomas, which can then turn into a malignant tumor teratocarcinoma.However, putting teratocarcinoma cells into the embryo at the blastocyst stage, caused them to become incorporated in the inner cell mass and often produced a normal chimeric (i.e. composed of cells from different organisms) animal. This indicated that the cause of the teratoma is a dissonance - mutual miscommunication between young donor cells and surrounding adult cells (the recipient's so-called "niche).

In August 2006, Japanese researchers circumvented the need for an oocyte, as in SCNT. By reprograming mouse embryonic fibroblasts into pluripotent stem cells via the ectopic expression of four transcription factors, namely Oct4, Sox2, Klf4 and c-Myc, they proved that the overexpression of a small number of factors can push the cell to transition to a new stable state that is associated with changes in the activity of thousands of genes.

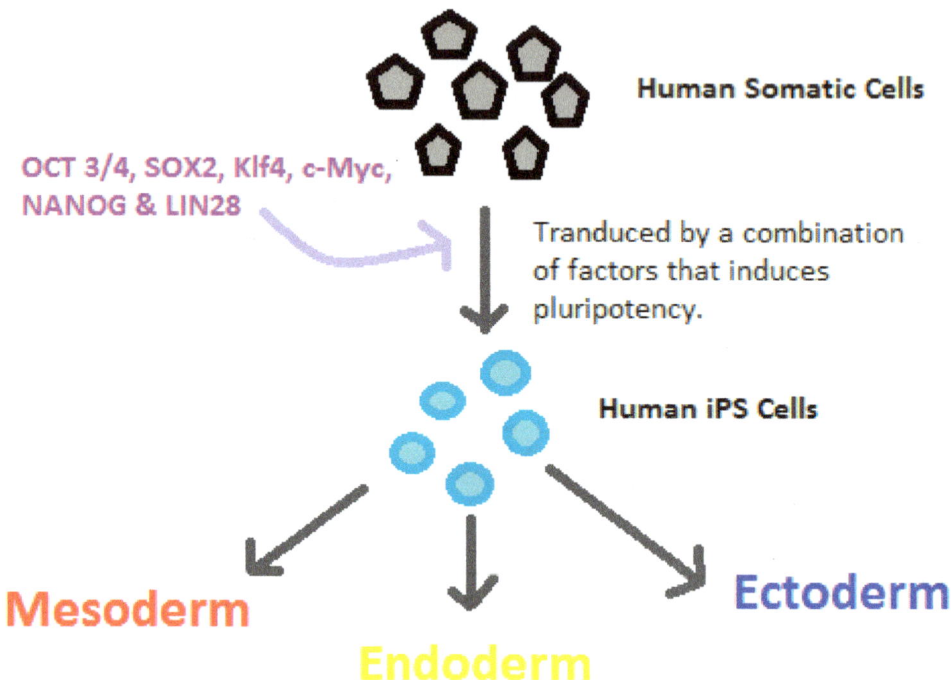

Human somatic cells are made pluripotent by transducing them with factors that induces pluripotency (OCT 3/4, SOX2, Klf4, c-Myc, NANOG and LIN28). This results in the production of IPS cells, which can differentiate into any cells of the three embryonic germ layers (Mesoderm, Endoderm, Ectoderm).

Reprogramming mechanisms are thus linked, rather than independent and are centered on a small number of genes.IPSC properties are very similar to ESCs. iPSCs have been shown to support the development of all-iPSC mice using a tetraploid (4n) embryo, the most stringent assay for developmental potential. However, some genetically normal iPSCs failed to produce all-iPSC mice because of aberrant epigenetic silencing of the imprinted Dlk1-Dio3 gene cluster.

An important advantage of iPSC over ESC is that they can be derived from adult cells, rather than from embryos. Therefore, it became possible to obtain iPSC from adult and even elderly patients.

Reprogramming somatic cells to iPSC leads to rejuvenation. It was found that reprogramming leads to telomere lengthening and subsequent shortening after their differentiation back into fibroblast-like derivatives. Thus, reprogramming leads to the restoration of embryonic telomere length, and hence increases the potential number of cell divisions otherwise limited by the Hayflick limit.

However, because of the dissonance between rejuvenated cells and the surrounding niche of the recipient›s older cells, the injection of his own iPSC usually leads to an immune response, which can be used for medical purposes, or the formation of tumors such as teratoma. The reason has been hypothesized to be that some cells differentiated from ESC and iPSC in vivo continue to synthesize embryonic protein isoforms. So, the immune system might detect and attack cells that are not cooperating properly.

A small molecule called MitoBloCK-6 can force the pluripotent stem cells to die by triggering apoptosis (via cytochrome c release across the mitochondrial outer membrane) in human pluripotent stem cells, but not in differentiated cells. Shortly after differentiation, daughter cells became resistant to death. When MitoBloCK-6 was introduced to differentiated cell lines, the cells remained healthy. The key to their survival, was hypothesized to be due to the changes undergone by pluripotent stem cell mitochondria in the process of cell differentiation. This ability of MitoBloCK-6 to separate the pluripotent and differentiated cell lines has the potential to reduce the risk of teratomas and other problems in regenerative medicine.

In 2012 other small molecules (selective cytotoxic inhibitors of human pluripotent stem cells—hPSCs) were identified that prevented human pluripotent stem cells from forming teratomas in mice. The most potent and selective compound of them (PluriSIn #1) inhibits stearoyl-coA desaturase (the key enzyme in oleic acid biosynthesis), which finally results in apoptosis. With the help of this molecule the undifferentiated cells can be selectively removed from culture. An efficient strategy to selectively eliminate pluripotent cells with teratoma potential is targeting pluripotent stem cell-specific antiapoptotic factor(s) (i.e., survivin or Bcl10). A single treatment with chemical survivin inhibitors (e.g., quercetin or YM155) can induce selective and complete cell death of undifferentiated hPSCs and is claimed to be sufficient to prevent teratoma formation after transplantation. However, it is unlikely that any kind of preliminary clearance, is able to secure the replanting iPSC or ESC. After the selective removal of pluripotent cells, they re-emerge quickly by reverting differentiated cells into stem cells, which leads to tumors. This may be due to the disorder of let-7 regulation of its target Nr6a1 (also known as Germ cell nuclear factor - GCNF), an embryonic transcriptional repressor of pluripotency genes that regulates gene expression in adult fibroblasts following micro-RNA miRNA loss.

Teratoma formation by pluripotent stem cells may be caused by low activity of PTEN enzyme, reported to promote the survival of a small population (0,1-5% of total population) of highly tumorigenic, aggressive, teratoma-initiating embryonic-like carcinoma cells during differentiation. The survival of these teratoma-initiating cells is associated with failed repression of Nanog as well as a propensity for increased glucose and cholesterol metabolism. These teratoma-initiating cells also expressed a lower ratio of p53/p21 when compared to non-tumorigenic cells. In connection with the above safety problems, the use iPSC for cell therapy is still limited. However, they can be used for a variety of other purposes - including the modeling of disease, screening (selective selection) of drugs, toxicity testing of various drugs.

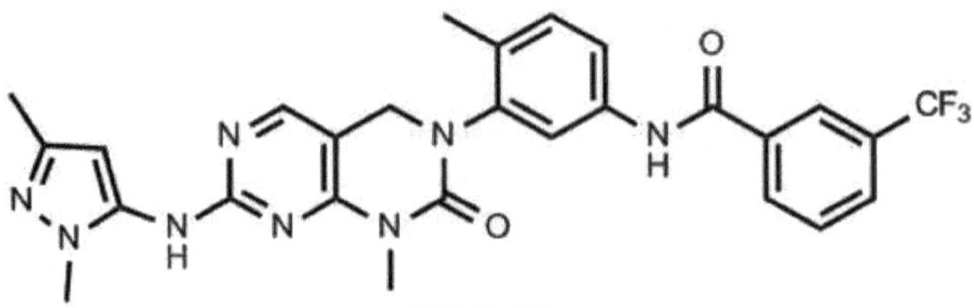

Pluripotin

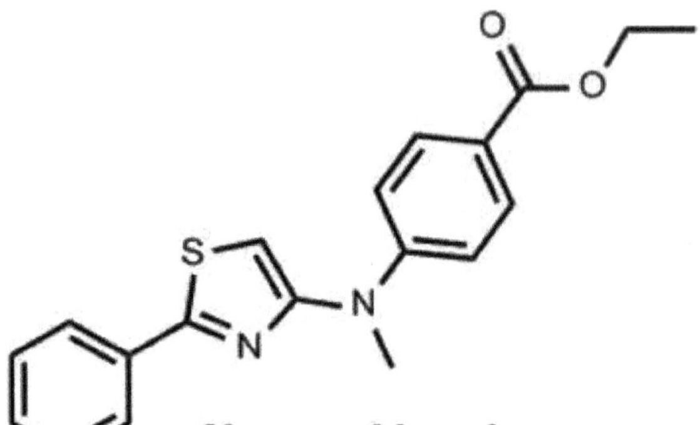

Neuropathioazol

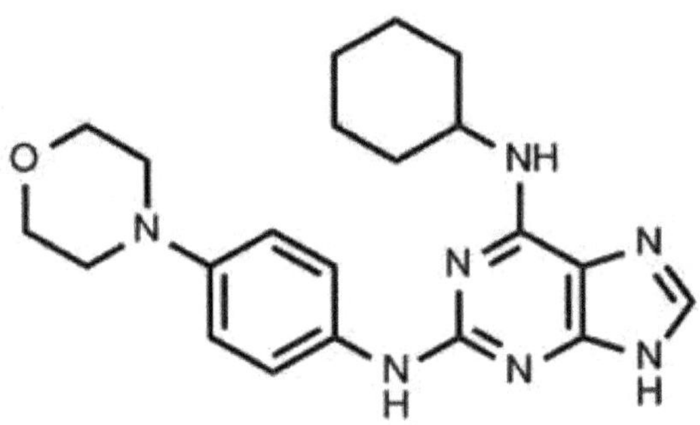

Reversine

Small molecule modulators of stem-cell fate.

It is interesting to note that the tissue grown from iPSCs, placed in the "chimeric" embryos in the early stages of mouse development, practically do not cause an immune response (after the embryos have grown into adult mice) and are suitable for autologous transplantation At the same time, full reprogramming of adult cells in vivo within tissues by transitory induction of the four factors Oct4, Sox2, Klf4 and c-Myc in mice results in teratomas emerging from multiple organs. Furthermore, partial reprogramming of cells toward pluripotency in vivo in mice demonstrates that incomplete reprogramming entails epigenetic changes (failed repression of Polycomb targets and altered DNA methylation) in cells that drive cancer development.

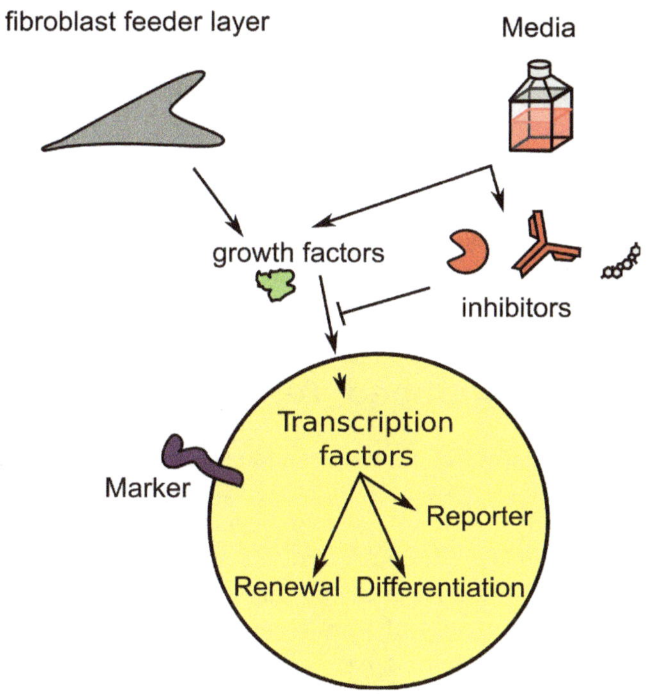

Cell culture example of a small molecule as a tool instead of a protein. in cell culture to obtain a pancreatic lineage from mesodermal stem cells the retinoic acid signalling pathway must be activated while the sonic hedgehog pathway inhibited, which can be done by adding to the media anti-shh antibodies, Hedgehog interacting protein or cyclopamine, the first two are protein and the last a small molecule.

Mogrify Algorithm

Determining the unique set of cellular factors that is needed to be manipulated for each cell conversion is a long and costly process that involved much trial and error. As a result, this first step of identifying the key set of cellular factors for cell conversion is the major obstacle researchers face in the field of cell reprogramming. An international team of researchers have developed an algorithm, called Mogrify(1), that can predict the optimal set of cellular factors required to convert one human cell type to another. When tested, Mogrify was able to accurately predict the set of cellular factors required for previously published cell conversions correctly. To further validate Mogrify's predictive ability, the team conducted two novel cell conversions in the laboratory using human cells and these were successful in both attempts solely using the predictions of Mogrify. Mogrify has been made available online for other researchers and scientists.

Chemical Inducement

By using solely small molecules, Deng Hongkui and colleagues demonstrated that endogenous "master genes" are enough for cell fate reprogramming. They induced a pluripotent state in adult cells from mice using seven small-molecule compounds. The effectiveness of the method is quite high: it was able to convert 0.02% of the adult tissue cells into iPSCs, which is comparable to the gene insertion conversion rate. The authors note that the mice generated from CiPSCs were "100% viable and apparently healthy for up to 6 months". So, this chemical reprogramming strategy has potential use in generating functional desirable cell types for clinical applications.

In 2015th year a robust chemical reprogramming system was established with a yield up to 1,000-fold greater than that of the previously reported protocol. So, chemical reprogramming became a promising approach to manipulate cell fates.

Differentiation from Induced Teratoma

The fact that human iPSCs capable of forming teratomas not only in humans but also in some animal body, in particular in mice or pigs, allowed to develop a method for differentiation of iPSCs in vivo. For this purpose, iPSCs with an agent for inducing differentiation into target cells are injected to genetically modified pig or mouse that has suppressed immune system activation on human cells. The formed teratoma is cut out and used for the isolation of the necessary differentiated human cells by means of monoclonal antibody to tissue-specific markers on the surface of these cells. This method has been successfully used for the production of functional myeloid, erythroid and lymphoid human cells suitable for transplantation (yet only to mice). Mice engrafted with human iPSC teratoma-derived hematopoietic cells produced human B and T cells capable of functional immune responses. These results offer hope that in vivo generation of patient customized cells is feasible, providing materials that could be useful for transplantation, human antibody generation and drug screening applications. Using MitoBloCK-6 and/or PluriSIn # 1 the differentiated progenitor cells can be further purified from teratoma forming pluripotent cells. The fact, that the differentiation takes place even in the teratoma niche, offers hope that the resulting cells are sufficiently stable to stimuli able to cause their transition back to the dedifferentiated (pluripotent) state and therefore safe. A similar in vivo differentiation system, yielding engraftable hematopoietic stem cells from mouse and human iPSCs in teratoma-bearing animals in combination with a maneuver to facilitate hematopoiesis, was described by Suzuki et al.They noted that neither leukemia nor tumors were observed in recipients after intravenous injection of iPSC-derived hematopoietic stem cells into irradiated recipients. Moreover, this injection resulted in multilineage and long-term reconstitution of the hematolymphopoietic system in serial transfers. Such system provides a useful tool for practical application of iPSCs in the treatment of hematologic and immunologic diseases.

For further development of this method animal in which is grown the human cell graft, for example mouse, must have so modified genome that all its cells express and have on its surface human SIRPα. To prevent rejection after transplantation to the patient of the allogenic organ or tissue, grown from the pluripotent stem cells in vivo in the animal, these cells should express two molecules: CTLA4-Ig, which disrupts T cell costimulatory pathways and PD-L1, which activates T cell inhibitory pathway.

Differentiated Cell Types

Retinal Cells

In the near-future, clinical trials designed to demonstrate the safety of the use of iPSCs for cell therapy of the people with age-related macular degeneration, a disease causing blindness through retina damaging, will begin. There are several articles describing methods for producing retinal cells from iPSCs and how to use them for cell therapy. Reports of iPSC-derived retinal pigmented epithelium transplantation showed enhanced visual-guided behaviors of experimental animals for 6 weeks after transplantation. However, clinical trials have been successful: ten patients suffering from retinitis pigmentosa have had their eyesight restored—including a woman who had only 17 percent of her vision left.

Lung and Airway Epithelial Cells

Chronic lung diseases such as idiopathic pulmonary fibrosis and cystic fibrosis or chronic obstructive pulmonary disease and asthma are leading causes of morbidity and mortality worldwide with a considerable human, societal and financial burden. So there is an urgent need for effective cell therapy and lung tissue engineering. Several protocols have been developed for generation of the most cell types of the respiratory system, which may be useful for deriving patient-specific therapeutic cells.

Reproductive Cells

Some lines of iPSCs have the potentiality to differentiate into male germ cells and oocyte-like cells in an appropriate niche (by culturing in retinoic acid and porcine follicular fluid differentiation medium or seminiferous tubule transplantation). Moreover, iPSC transplantation make a contribution to repairing the testis of infertile mice, demonstrating the potentiality of gamete derivation from iPSCs in vivo and in vitro.

Induced progenitor Stem Cells

Direct Transdifferentiation

The risk of cancer and tumors creates the need to develop methods for safer cell lines suitable for clinical use. An alternative approach is so-called "direct reprogramming" - transdifferentiation of cells without passing through the pluripotent state. The basis for this approach was that 5-azacytidine - a DNA demethylation reagent - can cause the formation of myogenic, chondrogenic and adipogeni clones in the immortal cell line of mouse embryonic fibroblasts and that the activation of a single gene, later named MyoD1, is sufficient for such reprogramming. Compared with iPSC whose reprogramming requires at least two weeks, the formation of induced progenitor cells sometimes occurs within a few days and the efficiency of reprogramming is usually many times higher. This reprogramming does not always require cell division. The cells resulting from such reprogramming are more suitable for cell therapy because they do not form teratomas. For example, Chandrakanthan et al., & Pimanda describe the generation of tissue-regenerative multipotent stem cells (iMS cells) by treating mature bone and fat cells transiently with a growth factor (platelet-derived growth factor–AB (PDGF-AB)) and 5-Azacytidine. These authors claim that: Unlike primary mesenchymal stem cells, which are used with little objective evidence in clinical practice to promote tissue repair, iMS cells contribute directly to in vivo tissue regeneration in a context-dependent manner without forming tumors and so has significant scope for application in tissue regeneration.

Single Transcription Factor Transdifferentiation

Originally only early embryonic cells could be coaxed into changing their identity. Mature cells are resistant to changing their identity once they've committed to a specific kind. However, brief expression of a single transcription factor, the ELT-7 GATA factor, can convert the identity of fully differentiated, specialized non-endodermal cells of the pharynx into fully differentiated intestinal cells in intact larvae and adult roundworm *Caenorhabditis elegans* with no requirement for a dedifferentiated intermediate.

Transdifferentiation with CRISPR-Mediated Activator

The cell fate can be effectively manipulated by epigenome editing. In particular, by directly activating of specific endogenous gene expression with CRISPR-mediated activator. When dCas9 (that has been modified so that it no longer cuts DNA, but still can be guided to specific sequences and to bind to them) is combined with transcription activators, it can precisely manipulate endogenous gene expression. Using this method, Wei et al., enhanced the expression of endogenous Cdx2 and Gata6 genes by CRISPR-mediated activators, thus directly converted mouse embryonic stem cells into two extraembryonic lineages, i.e., typical trophoblast stem cells and extraembryonic endoderm cells. An analogous approach was used to induce activation of the endogenous Brn2, Ascl1, and Mytl1 genes to convert mouse embryonic fibroblasts to induced neuronal cells. Thus, transcriptional activation and epigenetic remodeling of endogenous master transcription factors are sufficient for conversion between cell types. The rapid and sustained activation of endogenous genes in their native chromatin context by this approach may facilitate reprogramming with transient methods that avoid genomic integration and provides a new strategy for overcoming epigenetic barriers to cell fate specification.

Phased Process Modeling Regeneration

Another way of reprogramming is the simulation of the processes that occur during amphibian limb regeneration. In urodele amphibians, an early step in limb regeneration is skeletal muscle fiber dedifferentiation into a cellulate that proliferates into limb tissue. However, sequential small molecule treatment of the muscle fiber with myoseverin, reversine (the aurora B kinase inhibitor) and some other chemicals: BIO (glycogen synthase-3 kinase inhibitor), lysophosphatidic acid (pleiotropic activator of G-protein-coupled receptors), SB203580 (p38 MAP kinase inhibitor), or SQ22536 (adenylyl cyclase inhibitor) causes the formation of new muscle cell types as well as other cell types such as precursors to fat, bone and nervous system cells.

Antibody-Based Transdifferentiation

The researchers discovered that GCSF-mimicking antibody can activate a growth-stimulating receptor on marrow cells in a way that induces marrow stem cells that normally develop into white blood cells to become neural progenitor cells. The technique enables researchers to search large libraries of antibodies and quickly select the ones with a desired biological effect.

Conditionally Reprogrammed Cells

Schlegel and Liu demonstrated that the combination of feeder cells and a Rho kinase inhibitor (Y-27632) induces normal and tumor epithelial cells from many tissues to proliferate indefinitely in vitro. This process occurs without the need for transduction of exogenous viral or cellular genes. These cells have been termed Conditionally Reprogrammed Cells (CRC). The induction of CRCs is rapid and results from reprogramming of the entire cell population. CRCs do not express high levels of proteins characteristic of iPSCs or embryonic stem cells (ESCs) (e.g., Sox2, Oct4, Nanog, or Klf4). This induction of CRCs is reversible and removal of Y-27632 and feeders allows the cells to differentiate normally. CRC technology can generate 2×10^6 cells in 5 to 6 days from needle biopsies and can generate cultures from cryopreserved tissue and from fewer than four viable cells. CRCs retain a normal karyotype and remain nontumorigenic. This technique also efficiently establishes cell cultures from human and rodent tumors.

The ability to rapidly generate many tumor cells from small biopsy specimens and frozen tissue provides significant opportunities for cell-based diagnostics and therapeutics (including chemosensitivity testing) and greatly expands the value of biobanking. Using CRC technology, researchers were able to identify an effective therapy for a patient with a rare type of lung tumor. Engleman›s groupdescribes a pharmacogenomic platform that facilitates rapid discovery of drug combinations that can overcome resistance using CRC system. In addition, the CRC method allows for the genetic manipulation of epithelial cells ex vivo and their subsequent evaluation in vivo in the same host. While initial studies revealed that co-culturing epithelial cells with Swiss 3T3 cells J2 was essential for CRC induction, with transwell culture plates, physical contact between feeders and epithelial cells is not required for inducing CRCs and more importantly that irradiation of the feeder cells is required for this induction. Consistent with the transwell experiments, conditioned medium induces and maintains CRCs, which is accompanied by a concomitant increase of cellular telomerase activity. The activity of the conditioned medium correlates directly with radiation-induced feeder cell apoptosis. Thus, conditional reprogramming of epithelial cells is mediated by a combination of Y-27632 and a soluble factor(s) released by apoptotic feeder cells.

Riegel et al. demonstrate that mouse ME cells isolated from normal mammary glands or from mouse mammary tumor virus (MMTV)-Neu–induced mammary tumors, can be cultured indefinitely as conditionally reprogrammed cells (CRCs). Cell surface progenitor-associated markers are rapidly induced in normal mouse ME-CRCs relative to ME cells. However, the expression of certain mammary progenitor subpopulations, such as CD49f+

ESA+ CD44+, drops significantly in later passages. Nevertheless, mouse ME-CRCs grown in a three-dimensional extracellular matrix gave rise to mammary acinar structures. ME-CRCs isolated from MMTV-Neu transgenic mouse mammary tumors express high levels of HER2/neu, as well as tumor-initiating cell markers, such as CD44+, CD49f+ and ESA+ (EpCam). These patterns of expression are sustained in later CRC passages. Early and late passage ME-CRCs from MMTV-Neu tumors that were implanted in the mammary fat pads of syngeneic or nude mice developed vascular tumors that metastasized within 6 weeks of transplantation. Importantly, the histopathology of these tumors was indistinguishable from that of the parental tumors that develop in the MMTV-Neu mice. Application of the CRC system to mouse mammary epithelial cells provides an attractive model system to study the genetics and phenotype of normal and transformed mouse epithelium in a defined culture environment and in vivo transplant studies.

A different approach to CRC is to inhibit CD47—a membrane protein that is the thrombospondin-1 receptor. Loss of CD47 permits sustained proliferation of primary murine endothelial cells, increases asymmetric division and enables these cells to spontaneously reprogram to form multipotent embryoid body-like clusters. CD47 knockdown acutely increases mRNA levels of c-Myc and other stem cell transcription factors in cells in vitro and in vivo. Thrombospondin-1 is a key environmental signal that inhibits stem cell self-renewal via CD47. Thus, CD47 antagonists enable cell self-renewal and reprogramming by overcoming negative regulation of c-Myc and other stem cell transcription factors.In vivo blockade of CD47 using an antisense morpholino increases survival of mice exposed to lethal total body irradiation due to increased proliferative capacity of bone marrow-derived cells and radioprotection of radiosensitive gastrointestinal tissues.

Lineage-Specific Enhancers

Differentiated macrophages can self-renew in tissues and expand long-term in culture. Under certain conditions macrophages can divide without losing features they have acquired while specializing into immune cells - which is usually not possible with differentiated cells. The macrophages achieve this by activating a gene network similar to one found in embryonic stem cells. Single-cell analysis revealed that, *in vivo*, proliferating macrophages can derepress a macrophage-specific enhancer repertoire associated with a gene network controlling self-renewal. This happened when concentrations of two transcription factors named MafB and c-Maf were naturally low or were inhibited for a short time. Genetic manipulations that turned off MafB and c-Maf in the macrophages caused the cells to start a self-renewal program. The similar network also controls embryonic stem cell self-renewal but is associated with distinct embryonic stem cell-specific enhancers.

Hence macrophages isolated from MafB- and c-Maf-double deficient mice divide indefinitely; the self-renewal depends on c-Myc and Klf4.

Indirect Lineage Conversion

Indirect lineage conversion is a reprogramming methodology in which somatic cells transition through a plastic intermediate state of partially reprogrammed cells (pre-iPSC), induced by brief exposure to reprogramming factors, followed by differentiation in a specially developed chemical environment (artificial niche).

This method could be both more efficient and safer, since it does not seem to produce tumors or other undesirable genetic changes and results in much greater yield than other methods. However, the safety of these cells remains questionable. Since lineage conversion from pre-iPSC relies on the use of iPSC reprogramming conditions, a fraction of the cells could acquire pluripotent properties if they do not stop the de-differentation process in vitro or due to further de-differentiation in vivo.

Outer Membrane Glycoprotein

A common feature of pluripotent stem cells is the specific nature of protein glycosylation of their outer membrane. That distinguishes them from most nonpluripotent cells, although not white blood cells.The glycans on the stem cell surface respond rapidly to alterations in cellular state and signaling and are therefore ideal for identifying even minor changes in cell populations. Many stem cell markers are based on cell surface glycan epitopes including the widely used markers SSEA-3, SSEA-4, Tra 1-60 and Tra 1-81. Suila Heli et al. speculate that in human stem cells extracellular O-GlcNAc and extracellular O-LacNAc, play a crucial role in the fine tuning of Notch signaling pathway - a highly conserved cell signaling system, that regulates cell fate specification, differentiation, left–right asymmetry, apoptosis, somitogenesis, angiogenesis and plays a key role in stem cell proliferation (reviewed by Perdigoto and Bardin and Jafar-Nejad et al.)

Changes in outer membrane protein glycosylation are markers of cell states connected in some way with pluripotency and differentiation. The glycosylation change is apparently not just the result of the initialization of gene expression, but perform as an important gene regulator involved in the acquisition and maintenance of the undifferentiated state.

For example, activation of glycoprotein ACA, linking glycosylphosphatidylinositol on the surface of the progenitor cells in human peripheral blood, induces increased expression of genes Wnt, Notch-1, BMI1 and HOXB4 through a signaling cascade PI3K/Akt/mTor/PTEN and promotes the formation of a self-renewing population of hematopoietic stem cells.

Furthermore, dedifferentiation of progenitor cells induced by ACA-dependent signaling pathway leads to ACA-induced pluripotent stem cells, capable of differentiating in vitro into cells of all three germ layers. The study of lectins› ability to maintain a culture of pluripotent human stem cells has led to the discovery of lectin Erythrina crista-galli (ECA), which can serve as a simple and highly effective matrix for the cultivation of human pluripotent stem cells.

Reprogramming through a Physical Approach

Cell adhesion protein E-cadherin is indispensable for a robust pluripotent phenotype. During reprogramming for iPS cell generation, N-cadherin can replace function of E-cadherin. These functions of cadherins are not directly related to adhesion because sphere morphology helps maintaining the "stemness" of stem cells. Moreover, sphere formation, due to forced growth of cells on a low attachment surface, sometimes induces reprogramming. For example, neural progenitor cells can be generated from fibroblasts directly through a physical approach without introducing exogenous reprogramming factors.

Physical cues, in the form of parallel microgrooves on the surface of cell-adhesive substrates, can replace the effects of small-molecule epigenetic modifiers and significantly improve reprogramming efficiency. The mechanism relies on the mechanomodulation of the cells› epigenetic state. Specifically, decreased histone deacetylase activity and upregulation of the expression of WD repeat domain 5 (WDR5)—a subunit of H3 methyltranferase—by microgrooved surfaces lead to increased histone H3 acetylation and methylation. Nanofibrous scaffolds with aligned fibre orientation produce effects similar to those produced by microgrooves, suggesting that changes in cell morphology may be responsible for modulation of the epigenetic state.

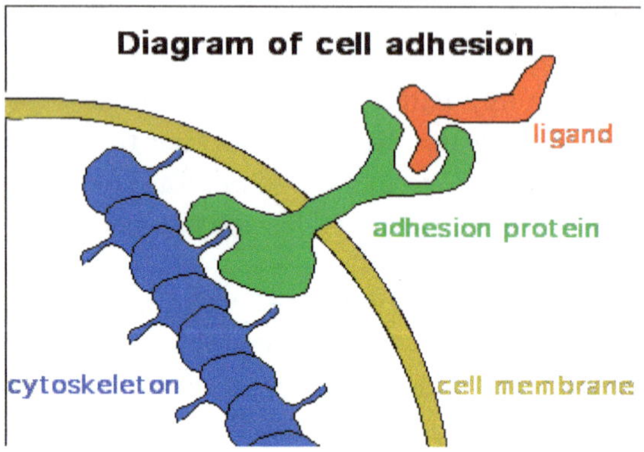

Role of cell adhesions in neural development. Image courtesy of Wikipedia user JWSchmidt under the GNU Free Documentation License.

Substrate rigidity is an important biophysical cue influencing neural induction and subtype specification. For example, soft substrates promote neuroepithelial conversion while inhibiting neural crest differentiation of hESCs in a BMP4-dependent manner. Mechanistic studies revealed a multi-targeted mechanotransductive process involving mechanosensitive Smad phosphorylation and nucleocytoplasmic shuttling, regulated by rigidity-dependent Hippo/YAP activities and actomyosin cytoskeleton integrity and contractility.

Mouse embryonic stem cells (mESCs) undergo self-renewal in the presence of the cytokine leukemia inhibitory factor (LIF). Following LIF withdrawal, mESCs differentiate, accompanied by an increase in cell–substratum adhesion and cell spreading. Restricted cell spreading in the absence of LIF by either culturing mESCs on chemically defined, weakly adhesive biosubstrates, or by manipulating the cytoskeleton allowed the cells to remain in an undifferentiated and pluripotent state. The effect of restricted cell spreading on mESC self-renewal is not mediated by increased intercellular adhesion, as inhibition of mESC adhesion using a function blocking anti E-cadherin antibody or siRNA does not promote differentiation. Possible mechanisms of stem cell fate predetermination by physical interactions with the extracellular matrix have been described.

A new method has been developed that turns cells into stem cells faster and more efficiently by ‹squeezing› them using 3D microenvironment stiffness and density of the surrounding gel. The technique can be applied to a large number of cells to produce stem cells for medical purposes on an industrial scale.

Cells involved in the reprogramming process change morphologically as the process proceeds. This results in physical difference in adhesive forces among cells. Substantial differences in ‹adhesive signature› between pluripotent stem cells, partially reprogrammed cells, differentiated progeny and somatic cells allowed to develop separation process for isolation of pluripotent stem cells in microfluidic devices, which is:

- fast (separation takes less than 10 minutes);
- efficient (separation results in a greater than 95 percent pure iPS cell culture);
- innocuous (cell survival rate is greater than 80 percent and the resulting cells retain normal transcriptional profiles, differentiation potential and karyotype).

Stem cells possess mechanical memory (they remember past physical signals)—with the Hippo signaling pathway factors: Yes-associated protein (YAP) and transcriptional coactivator with PDZ-binding domain (TAZ) acting as an intracellular mechanical rheostat—that stores information from past physical environments and influences the cells' fate.

Neural Stem Cells

Stroke and many neurodegenerative disorders such as Parkinson's disease, Alzheimer's disease, amyotrophic lateral sclerosis need cell replacement therapy. The successful use of converted neural cells (cNs) in transplantations open a new avenue to treat such diseases. Nevertheless, induced neurons (iNs), directly converted from fibroblasts are terminally committed and exhibit very limited proliferative ability that may not provide enough autologous donor cells for transplantation. Self-renewing induced neural stem cells (iNSCs) provide additional advantages over iNs for both basic research and clinical applications.

For example, under specific growth conditions, mouse fibroblasts can be reprogrammed with a single factor, Sox2, to form iNSCs that self-renew in culture and after transplantation can survive and integrate without forming tumors in mouse brains. INSCs can be derived from adult human fibroblasts by non-viral techniques, thus offering a safe method for autologous transplantation or for the development of cell-based disease models.

Neural chemically induced progenitor cells (ciNPCs) can be generated from mouse tail-tip fibroblasts and human urinary somatic cells without introducing exogenous factors, but - by a chemical cocktail, namely VCR (V, VPA, an inhibitor of HDACs; C, CHIR99021, an inhibitor of GSK-3 kinases and R, RepSox, an inhibitor of TGF beta signaling pathways), under a physiological hypoxic condition. Alternative cocktails with inhibitors of histone deacetylation, glycogen synthase kinase and TGF-β pathways (where: sodium butyrate (NaB) or Trichostatin A (TSA) could replace VPA, Lithium chloride (LiCl) or lithium carbonate (Li2CO3) could substitute CHIR99021, or Repsox may be replaced with SB-431542 or Tranilast) show similar efficacies for ciNPC induction. Zhang, et al., also report highly efficient reprogramming of mouse fibroblasts into induced neural stem cell-like cells (ciNSLCs) using a cocktail of nine components.

Multiple methods of direct transformation of somatic cells into induced neural stem cells have been described.

Proof of principle experiments demonstrate that it is possible to convert transplanted human fibroblasts and human astrocytes directly in the brain that are engineered to express inducible forms of neural reprogramming genes, into neurons, when reprogramming genes (Ascl1, Brn2a and Myt1l) are activated after transplantation using a drug.

Astrocytes—the most common neuroglial brain cells, which contribute to scar formation in response to injury—can be directly reprogrammed in vivo to become functional neurons that formed networks in mice without the need of cell transplantation. The researchers followed the mice for nearly a year to look for signs of tumor formation and reported finding none. The same researchers have turned scar-forming astrocytes into progenitor cells called neuroblasts that regenerated into neurons in the injured adult spinal cord.

Oligodendrocyte Precursor Cells

Without myelin to insulate neurons, nerve signals quickly lose power. Diseases that attack myelin, such as multiple sclerosis, result in nerve signals that cannot propagate to nerve endings and as a consequence lead to cognitive, motor and sensory problems. Transplantation of oligodendrocyte precursor cells (OPCs), which can successfully create myelin sheaths around nerve cells, is a promising potential therapeutic response. Direct lineage conversion of mouse and rat fibroblasts into oligodendroglial cells provides a potential source of OPCs. Conversion by forced expression of both eight or of the three transcription factors Sox10, Olig2 and Zfp536, may provide such cells.

Cardiomyocytes

Cell-based in vivo therapies may provide a transformative approach to augment vascular and muscle growth and to prevent non-contractile scar formation by delivering transcription factors or microRNAs to the heart. Cardiac fibroblasts, which represent 50% of the cells in the mammalian heart, can be reprogrammed into cardiomyocyte-like cells in vivo by local delivery of cardiac core transcription factors (GATA4, MEF2C, TBX5 and for improved reprogramming plus ESRRG, MESP1, Myocardin and ZFPM2) after coronary ligation. These results implicated therapies that can directly remuscularize the heart without cell transplantation. However, the efficiency of such reprogramming turned out to be very low and the phenotype of received cardiomyocyte-like cells does not resemble those of a mature normal cardiomyocyte. Furthermore, transplantation of cardiac transcription factors into injured murine hearts resulted in poor cell survival and minimal expression of cardiac genes.

Meanwhile, advances in the methods of obtaining cardiac myocytes in vitro occurred. Efficient cardiac differentiation of human iPS cells gave rise to progenitors that were retained within infarcted rat hearts and reduced remodeling of the heart after ischemic damage.

The team of scientists, who were led by Sheng Ding, used a cocktail of nine chemicals (9C) for transdifferentiation of human skin cells into beating heart cells. With this method, more than 97% of the cells began beating, a characteristic of fully developed, healthy heart cells. The chemically induced cardiomyocyte-like cells (ciCMs) uniformly contracted and resembled human cardiomyocytes in their transcriptome, epigenetic, and electrophysiological properties. When transplanted into infarcted mouse hearts, 9C-treated fibroblasts were efficiently converted to ciCMs and developed into healthy-looking heart muscle cells within the organ. This chemical reprogramming approach, after further optimization, may offer an easy way to provide the cues that induce heart muscle to regenerate locally.

In another study, ischemic cardiomyopathy in the murine infarction model was targeted by iPS cell transplantation. It synchronized failing ventricles, offering a regenerative strategy to achieve resynchronization and protection from decompensation by dint of improved left ventricular conduction and contractility, reduced scarring and reversal of structural remodelling. One protocol generated populations of up to 98% cardiomyocytes from hPSCs simply by modulating the canonical Wnt signaling pathway at defined time points in during differentiation, using readily accessible small molecule compounds.

Discovery of the mechanisms controlling the formation of cardiomyocytes led to the development of the drug ITD-1, which effectively clears the cell surface from TGF-β receptor type II and selectively inhibits intracellular TGF-β signaling. It thus selectively enhances the differentiation of uncommitted mesoderm to cardiomyocytes, but not to vascular smooth muscle and endothelial cells.

One project seeded decellularized mouse hearts with human iPSC-derived multipotential cardiovascular progenitor cells. The introduced cells migrated, proliferated and differentiated in situ into cardiomyocytes, smooth muscle cells and endothelial cells to reconstruct the hearts. In addition, the heart›s extracellular matrix (the substrate of heart scaffold) signalled the human cells into becoming the specialised cells needed for proper heart function. After 20 days of perfusion with growth factors, the engineered heart tissues started to beat again and were responsive to drugs.

Reprogramming of cardiac fibroblasts into induced cardiomyocyte-like cells (iCMs) *in situ* represents a promising strategy for cardiac regeneration. Mice exposed *in vivo*, to three cardiac transcription factors GMT (Gata4, Mef2c, Tbx5) and the small-molecules: SB-431542 (the transforming growth factor (TGF)-β inhibitor), and XAV939 (the WNT inhibitor) for 2 weeks after myocardial infarction showed significantly improved reprogramming (reprogramming efficiency increased eight-fold) and cardiac function compared to those exposed to only GMT.

Rejuvenation of the Muscle Stem Cell

The elderly often suffer from progressive muscle weakness and regenerative failure owing in part to elevated activity of the p38α and p38β mitogen-activated kinase pathway in senescent skeletal muscle stem cells. Subjecting such stem cells to transient inhibition of p38α and p38β in conjunction with culture on soft hydrogel substrates rapidly expands and rejuvenates them that result in the return of their strength.

In geriatric mice, resting satellite cells lose reversible quiescence by switching to an irreversible pre-senescence state, caused by derepression of p16INK4a (also called Cdkn2a). On injury, these cells fail to activate and expand, even in a youthful environment. p16INK4a silencing in geriatric satellite cells restores quiescence and muscle regenerative functions.

Myogenic progenitors for potential use in disease modeling or cell-based therapies targeting skeletal muscle could also be generated directly from induced pluripotent stem cells using free-floating spherical culture (EZ spheres) in a culture medium supplemented with high concentrations (100 ng/ml) of fibroblast growth factor-2 (FGF-2) and epidermal growth factor.

Hepatocytes

Unlike current protocols for deriving hepatocytes from human fibroblasts, Saiyong Zhu et al., (2014)did not generate iPSCs but, using small molecules, cut short reprogramming to pluripotency to generate an induced multipotent progenitor cell (iMPC) state from which endoderm progenitor cells and subsequently hepatocytes (iMPC-Heps) were efficiently differentiated. After transplantation into an immune-deficient mouse model of human liver failure, iMPC-Heps proliferated extensively and acquired levels of hepatocyte function similar to those of human primary adult hepatocytes. iMPC-Heps did not form tumours, most probably because they never entered a pluripotent state.

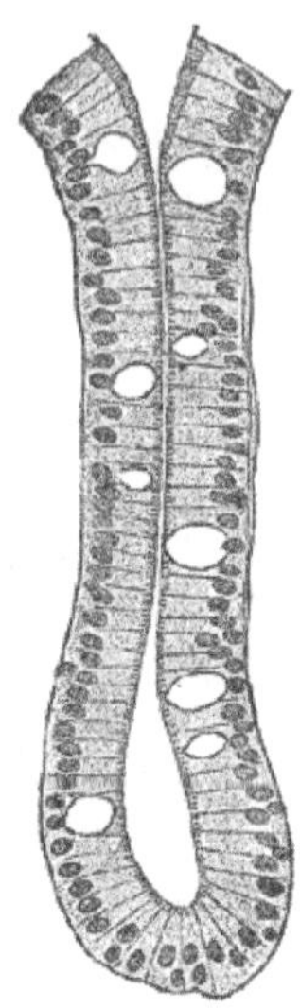

An intestinal crypt - an accessible and abundant source of intestinal epithelial cells for conversion into β-like cells.

These results establish the feasibility of significant liver repopulation of mice with human hepatocytes generated in vitro, which removes a long-standing roadblock on the path to autologous liver cell therapy.

Cocktail of small molecules, Y-27632, A-83-01 (a TGFβ kinase/activin receptor like kinase (ALK5) inhibitor), and CHIR99021 (potent inhibitor of GSK-3), can convert rat and mouse mature hepatocytes in vitro into proliferative bipotent cells - CLiPs (chemically induced liver progenitors). CLiPs can differentiate into both mature hepatocytes and biliary epithelial cells that can form functional ductal structures. In long-term culture CLiPs did not lose their proliferative capacity and their hepatic differentiation ability, and can repopulate chronically injured liver tissue.

Insulin-Producing Cells

Complications of Diabetes mellitus such as cardiovascular diseases, retinopathy, neuropathy, nephropathy and peripheral circulatory diseases depend on sugar dysregulation due to lack of insulin from pancreatic beta cells and can be lethal if they are not treated. One of the promising approaches to understand and cure diabetes is to use pluripotent stem cells (PSCs), including embryonic stem cells (ESCs) and induced PCSs (iPSCs). Unfortunately, human PSC-derived insulin-expressing cells resemble human fetal β cells rather than adult β cells. In contrast to adult β cells, fetal β cells seem functionally immature, as indicated by increased basal glucose secretion and lack of glucose stimulation and confirmed by RNA-seq of whose transcripts.

An alternative strategy is the conversion of fibroblasts towards distinct endodermal progenitor cell populations and, using cocktails of signalling factors, successful differentiation of these endodermal progenitor cells into functional beta-like cells both in vitro and in vivo.

Overexpression of the three transcription factors, **PDX1** (required for pancreatic bud outgrowth and beta-cell maturation), **NGN3** (required for endocrine precursor cell formation) and **MAFA** (for beta-cell maturation) combination (called PNM) can lead to the transformation of some cell types into a beta cell-like state. An accessible and abundant source of functional insulin-producing cells is intestine. PMN expression in human intestinal organoids stimulates the conversion of intestinal epithelial cells into β-like cells possibly acceptable for transplantation.

NEPHRON PROGENITORS

Adult proximal tubule cells were directly transcriptionally reprogrammed to nephron progenitors of the embryonic kidney, using a pool of six genes of instructive transcription factors (SIX1, SIX2, OSR1, Eyes absent homolog 1(EYA1), Homeobox A11 (HOXA11) and Snail homolog 2 (SNAI2)) that activated genes consistent with a cap mesenchyme/nephron progenitor phenotype in the adult proximal tubule cell line. The generation of such cells may lead to cellular therapies for adult renal disease. Embryonic kidney organoids placed into adult rat kidneys can undergo onward development and vascular development.

Blood Vessel Cells

As blood vessels age, they often become abnormal in structure and function, thereby contributing to numerous age-associated diseases including myocardial infarction, ischemic stroke and atherosclerosis of arteries supplying the heart, brain and lower extremities. So, an important goal is to stimulate vascular growth for the collateral circulation to prevent the exacerbation of these diseases. Induced Vascular Progenitor Cells (iVPCs) are useful for cell-based therapy designed to stimulate coronary collateral growth. They were generated by partially reprogramming endothelial cells. The vascular commitment of iVPCs is related to the epigenetic memory of endothelial cells, which engenders them as cellular components of growing blood vessels. That is why, when iVPCs were implanted into myocardium, they engrafted in blood vessels and increased coronary collateral flow better than iPSCs, mesenchymal stem cells, or native endothelial cells.

Ex vivo genetic modification can be an effective strategy to enhance stem cell function. For example, cellular therapy employing genetic modification with Pim-1 kinase (a downstream effector of Akt, which positively regulates neovasculogenesis) of bone marrow–derived cells or human cardiac progenitor cells, isolated from failing myocardium results in durability of repair, together with the improvement of functional parameters of myocardial hemodynamic performance.

Stem cells extracted from fat tissue after liposuction may be coaxed into becoming progenitor smooth muscle cells (iPVSMCs) found in arteries and veins.

The 2D culture system of human iPS cells in conjunction with triple marker selection (CD34 (a surface glycophosphoprotein expressed on developmentally early embryonic fibroblasts), NP1 (receptor - neuropilin 1) and KDR (kinase insert domain-containing receptor)) for the isolation of vasculogenic precursor cells from human iPSC, generated endothelial cells that, after transplantation, formed stable, functional mouse blood vessels in vivo, lasting for 280 days.

To treat infarction, it is important to prevent the formation of fibrotic scar tissue. This can be achieved in vivo by transient application of paracrine factors that redirect native heart progenitor stem cell contributions from scar tissue to cardiovascular tissue. For example, in a mouse myocardial infarction model, a single intramyocardial injection of human vascular endothelial growth factor A mRNA (VEGF-A modRNA), modified to escape the body's normal defense system, results in long-term improvement of heart function due to mobilization and redirection of epicardial progenitor cells toward cardiovascular cell types.

Blood Stem Cells

Red Blood Cells

RBC transfusion is necessary for many patients. However, to date the supply of RBCs remains labile. In addition, transfusion risks infectious disease transmission. A large supply of safe RBCs generated in vitro would help to address this issue. Ex vivo erythroid cell generation may provide alternative transfusion products to meet present and future clinical requirements. Red blood cells (RBC)s generated in vitro from mobilized CD34 positive cells have normal survival when transfused into an autologous recipient. RBC produced in vitro contained exclusively fetal hemoglobin (HbF), which rescues the functionality of these RBCs. In vivo the switch of fetal to adult hemoglobin was observed after infusion of nucleated erythroid precursors derived from iPSCs. Although RBCs do not have nuclei and therefore can not form a tumor, their immediate erythroblasts precursors have nuclei. The terminal maturation of erythroblasts into functional RBCs requires a complex remodeling process that ends with extrusion of the nucleus and the formation of an enucleated RBC. Cell reprogramming often disrupts enucleation. Transfusion of in vitro-generated RBCs or erythroblasts does not sufficiently protect against tumor formation.

The aryl hydrocarbon receptor (AhR) pathway (which has been shown to be involved in the promotion of cancer cell development) plays an important role in normal blood cell development. AhR activation in human hematopoietic progenitor cells (HPs) drives an unprecedented expansion of HPs, megakaryocyte- and erythroid-lineage cells. See also Concise Review: The SH2B3 gene encodes a negative regulator of cytokine signaling and naturally occurring loss-of-function variants in this gene increase RBC counts in vivo. Targeted suppression of SH2B3 in primary human hematopoietic stem and progenitor cells enhanced the maturation and overall yield of in-vitro-derived RBCs. Moreover, inactivation of SH2B3 by CRISPR/Cas9 genome editing in human pluripotent stem cells allowed enhanced erythroid cell expansion with preserved differentiation. (See also overview.)

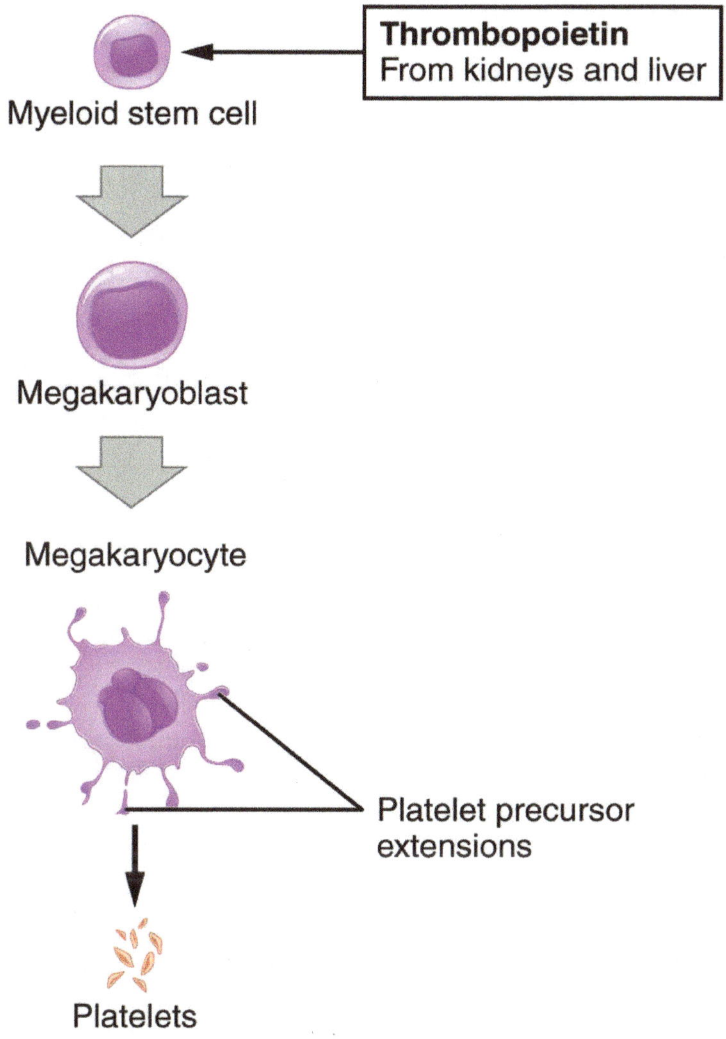

Platelets extruded from megakaryocytes.

Platelets

Platelets help prevent hemorrhage in thrombocytopenic patients and patients with thrombocythemia. A significant problem for multitransfused patients is refractoriness to platelet transfusions. Thus, the ability to generate platelet products ex vivo and platelet products lacking HLA antigens in serum-free media would have clinical value. An RNA interference-based mechanism used a lentiviral vector to express short-hairpin RNAi targeting β2-microglobulin transcripts in CD34-positive cells. Generated platelets demonstrated an 85% reduction in class I HLA antigens. These platelets appeared to have normal function in vitro

One clinically-applicable strategy for the derivation of functional platelets from human iPSC involves the establishment of stable immortalized megakaryocyte progenitor cell lines (imMKCLs) through doxycycline-dependent overexpression of BMI1 and BCL-XL. The resulting imMKCLs can be expanded in culture over extended periods (4–5 months), even after cryopreservation. Halting the overexpression (by the removal of doxycycline from the medium) of c-MYC, BMI1 and BCL-XL in growing imMKCLs led to the production of CD42b+ platelets with functionality comparable to that of native platelets on the basis of a range of assays in vitro and in vivo. Thomas et al., describe a forward programming strategy relying on the concurrent exogenous expression of 3 transcription factors: GATA1, FLI1 and TAL1. The forward programmed megakaryocytes proliferate and differentiate in culture for several months with megakaryocyte purity over 90% reaching up to $2x10^5$ mature megakaryocytes per input hPSC. Functional platelets are generated throughout the culture allowing the prospective collection of several transfusion units from as few as one million starting hPSCs. See also overview

Immune Cells

A specialised type of white blood cell, known as cytotoxic T lymphocytes (CTLs), are produced by the immune system and are able to recognise specific markers on the surface of various infectious or tumour cells, causing them to launch an attack to kill the harmful cells. Thence, immunotherapy with functional antigen-specific T cells has potential as a therapeutic strategy for combating many cancers and viral infections. However, cell sources are limited, because they are produced in small numbers naturally and have a short lifespan.

A potentially efficient approach for generating antigen-specific CTLs is to revert mature immune T cells into iPSCs, which possess indefinite proliferative capacity in vitro and after their multiplication to coax them to redifferentiate back into T cells.

Another method combines iPSC and chimeric antigen receptor (CAR) technologies to generate human T cells targeted to CD19, an antigen expressed by malignant B cells, in tissue culture. This approach of generating therapeutic human T cells may be useful for cancer immunotherapy and other medical applications.

Invariant natural killer T (iNKT) cells have great clinical potential as adjuvants for cancer immunotherapy. iNKT cells act as innate T lymphocytes and serve as a bridge between the innate and acquired immune systems. They augment anti-tumor responses by producing interferon-gamma (IFN-γ). The approach of collection, reprogramming/dedifferentiation, re-differentiation and injection has been proposed for related tumor treatment.

Dendritic cells (DC) are specialized to control T-cell responses. DC with appropriate genetic modifications may survive long enough to stimulate antigen-specific CTL and after that be completely eliminated. DC-like antigen-presenting cells obtained from human induced pluripotent stem cells can serve as a source for vaccination therapy.

CCAAT/enhancer binding protein-α (C/EBPα) induces transdifferentiation of B cells into macrophages at high efficiencies and enhances reprogramming into iPS cells when co-expressed with transcription factors Oct4, Sox2, Klf4 and Myc. with a 100-fold increase in iPS cell reprogramming efficiency, involving 95% of the population. Furthermore, C/EBPa can convert selected human B cell lymphoma and leukemia cell lines into macrophage-like cells at high efficiencies, impairing the cells' tumor-forming capacity.

Thymic Epithelial Cells Rejuvenation

The thymus is the first organ to deteriorate as people age. This shrinking is one of the main reasons the immune system becomes less effective with age. Diminished expression of the thymic epithelial cell transcription factor FOXN1 has been implicated as a component of the mechanism regulating age-related involution.

Clare Blackburn and colleagues show that established age-related thymic involution can be reversed by forced upregulation of just one transcription factor - FOXN1 in the thymic epithelial cells in order to promote rejuvenation, proliferation and differentiation of these cells into fully functional thymic epithelium. This rejuvenation and increased proliferation was accompanied by upregulation of genes that promote cell cycle progression (cyclin D1, ΔNp63, FgfR2IIIb) and that are required in the thymic epithelial cells to promote specific aspects of T cell development (Dll4, Kitl, Ccl25, Cxcl12, Cd40, Cd80, Ctsl, Pax1).

Mesenchymal Stem Cells

Induction

Mesenchymal stem/stromal cells (MSCs) are under investigation for applications in cardiac, renal, neural, joint and bone repair, as well as in inflammatory conditions and hemopoietic cotransplantation. This is because of their immunosuppressive properties and ability to differentiate into a wide range of mesenchymal-lineage tissues. MSCs are typically harvested from adult bone marrow or fat, but these require painful invasive procedures and are low-frequency sources, making up only 0.001%– 0.01% of bone marrow cells and 0.05% in liposuction aspirates. Of concern for autologous use, in particular in the elderly most in need of tissue repair, MSCs decline in quantity and quality with age.

IPSCs could be obtained by the cells rejuvenation of even centenarians. Because iPSCs can be harvested free of ethical constraints and culture can be expanded indefinitely, they are an advantageous source of MSCs. IPSC treatment with SB-431542 leads to rapid and uniform MSC generation from human iPSCs. (SB-431542 is an inhibitor of activin/TGF- pathways by blocking phosphorylation of ALK4, ALK5 and ALK7 receptors.) These iPS-MSCs may lack teratoma-forming ability, display a normal stable karyotype in culture and exhibit growth and differentiation characteristics that closely resemble those of primary MSCs. It has potential for in vitro scale-up, enabling MSC-based therapies. MSC derived from iPSC have the capacity to aid periodontal regeneration and are a promising source of readily accessible stem cells for use in the clinical treatment of periodontitis.

Besides cell therapy in vivo, the culture of human mesenchymal stem cells can be used in vitro for mass-production of exosomes, which are ideal vehicles for drug delivery.

Dedifferentiated Adipocytes

Adipose tissue, because of its abundance and relatively less invasive harvest methods, represents a source of mesenchymal stem cells (MSCs). Unfortunately, liposuction aspirates are only 0.05% MSCs. However, a large amount of mature adipocytes, which in general have lost their proliferative abilities and therefore are typically discarded, can be easily isolated from the adipose cell suspension and dedifferentiated into lipid-free fibroblast-like cells, named dedifferentiated fat (DFAT) cells. DFAT cells re-establish active proliferation ability and express multipotent capacities. Compared with adult stem cells, DFAT cells show unique advantages in abundance, isolation and homogeneity. Under proper induction culture in vitro or proper environment in vivo, DFAT cells could demonstrate adipogenic, osteogenic, chondrogenic and myogenic potentials. They could also exhibit perivascular characteristics and elicit neovascularization.

Chondrogenic Cells

Cartilage is the connective tissue responsible for frictionless joint movement. Its degeneration ultimately results in complete loss of joint function in the late stages of osteoarthritis. As an avascular and hypocellular tissue, cartilage has a limited capacity for self-repair. Chondrocytes are the only cell type in cartilage, in which they are surrounded by the extracellular matrix that they secrete and assemble.

One method of producing cartilage is to induce it from iPS cells. Alternatively, it is possible to convert fibroblasts directly into induced chondrogenic cells (iChon) without an intermediate iPS cell stage, by inserting three reprogramming factors (c-MYC, KLF4 and SOX9). Human iChon cells expressed marker genes for chondrocytes (type II collagen) but not fibroblasts.

Implanted into defects created in the articular cartilage of rats, human iChon cells survived to form cartilaginous tissue for at least four weeks, with no tumors. The method makes use of c-MYC, which is thought to have a major role in tumorigenesis and employs a retrovirus to introduce the reprogramming factors, excluding it from unmodified use in human therapy.

SOURCES OF CELLS FOR REPROGRAMMING

The most frequently used sources for reprogramming are blood cells and fibroblasts, obtained by biopsy of the skin, but taking cells from urine is less invasive. The latter method does not require a biopsy or blood sampling. As of 2013, urine-derived stem cells had been differentiated into endothelial, osteogenic, chondrogenic, adipogenic, skeletal myogenic and neurogenic lineages, without forming teratomas. Therefore, their epigenetic memory is suited to reprogramming into iPS cells. However, few cells appear in urine, only low conversion efficiencies had been achieved and the risk of bacterial contamination is relatively high.

Another promising source of cells for reprogramming are mesenchymal stem cells derived from human hair follicles.

The origin of somatic cells used for reprogramming may influence the efficiency of reprogramming, the functional properties of the resulting induced stem cells and the ability to form tumors.

IPSCs retain an epigenetic memory of their tissue of origin, which impacts their differentiation potential. This epigenetic memory does not necessarily manifest itself at the pluripotency stage – iPSCs derived from different tissues exhibit proper morphology, express pluripotency markers and are able to differentiate into the three embryonic layers in vitro and in vivo. However, this epigenetic memory may manifest during re-differentiation into specific cell types that require the specific loci bearing residual epigenetic marks.

ADULT STEM CELL

Adult stem cells are undifferentiated cells, found throughout the body after development, that multiply by cell division to replenish dying cells and regenerate damaged tissues. More accurately known as **somaticstem cells** (from Greek Σωματικός, meaning *of the body*), because they are usually more plentiful in juvenile (child) than in adult animal and human bodies.

Scientific interest in adult stem cells is centered on their ability to divide or *self-renew* indefinitely, and generate all the cell types of the organ from which they originate, potentially regenerating the entire organ from a few cells. Unlike embryonic stem cells, the use of human adult stem cells in research and therapy is not considered to be controversial, as they are derived from adult tissue samples rather than human embryos designated for scientific research. They have mainly been studied in humans and model organisms such as mice and rats.

Defining Properties

A stem cell possesses two properties:

- ***Self-renewal***, which is the ability to go through numerous cycles of cell division while still maintaining its undifferentiated state.
- ***multipotency*** or ***multidifferentiative potential***, which is the ability to generate progeny of several distinct cell types, (for example glial cells and neurons) as opposed to unipotency, which is the term for cells that are restricted to producing a single-cell type. However, some researchers do not consider multipotency to be essential, and believe that unipotent self-renewing stem cells can exist. These properties can be illustrated with relative ease *in vitro*, using methods such as clonogenic assays, where the progeny of a single cell is characterized. However, it is known that *in vitro* cell culture conditions can alter the behavior of cells, proving that a particular subpopulation of cells possesses stem cell properties *in vivo* is challenging, and so considerable debate exists as to whether some proposed stem cell populations in the adult are indeed stem cells.

Lineage

To ensure self-renewal, stem cells undergo two types of cell division (see *Stem cell division and differentiation* diagram). Symmetric division gives rise to two identical daughter cells, both endowed with stem cell properties, whereas asymmetric division produces only one stem cell and a progenitor cell with limited self-renewal potential. Progenitors can go through several rounds of cell division before finally differentiating into a mature cell. It is believed that the molecular distinction between symmetric and asymmetric divisions lies in differential segregation of cell membrane proteins (such as receptors) between the daughter cells.

Multidrug Resistance

Adult stem cells express transporters of the ATP-binding cassette family that actively pump a diversity of organic molecules out of the cell. Many pharmaceuticals are exported by these transporters conferring multidrug resistance onto the cell. This complicates the design of drugs, for instance neural stem cell targeted therapies for the treatment of clinical depression.

Signaling Pathways

Adult stem cell research has been focused on uncovering the general molecular mechanisms that control their self-renewal and differentiation.

- Notch

The Notch pathway has been known to developmental biologists for decades. Its role in control of stem cell proliferation has now been demonstrated for several cell types including haematopoietic, neural, and mammary stem cells.

- Wnt

These developmental pathways are also strongly implicated as stem cell regulators.

- TGFβ

The TGFβ family of cytokines regulate the stemness of both normal and cancer stem cells.

Plasticity

Discoveries in recent years have suggested that adult stem cells might have the ability to differentiate into cell types from different germ layers. For instance, neural stem cells from the brain, which are derived from ectoderm, can differentiate into ectoderm, mesoderm, and endoderm. Stem cells from the bone marrow, which is derived from mesoderm, can differentiate into liver, lung, GI tract and skin, which are derived from endoderm and mesoderm. This phenomenon is referred to as stem cell transdifferentiation or plasticity. It can be induced by modifying the growth medium when stem cells are cultured *in vitro* or transplanting them to an organ of the body different from the one they were originally isolated from. There is yet no consensus among biologists on the prevalence and physiological and therapeutic relevance of stem cell plasticity. More recent findings suggest that pluripotent stem cells may reside in blood and adult tissues in a dormant state. These cells are referred to as "Blastomere Like Stem Cells" (Am Surg. 2007 Nov;73:1106-10) and very small embryonic like - VSEL stem cells, and display pluripotency in vitro. As BLSC›s and VSEL cells are present in virtually all adult tissues, including lung, brain, kidneys, muscles, and pancreas Co-purification of BLSC›s and VSEL cells with other populations of adult stem cells may explain the apparent pluripotency of adult stem cell populations. However, recent studies have shown that both human and murine VSEL cells lack stem cell characteristics and are not pluripotent.

Aging

Stem cell function becomes impaired with age, and this contributes to progressive deterioration of tissue maintenance and repair. A likely important cause of increasing stem cell dysfunction is age-dependent accumulation of DNA damage in both stem cells and the cells that comprise the stem cell environment. (See also DNA damage theory of aging.)

Types

Hematopoietic Stem Cells

Hematopoietic stem cells are found in the bone marrow and umbilical cord blood and give rise to all the blood cell types.

Mammary Stem Cells

Mammary stem cells provide the source of cells for growth of the mammary gland during puberty and gestation and play an important role in carcinogenesis of the breast. Mammary stem cells have been isolated from human and mouse tissue as well as from cell lines derived from the mammary gland. Single such cells can give rise to both the luminal and myoepithelial cell types of the gland, and have been shown to have the ability to regenerate the entire organ in mice.

Intestinal stem cells

Intestinal stem cells divide continuously throughout life and use a complex genetic program to produce the cells lining the surface of the small and large intestines. Intestinal stem cells reside near the base of the stem cell niche, called the crypts of Lieberkuhn. Intestinal stem cells are probably the source of most cancers of the small intestine and colon.

Mesenchymal Stem Cells

Mesenchymal stem cells (MSCs) are of stromal origin and may differentiate into a variety of tissues. MSCs have been isolated from placenta, adipose tissue, lung, bone marrow and blood, Wharton›s jelly from the umbilical cord, and teeth (perivascular niche of dental pulp and periodontal ligament).MSCs are attractive for clinical therapy due to their ability to differentiate, provide trophic support, and modulate innate immune response. These cells have the ability to differentiate into various cell types such as osteoblasts, chondroblasts, adypocytes, neuroectodermal cells, and hepatocytes. Bioactive mediators that favor local cell growth are also secreted by MSCs. Anti-inflammatory effects on the local microenvironment, which promote tissue healing, are also observed. The inflammatory response can be modulated by adipose-derived regenerative cells (ADRC) including mesenchymal stem cells and regulatory T-lymphocytes. The mesenchymal stem cells thus alter the outcome of the immune response by changing the cytokine secretion of dendritic and T-cell subsets. This results in a shift from a pro-inflammatory environment to an anti-inflammatory or tolerant cell environment.

Endothelial Stem Cells

Endothelial stem cells are one of the three types of multipotent stem cells found in the bone marrow. They are a rare and controversial group with the ability to differentiate into endothelial cells, the cells that line blood vessels.

Neural Stem Cells

The existence of stem cells in the adult brain has been postulated following the discovery that the process of neurogenesis, the birth of new neurons, continues into adulthood in rats. The presence of stem cells in the mature primate brain was first reported in 1967. It has since been shown that new neurons are generated in adult mice, songbirds and primates, including humans. Normally, adult neurogenesis is restricted to two areas of the brain – the subventricular zone, which lines the lateral ventricles, and the dentate gyrus of the hippocampal formation. Although the generation of new neurons in the hippocampus is well established, the presence of true self-renewing stem cells there has been debated. Under certain circumstances, such as following tissue damage in ischemia, neurogenesis can be induced in other brain regions, including the neocortex.

Neural stem cells are commonly cultured *in vitro* as so called neurospheres – floating heterogeneous aggregates of cells, containing a large proportion of stem cells. They can be propagated for extended periods of time and differentiated into both neuronal and glia cells, and therefore behave as stem cells. However, some recent studies suggest that this behaviour is induced by the culture conditions in progenitor cells, the progeny of stem cell division that normally undergo a strictly limited number of replication cycles *in vivo*. Furthermore, neurosphere-derived cells do not behave as stem cells when transplanted back into the brain.

Neural stem cells share many properties with haematopoietic stem cells (HSCs). Remarkably, when injected into the blood, neurosphere-derived cells differentiate into various cell types of the immune system.

Olfactory Adult Stem Cells

Olfactory adult stem cells have been successfully harvested from the human olfactory mucosa cells, which are found in the lining of the nose and are involved in the sense of smell. If they are given the right chemical environment these cells have the same ability as embryonic stem cells to develop into many different cell types. Olfactory stem cells hold the potential for therapeutic applications and, in contrast to neural stem cells, can be harvested with ease without harm to the patient. This means they can be easily obtained from all individuals, including older patients who might be most in need of stem cell therapies.

Neural Crest Stem Cells

Hair follicles contain two types of stem cells, one of which appears to represent a remnant of the stem cells of the embryonic neural crest. Similar cells have been found in the gastrointestinal tract, sciatic nerve, cardiac outflow tract and spinal and sympathetic ganglia. These cells can generate neurons, Schwann cells, myofibroblast, chondrocytes and melanocytes.

Testicular Cells

Multipotent stem cells with a claimed equivalency to embryonic stem cells have been derived from spermatogonial progenitor cells found in the testicles of laboratory mice by scientists in Germany and the United States, and, a year later, researchers from Germany and the United Kingdom confirmed the same capability using cells from the testicles of humans. The extracted stem cells are known as human adult germline stem cells (GSCs)

Multipotent stem cells have also been derived from germ cells found in human testicles.

Adult stem cell therapies

Stem-cell therapy

The therapeutic potential of adult stem cells is the focus of much scientific research, due to their ability to be harvested from the patient. In common with embryonic stem cells, adult stem cells have the ability to differentiate into more than one cell type, but unlike the former they are often restricted to certain types or "lineages". The ability of a differentiated stem cell of one lineage to produce cells of a different lineage is called transdifferentiation. Some types of adult stem cells are more capable of transdifferentiation than others, but for many there is no evidence that such a transformation is possible. Consequently, adult stem therapies require a stem cell source of the specific lineage needed, and harvesting and/or culturing them up to the numbers required is a challenge. Additionally, cues from the immediate environment (including how stiff or porous the surrounding structure/extracellular matrix is) can alter or enhance the fate and differentiation of the stem cells.

Sources

Pluripotent stem cells, i.e. cells that can give rise to any fetal or adult cell type, can be found in a number of tissues, including umbilical cord blood. Using genetic reprogramming, pluripotent stem cells equivalent to embryonic stem cells have been derived from human adult skin tissue.Other adult stem cells are multipotent, meaning they are restricted in the types of cell they can become, and are generally referred to by their tissue origin (such as mesenchymal stem cell, adipose-derived stem cell, endothelial stem cell, etc.). A great deal of adult stem cell research has focused on investigating their capacity to divide or self-renew indefinitely, and their potential for differentiation. In mice, pluripotent stem cells can be directly generated from adult fibroblast cultures.

Clinical Applications

Adult stem cell treatments have been used for many years to successfully treat leukemia and related bone/blood cancers utilizing bone marrow transplants. The use of adult stem cells in research and therapy is not considered as controversial as the use of embryonic stem cells, because the production of adult stem cells does not require the destruction of an embryo.

Early regenerative applications of adult stem cells has focused on intravenous delivery of blood progenitors known as Hematopetic Stem Cells (HSC›s). CD34+ hematopoietic Stem Cells have been clinically applied to treat various diseases including spinal cord injury, liver cirrhosis and Peripheral Vascular disease. Research has shown that CD34+ hematopoietic Stem

Cells are relatively more numerous in men than in women of reproductive age group among spinal cord Injury victims. Other early commercial applications have focused on Mesenchymal Stem Cells (MSCs). For both cell lines, direct injection or placement of cells into a site in need of repair may be the preferred method of treatment, as vascular delivery suffers from a "pulmonary first pass effect" where intravenous injected cells are sequestered in the lungs. Clinical case reports in orthopedic applications have been published. Wakitani has published a small case series of nine defects in five knees involving surgical transplantation of mesenchymal stem cells with coverage of the treated chondral defects. Centeno et al. have reported high field MRI evidence of increased cartilage and meniscus volume in individual human clinical subjects as well as a large n=227 safety study. Many other stem cell based treatments are operating outside the US, with much controversy being reported regarding these treatments as some feel more regulation is needed as clinics tend to exaggerate claims of success and minimize or omit risks.

Adult Stem Cells and Cancer

In recent years, acceptance of the concept of adult stem cells has increased. There is now a hypothesis that stem cells reside in many adult tissues and that these unique reservoirs of cells not only are responsible for the normal reparative and regenerative processes but are also considered to be a prime target for genetic and epigenetic changes, culminating in many abnormal conditions including cancer. (See cancer stem cell for more details.)

REFERENCES

1. Yamanaka, S.; Blau, H. M. (2010). "Nuclear reprogramming to a pluripotent state by three approaches". Nature. 465 (7299): 704–12. doi:10.1038/nature09229. PMC 2901154 . PMID 20535199.
2. Gurdon J. B. and Ian Wilmut (2011) Nuclear Transfer to Eggs and Oocytes Cold Spring Harb Perspect Biol; 3: a002659
3. Tachibana, M.; Amato, P.; Sparman, M.; Gutierrez, N. M.; Tippner-Hedges, R.; Ma, H.; Kang, E.; Fulati, A.; Lee, H. S.; Sritanaudomchai, H.; Masterson, K.; Larson, J.; Eaton, D.; Sadler-Fredd, K.; Battaglia, D.; Lee, D.; Wu, D.; Jensen, J.; Patton, P.; Gokhale, S.; Stouffer, R. L.; Wolf, D.; Mitalipov, S. (2013). "Human Embryonic Stem Cells Derived by Somatic Cell Nuclear Transfer". Cell. 153 (6): 1228–38. doi:10.1016/j.cell.2013.05.006. PMID 23683578.
4. Noggle, S.; Fung, H. L.; Gore, A.; Martinez, H.; Satriani, K. C.; Prosser, R.; Oum, K.; Paull, D.; Druckenmiller, S.; Freeby, M.; Greenberg, E.; Zhang, K.; Goland, R.; Sauer, M. V.; Leibel, R. L.; Egli, D. (2011). "Human oocytes reprogram somatic cells to a pluripotent state". Nature. 478 (7367): 70–5. doi:10.1038/nature10397. PMID 21979046.
5. Pan, G.; Wang, T.; Yao, H.; Pei, D. (2012). "Somatic cell reprogramming for regenerative medicine: SCNT vs. IPS cells". BioEssays. 34 (6): 472–6. doi:10.1002/bies.201100174. PMID 22419173.
6. Do, J. T.; Han, D. W.; Gentile, L; Sobek-Klocke, I; Stehling, M; Lee, H. T.;

Schöler, H. R. (2007). "Erasure of cellular memory by fusion with pluripotent cells". Stem Cells. 25 (4): 1013–20. doi:10.1634/stemcells.2006-0691. PMID 17218392.

7. b Takahashi, K.; Tanabe, K.; Ohnuki, M.; Narita, M.; Ichisaka, T.; Tomoda, K.; Yamanaka, S. (2007). "Induction of Pluripotent Stem Cells from Adult Human Fibroblasts by Defined Factors". Cell. 131 (5): 861–872. doi:10.1016/j.cell.2007.11.019. PMID 18035408.
8. Wang, W.; Yang, J.; Liu, H.; Lu, D.; Chen, X.; Zenonos, Z.; Campos, L. S.; Rad, R.; Guo, G.; Zhang, S.; Bradley, A.; Liu, P. (2011). "Rapid and efficient reprogramming of somatic cells to induced pluripotent stem cells by retinoic acid receptor gamma and liver receptor homolog 1". Proceedings of the National Academy of Sciences. 108 (45): 18283–18288. doi:10.1073/pnas.1100893108.
9. Lapasset, L.; Milhavet, O.; Prieur, A.; Besnard, E.; Babled, A.; Ait-Hamou, N.; Leschik, J.; Pellestor, F.; Ramirez, J. -M.; De Vos, J.; Lehmann, S.; Lemaitre, J. -M. (2011). "Rejuvenating senescent and centenarian human cells by reprogramming through the pluripotent state". Genes & Development. 25 (21): 2248–2253. doi:10.1101/gad.173922.111.
10. Zhou, H.; Wu, S.; Joo, J. Y.; Zhu, S.; Han, D. W.; Lin, T.; Trauger, S.; Bien, G.; Yao, S.; Zhu, Y.; Siuzdak, G.; Schöler, H. R.; Duan, L.; Ding, S. (2009). "Generation of Induced Pluripotent Stem Cells Using Recombinant Proteins". Cell Stem Cell. 4 (5): 381–4. doi:10.1016/j.stem.2009.04.005. PMID 19398399.
11. Li, Z.; Rana, T. M. (2012). "Using MicroRNAs to Enhance the Generation of Induced Pluripotent Stem Cells". Current Protocols in Stem Cell Biology. doi:10.1002/9780470151808.sc04a04s20. ISBN 0470151803.
12. Anokye-Danso, F.; Trivedi, C. M.; Juhr, D.; Gupta, M.; Cui, Z.; Tian, Y.; Zhang, Y.; Yang, W.; Gruber, P. J.; Epstein, J. A.; Morrisey, E. E. (2011). "Highly Efficient miRNA-Mediated Reprogramming of Mouse and Human Somatic Cells to Pluripotency". Cell Stem Cell. 8 (4): 376–88. doi:10.1016/j.stem.2011.03.001. PMID 21474102.
13. Miyoshi, N.; Ishii, H.; Nagano, H.; Haraguchi, N.; Dewi, D. L.; Kano, Y.; Nishikawa, S.; Tanemura, M.; Mimori, K.; Tanaka, F.; Saito, T.; Nishimura, J.; Takemasa, I.; Mizushima, T.; Ikeda, M.; Yamamoto, H.; Sekimoto, M.; Doki, Y.; Mori, M. (2011). "Reprogramming of Mouse and Human Cells to Pluripotency Using Mature MicroRNAs". Cell Stem Cell. 8 (6): 633–8. doi:10.1016/j.stem.2011.05.001. PMID 21620789.
14. Jayawardena, T. M.; Egemnazarov, B.; Finch, E. A.; Zhang, L.; Payne, J. A.; Pandya, K.; Zhang, Z.; Rosenberg, P.; Mirotsou, M.; Dzau, V. J. (2012). "MicroRNA-Mediated in Vitro and in Vivo Direct Reprogramming of Cardiac Fibroblasts to Cardiomyocytes". Circulation Research. 110 (11): 1465–73. doi:10.1161/CIRCRESAHA.112.269035. PMID 22539765.
15. Bao, X.; Zhu, X.; Liao, B.; Benda, C.; Zhuang, Q.; Pei, D.; Qin, B.; Esteban, M. A. (2013). "MicroRNAs in somatic cell reprogramming". Current Opinion in

Cell Biology. 25 (2): 208–14. doi:10.1016/j.ceb.2012.12.004. PMID 23332905.

16. Yoshioka, N.; Gros, E.; Li, H. R.; Kumar, S.; Deacon, D. C.; Maron, C.; Muotri, A. R.; Chi, N. C.; Fu, X. D.; Yu, B. D.; Dowdy, S. F. (2013). "Efficient Generation of Human iPSCs by a Synthetic Self-Replicative RNA". Cell Stem Cell. 13 (2): 246–54. doi:10.1016/j.stem.2013.06.001. PMID 23910086.
17. Hou, P.; Li, Y.; Zhang, X.; Liu, C.; Guan, J.; Li, H.; Zhao, T.; Ye, J.; Yang, W.; Liu, K.; Ge, J.; Xu, J.; Zhang, Q.; Zhao, Y.; Deng, H. (2013). "Pluripotent Stem Cells Induced from Mouse Somatic Cells by Small-Molecule Compounds". Science. 341 (6146): 651–4. doi:10.1126/science.1239278. PMID 23868920.
18. Stadtfeld, M.; Apostolou, E.; Ferrari, F.; Choi, J.; Walsh, R. M.; Chen, T.; Ooi, S. S. K.; Kim, S. Y.; Bestor, T. H.; Shioda, T.; Park, P. J.; Hochedlinger, K. (2012). "Ascorbic acid prevents loss of Dlk1-Dio3 imprinting and facilitates generation of all–iPS cell mice from terminally differentiated B cells". Nature Genetics. 44 (4): 398–405, S1–2. doi:10.1038/ng.1110. PMID 22387999.
19. Pandian, G. N.; Sugiyama, H. (2012). "Programmable genetic switches to control transcriptional machinery of pluripotency". Biotechnology Journal. 7 (6): 798–809. doi:10.1002/biot.201100361. PMID 22588775.
20. De Robertis, Edward M. (2006). "Spemanns organizer and self-regulation in amphibian embryos". Nature Reviews Molecular Cell Biology. 7: 296–302. doi:10.1038/nrm1855. PMC 2464568 . PMID 16482093.
21. Slack, J. M. W. (2009). "Metaplasia and somatic cell reprogramming". The Journal of Pathology. 217 (2): 161–8. doi:10.1002/path.2442. PMID 18855879.
22. Wei, G.; Schubiger, G.; Harder, F.; Müller, A. M. (2000). "Stem Cell Plasticity in Mammals and Transdetermination in Drosophila: Common Themes?". Stem Cells. 18 (6): 409–14. doi:10.1634/stemcells.18-6-409. PMID 11072028.
23. Xu, Peng-Fei; Houssin, Nathalie; Ferri-Lagneau, Karine F.; Thisse, Bernard; Thisse, Christine (2014). "Construction of a Vertebrate Embryo from Two Opposing Morphogen Gradients". Science. 344 (6179): 87–89. doi:10.1126/science.1248252.
24. Stange, D. E.; Koo, B. K.; Huch, M.; Sibbel, G.; Basak, O.; Lyubimova, A.; Kujala, P.; Bartfeld, S.; Koster, J.; Geahlen, J. H.; Peters, P. J.; Van Es, J. H.; Van De Wetering, M.; Mills, J. C.; Clevers, H. (2013). "Differentiated Troy+ Chief Cells Act as Reserve Stem Cells to Generate All Lineages of the Stomach Epithelium". Cell. 155 (2): 357–68. doi:10.1016/j.cell.2013.09.008. PMC 4094146 . PMID 24120136.
25. Tata, P. R.; Mou, H.; Pardo-Saganta, A.; Zhao, R.; Prabhu, M.; Law, B. M.; Vinarsky, V.; Cho, J. L.; Breton, S.; Sahay, A.; Medoff, B. D.; Rajagopal, J. (2013). "Dedifferentiation of committed epithelial cells into stem cells in vivo". Nature. doi:10.1038/nature12777.
26. Kusaba, T.; Lalli, M.; Kramann, R.; Kobayashi, A.; Humphreys, B. D. (2013). "Differentiated kidney epithelial cells repair injured proximal tubule". Proceedings of the National Academy of Sciences. 111 (4): 1527–1532. doi:10.1073/

pnas.1310653110.

27. Sieweke, Michael H.; Allen, Judith E. (2013). "Beyond Stem Cells: Self-Renewal of Differentiated Macrophages". Science. 342 (6161): 1242974. doi:10.1126/science.1242974. PMID 24264994.

28. Soucie, E. L.; Weng, Z.; Geirsdóttir, L.; et al. (2016). "Lineage-specific enhancers activate self-renewal genes in macrophages and embryonic stem cells". Science. 351: aad5510. doi:10.1126/science.aad5510.

29. Sandoval-Guzmán, T.; Wang, H.; Khattak, S.; Schuez, M.; Roensch, K.; Nacu, E.; Tazaki, A.; Joven, A.; Tanaka, E. M.; Simon, A. S. (2014). "Fundamental Differences in Dedifferentiation and Stem Cell Recruitment during Skeletal Muscle Regeneration in Two Salamander Species". Cell Stem Cell. 14 (2): 174–87. doi:10.1016/j.stem.2013.11.007. PMID 24268695.

30. Kuroda, Y; Wakao, S; Kitada, M; Murakami, T; Nojima, M; Dezawa, M (2013). "Isolation, culture and evaluation of multilineage-differentiating stress-enduring (Muse) cells". Nat Protoc. 8 (7): 1391–415. doi:10.1038/nprot.2013.076. PMID 23787896.

31. Kuroda, Y.; Kitada, M.; Wakao, S.; et al. (2010). "Unique multipotent cells in adult human mesenchymal cell populations". PNAS. 107 (19): 8639–8643. doi:10.1073/pnas.0911647107. PMC 2889306 . PMID 20421459.

32. Ogura, F; Wakao, S; Kuroda, Y; Tsuchiyama, K; Bagheri, M; Heneidi, S; Chazenbalk, G; Aiba, S; Dezawa, M (2014). "Human Adipose Tissue Possesses a Unique Population of Pluripotent Stem Cells with Nontumorigenic and Low Telomerase Activities: Potential Implications in Regenerative Medicine". Stem Cells Dev. 23: 717–28. doi:10.1089/scd.2013.0473. PMID 24256547.

33. Heneidi, S; Simerman, AA; Keller, E; Singh, P; Li, X; et al. (2013). "Awakened by Cellular Stress: Isolation and Characterization of a Novel Population of Pluripotent Stem Cells Derived from Human Adipose Tissue". PLoS ONE. 8 (6): e64752. doi:10.1371/journal.pone.0064752. PMC 3673968 . PMID 23755141.

34. Shigemoto, T; Kuroda, Y; Wakao, S; Dezawa, M (2013). "A Novel Approach to Collecting Satellite Cells From Adult Skeletal Muscles on the Basis of Their Stress Tolerance". Stem Cells Trans Med. 2 (7): 488–498. doi:10.5966/sctm.2012-0130. PMC 3697816 . PMID 23748608.

35. Sisakhtnezhad, S.; Matin, M. M. (2012). "Transdifferentiation: A cell and molecular reprogramming process". Cell and Tissue Research. 348 (3): 379–96. doi:10.1007/s00441-012-1403-y. PMID 22526624.

36. Allyson J. Merrell & Ben Z. Stanger (2016). Adult cell plasticity in vivo: de-differentiation and transdifferentiation are back in style. Nature Reviews Molecular Cell Biology. doi:10.1038/nrm.2016.24

37. Dinnyes, Andras; Tian, Xiuchun Cindy; Oback, Bj¨orn (17 April 2013). Robert A. Meyers, ed. Nuclear Transfer for Cloning Animals. John Wiley & Sons. pp. 299–344. ISBN 978-3-527-66854-0.

38. Jullien, J.; Pasque, V.; Halley-Stott, R. P.; Miyamoto, K.; Gurdon, J. B. (2011). "Mechanisms of nuclear reprogramming by eggs and oocytes: A deterministic

process?". Nature Reviews Molecular Cell Biology. 12 (7): 453–9. doi:10.1038/nrm3140. PMID 21697902.

39. Campbell, K. H. S. (2002). "A background to nuclear transfer and its applications in agriculture and human therapeutic medicine". Journal of Anatomy. 200 (3): 267–275. doi:10.1046/j.1469-7580.2002.00035.x.
40. US 8,647,872 patent
41. Chung, Y. G.; Eum, J. H.; Lee, J. E.; Shim, S. H.; Sepilian, V.; Hong, S. W.; Lee, Y.; Treff, N. R.; Choi, Y. H.; Kimbrel, E. A.; Dittman, R. E.; Lanza, R.; Lee, D. R. (2014). "Human Somatic Cell Nuclear Transfer Using Adult Cells". Cell Stem Cell. 14 (6): 777–80. doi:10.1016/j.stem.2014.03.015. PMID 24746675.
42. Yang, H.; Shi, L.; Wang, B. A.; Liang, D.; Zhong, C.; Liu, W.; Nie, Y.; Liu, J.; Zhao, J.; Gao, X.; Li, D.; Xu, G. L.; Li, J. (2012). "Generation of Genetically Modified Mice by Oocyte Injection of Androgenetic Haploid Embryonic Stem Cells". Cell. 149 (3): 605–17. doi:10.1016/j.cell.2012.04.002. PMID 22541431.
43. Hayashi, K.; Ogushi, S.; Kurimoto, K.; Shimamoto, S.; Ohta, H.; Saitou, M. (2012). "Offspring from Oocytes Derived from in Vitro Primordial Germ Cell-like Cells in Mice". Science. 338 (6109): 971–975. doi:10.1126/science.1226889. PMID 23042295.
44. Kishigami, S.; Mizutani, E.; Ohta, H.; Hikichi, T.; Thuan, N. V.; Wakayama, S.; Bui, H. T.; Wakayama, T. (2006). "Significant improvement of mouse cloning technique by treatment with trichostatin a after somatic nuclear transfer". Biochemical and Biophysical Research Communications. 340 (1): 183–9. doi:10.1016/j.bbrc.2005.11.164. PMID 16356478.
45. Wakayama, S.; Kohda, T.; Obokata, H.; Tokoro, M.; Li, C.; Terashita, Y.; Mizutani, E.; Nguyen, V. T.; Kishigami, S.; Ishino, F.; Wakayama, T. (2013). "Successful Serial Recloning in the Mouse over Multiple Generations". Cell Stem Cell. 12 (3): 293–7. doi:10.1016/j.stem.2013.01.005. PMID 23472871.
46. Official website of the Presidential Commission for the Study of Bioethical Issues
47. Paull, D.; Emmanuele, V.; Weiss, K. A.; Treff, N.; Stewart, L.; Hua, H.; Zimmer, M.; Kahler, D. J.; Goland, R. S.; Noggle, S. A.; Prosser, R.; Hirano, M.; Sauer, M. V.; Egli, D. (2012). "Nuclear genome transfer in human oocytes eliminates mitochondrial DNA variants". Nature. 493 (7434): 632–7. doi:10.1038/nature11800. PMID 23254936.
48. Tachibana, M.; Amato, P.; Sparman, M.; Woodward, J.; Sanchis, D. M.; Ma, H.; Gutierrez, N. M.; Tippner-Hedges, R.; Kang, E.; Lee, H. S.; Ramsey, C.; Masterson, K.; Battaglia, D.; Lee, D.; Wu, D.; Jensen, J.; Patton, P.; Gokhale, S.; Stouffer, R.; Mitalipov, S. (2012). "Towards germline gene therapy of inherited mitochondrial diseases". Nature. 493 (7434): 627–31. doi:10.1038/nature11647. PMID 23103867.
49. Check Hayden, E. (2013). "Regulators weigh benefits of 'three-parent' fertilization". Nature. 502 (7471): 284–5. doi:10.1038/502284a. PMID 24132269.
50. Le, R.; Kou, Z.; Jiang, Y.; Li, M.; Huang, B.; Liu, W.; Li, H.; Kou, X.; He, W.; Rudolph, K. L.; Ju, Z.; Gao, S. (2014). "Enhanced Telomere Rejuvenation

in Pluripotent Cells Reprogrammed via Nuclear Transfer Relative to Induced Pluripotent Stem Cells". Cell Stem Cell. 14 (1): 27–39. doi:10.1016/j.stem.2013.11.005. PMID 24268696.

51. Cibelli, Jose; Lanza, Robert; Campbell, Keith H.S.; West, Michael D. (14 September 2002). Principles of Cloning. Academic Press. ISBN 978-0-08-049215-5.

52. Shinagawa, T.; Takagi, T.; Tsukamoto, D.; Tomaru, C.; Huynh, L. M.; Sivaraman, P.; Kumarevel, T.; Inoue, K.; Nakato, R.; Katou, Y.; Sado, T.; Takahashi, S.; Ogura, A.; Shirahige, K.; Ishii, S. (2014). "Histone Variants Enriched in Oocytes Enhance Reprogramming to Induced Pluripotent Stem Cells". Cell Stem Cell. 14 (2): 217–27. doi:10.1016/j.stem.2013.12.015. PMID 24506885.

53. Abad, M. A.; Mosteiro, L.; Pantoja, C.; Cañamero, M.; Rayon, T.; Ors, I.; Graña, O.; Megías, D.; Domínguez, O.; Martínez, D.; Manzanares, M.; Ortega, S.; Serrano, M. (2013). "Reprogramming in vivo produces teratomas and iPS cells with totipotency features". Nature. 502 (7471): 340–5. doi:10.1038/nature12586. PMID 24025773.

54. Naik, Gautam (2013-09-11). "New Promise for Stem Cells - WSJ.com". Online. wsj.com. Retrieved 2014-01-30.

55. Stevens, L. C. (1970). "The development of transplantable teratocarcinomas from intratesticular grafts of pre- and postimplantation mouse embryos". Developmental Biology. 21 (3): 364–82. doi:10.1016/0012-1606(70)90130-2. PMID 5436899.

56. Mintz, B; Cronmiller, C; Custer, R. P. (1978). "Somatic cell origin of teratocarcinomas". Proceedings of the National Academy of Sciences of the United States of America. 75 (6): 2834–8. doi:10.1073/pnas.75.6.2834. PMC 392659 . PMID 275854.

57. Mintz, B; Illmensee, K (1975). "Normal genetically mosaic mice produced from malignant teratocarcinoma cells". Proc Natl Acad Sci U S A. 72 (9): 3585–3589. doi:10.1073/pnas.72.9.3585.

58. Martin, G. R.; Evans, M. J. (1975). "Differentiation of clonal lines of teratocarcinoma cells: formation of embryoid bodies in vitro". Proc. Natl. Acad. Sci. USA. 72 (4): 1441–1445. doi:10.1073/pnas.72.4.1441.

59. Illmensee, K; Mintz, B (1976). "Totipotency and normal differentiation of single teratocarcinoma cells cloned by injection into blastocysts". Proceedings of the National Academy of Sciences of the United States of America. 73 (2): 549–53. doi:10.1073/pnas.73.2.549. PMC 335947 . PMID 1061157.

60. Martin, GR (1981). "Isolation of a pluripotent cell line from early mouse embryos cultured in medium conditioned by teratocarcinoma stem cells". Proc. Natl. Acad. Sci. USA. 78 (12): 7634–7638. doi:10.1073/pnas.78.12.7634. PMC 349323 . PMID 6950406.

61. Martin, G. R. (1980). "Teratocarcinomas and mammalian embryogenesis". Science. 209 (4458): 768–76. doi:10.1126/science.6250214. PMID 6250214.

62. Papaioannou, V. E.; Gardner, R. L.; McBurney, M. W.; Babinet, C; Evans, M. J. (1978). "Participation of cultured teratocarcinoma cells in mouse embryogenesis".

Journal of embryology and experimental morphology. 44: 93–104. PMID 650144.

63. GRAHAM, C. F. (January 1977). Teratocarcinoma cells and normal mouse embryogenesiseditor=Michael I. Sherman. MIT Press. ISBN 978-0-262-19158-6.
64. ILLMENSEE, K. (14 June 2012). L. B. Russell, ed. Reversion of malignancy and normalized differentiation of teratocarcinoma cells in chimeric mice. Springer London, Limited. pp. 3–24. ISBN 978-1-4684-3392-0.
65. Stuart, H. T.; Van Oosten, A. L.; Radzisheuskaya, A.; Martello, G.; Miller, A.; Dietmann, S.; Nichols, J.; Silva, J. C. R. (2014). "NANOG Amplifies STAT3 Activation and They Synergistically Induce the Naive Pluripotent Program". Current Biology. 24 (3): 340–6. doi:10.1016/j.cub.2013.12.040. PMID 24462001.
66. Choi, Jiho; Lee, Soohyun; Mallard, William; et al. (2015). "A comparison of genetically matched cell lines reveals the equivalence of human iPSCs and ESCs". Nature Biotechnology. 33: 1173–1181. doi:10.1038/nbt.3388.
67. Boland, M. J.; Hazen, J. L.; Nazor, K. L.; Rodriguez, A. R.; Gifford, W; Martin, G; Kupriyanov, S; Baldwin, K. K. (2009). "Adult mice generated from induced pluripotent stem cells". Nature. 461 (7260): 91–4. doi:10.1038/nature08310. PMID 19672243.
68. Kang, L.; Wang, J.; Zhang, Y.; Kou, Z.; Gao, S. (2009). "IPS Cells Can Support Full-Term Development of Tetraploid Blastocyst-Complemented Embryos". Cell Stem Cell. 5 (2): 135–8. doi:10.1016/j.stem.2009.07.001. PMID 19631602.
69. Yagi, T.; Kosakai, A.; Ito, D.; Okada, Y.; Akamatsu, W.; Nihei, Y.; Nabetani, A.; Ishikawa, F.; Arai, Y.; Hirose, N.; Okano, H.; Suzuki, N. (2012). "Establishment of Induced Pluripotent Stem Cells from Centenarians for Neurodegenerative Disease Research". PLoS ONE. 7 (7): e41572. doi:10.1371/journal.pone.0041572. PMC 3405135 . PMID 22848530.
70. Rohani, L.; Johnson, A. A.; Arnold, A.; Stolzing, A. (2014). "The aging signature: A hallmark of induced pluripotent stem cells?". Aging Cell. 13 (1): 2–7. doi:10.1111/acel.12182. PMC 4326871 . PMID 24256351.
71. Yehezkel, S; Rebibo-Sabbah, A; Segev, Y; Tzukerman, M; Shaked, R; Huber, I; Gepstein, L; Skorecki, K; Selig, S (2011). "Reprogramming of telomeric regions during the generation of human induced pluripotent stem cells and subsequent differentiation into fibroblast-like derivatives". Epigenetics. 6 (1): 63–75. doi:10.4161/epi.6.1.13390. PMC 3052915 . PMID 20861676.
72. West, M. D.; Vaziri, H (2010). "Back to immortality: The restoration of embryonic telomere length during induced pluripotency". Regenerative Medicine. 5 (4): 485–8. doi:10.2217/rme.10.51. PMID 20632849.
73. Marión, R. M.; Blasco, M. A. (2010). "Telomere rejuvenation during nuclear reprogramming". Current Opinion in Genetics & Development. 20 (2): 190–6. doi:10.1016/j.gde.2010.01.005. PMID 20176474.
74. Gourronc, F. A.; Klingelhutz, A. J. (2012). "Therapeutic opportunities: Telomere maintenance in inducible pluripotent stem cells". Mutation Research/Fundamental and Molecular Mechanisms of Mutagenesis. 730 (1–2): 98–105. doi:10.1016/j.mrfmmm.2011.05.008. PMC 3179558 . PMID 21605571.

75. Zhao, T.; Zhang, Z. N.; Rong, Z.; Xu, Y. (2011). "Immunogenicity of induced pluripotent stem cells". Nature. 474 (7350): 212–5. doi:10.1038/nature10135. PMID 21572395.

76. Dhodapkar, M. V.; Dhodapkar, K. M. (2011). "Spontaneous and therapy-induced immunity to pluripotency genes in humans: Clinical implications, opportunities and challenges". Cancer Immunology, Immunotherapy. 60 (3): 413–8. doi:10.1007/s00262-010-0944-8. PMC 3574640 . PMID 21104412.

77. Gutierrez-Aranda, I.; Ramos-Mejia, V.; Bueno, C.; Munoz-Lopez, M.; Real, P. J.; Mácia, A.; Sanchez, L.; Ligero, G.; Garcia-Parez, J. L.; Menendez, P. (2010). "Human Induced Pluripotent Stem Cells Develop Teratoma More Efficiently and Faster Than Human Embryonic Stem Cells Regardless the Site of Injection". Stem Cells. 28 (9): 1568–1570. doi:10.1002/stem.471. PMC 2996086 . PMID 20641038.

78. Chang, C. J.; Mitra, K.; Koya, M.; Velho, M.; Desprat, R.; Lenz, J.; Bouhassira, E. E. (2011). "Production of Embryonic and Fetal-Like Red Blood Cells from Human Induced Pluripotent Stem Cells". PLoS ONE. 6 (10): e25761. doi:10.1371/journal.pone.0025761. PMC 3192723 . PMID 22022444.

79. Dabir, D. V.; Hasson, S. A.; Setoguchi, K.; Johnson, M. E.; Wongkongkathep, P.; Douglas, C. J.; Zimmerman, J.; Damoiseaux, R.; Teitell, M. A.; Koehler, C. M. (2013). "A Small Molecule Inhibitor of Redox-Regulated Protein Translocation into Mitochondria". Developmental Cell. 25 (1): 81–92. doi:10.1016/j.devcel.2013.03.006. PMC 3726224 . PMID 23597483.

80. Ben-David, Uri; Gan, Qing-Fen; Golan-Lev, Tamar; et al. (2013). "Selective Elimination of Human Pluripotent Stem Cells by an Oleate Synthesis Inhibitor Discovered in a High-Throughput Screen". Cell Stem Cell. 12 (2): 167–179. doi:10.1016/j.stem.2012.11.015. PMID 23318055.

81. Lou, K. J. (2013). "Small molecules vs. Teratomas". Science-Business eXchange. 6 (7). doi:10.1038/scibx.2013.158.

82. Lee, M. -O.; Moon, S. H.; Jeong, H. -C.; Yi, J. -Y.; Lee, T. -H.; Shim, S. H.; Rhee, Y. -H.; Lee, S. -H.; Oh, S. -J.; Lee, M. -Y.; Han, M. -J.; Cho, Y. S.; Chung, H. -M.; Kim, K. -S.; Cha, H. -J. (2013). "Inhibition of pluripotent stem cell-derived teratoma formation by small molecules". Proceedings of the National Academy of Sciences. 110 (35): E3281. doi:10.1073/pnas.1303669110.

83. Tang, C; Weissman, I. L.; Drukker, M (2012). "The safety of embryonic stem cell therapy relies on teratoma removal". Oncotarget. 3 (1): 7–8. doi:10.18632/oncotarget.434. PMC 3292887 . PMID 22294556.

84. Chaffer, C. L.; Brueckmann, I.; Scheel, C.; Kaestli, A. J.; Wiggins, P. A.; Rodrigues, L. O.; Brooks, M.; Reinhardt, F.; Su, Y.; Polyak, K.; Arendt, L. M.; Kuperwasser, C.; Bierie, B.; Weinberg, R. A. (2011). "Normal and neoplastic nonstem cells can spontaneously convert to a stem-like state". Proceedings of the National Academy of Sciences. 108 (19): 7950–7955. doi:10.1073/pnas.1102454108.

85. "Residual Undifferentiated Cells During Differentiation of Induced Pluripotent

Stem Cells In Vitro and In Vivo". Stem Cells and Development. 21: 521–529. doi:10.1089/scd.2011.0131.

86. Gurtan, A. M.; Ravi, A.; Rahl, P. B.; Bosson, A. D.; Jnbaptiste, C. K.; Bhutkar, A.; Whittaker, C. A.; Young, R. A.; Sharp, P. A. (2013). "Let-7 represses Nr6a1 and a mid-gestation developmental program in adult fibroblasts". Genes & Development. 27 (8): 941–954. doi:10.1101/gad.215376.113.

87. Wang, H.; Wang, X.; Xu, X.; Zwaka, T. P.; Cooney, A. J. (2013). "Epigenetic Reprogramming of the Germ Cell Nuclear Factor Gene is Required for Proper Differentiation of Induced Pluripotent Cells". Stem Cells. 31 (12): 2659–66. doi:10.1002/stem.1367. PMID 23495137.

88. Lindgren, A. G.; Natsuhara, K.; Tian, E.; Vincent, J. J.; Li, X.; Jiao, J.; Wu, H.; Banerjee, U.; Clark, A. T. (2011). "Loss of Pten Causes Tumor Initiation Following Differentiation of Murine Pluripotent Stem Cells Due to Failed Repression of Nanog". PLoS ONE. 6 (1): e16478. doi:10.1371/journal.pone.0016478. PMC 3029365 . PMID 21304588.

89. Grad, I; Hibaoui, Y; Jaconi, M; Chicha, L; Bergström-Tengzelius, R; Sailani, M. R.; Pelte, M. F.; Dahoun, S; Mitsiadis, T. A.; Töhönen, V; Bouillaguet, S; Antonarakis, S. E.; Kere, J; Zucchelli, M; Hovatta, O; Feki, A (2011). "NANOG priming before full reprogramming may generate germ cell tumours". European cells & materials. 22: 258–74; discussio 274. PMID 22071697.

90. Okano, H.; Nakamura, M.; Yoshida, K.; Okada, Y.; Tsuji, O.; Nori, S.; Ikeda, E.; Yamanaka, S.; Miura, K. (2013). "Steps Toward Safe Cell Therapy Using Induced Pluripotent Stem Cells". Circulation Research. 112 (3): 523–33. doi:10.1161/CIRCRESAHA.111.256149. PMID 23371901.

91. Cunningham, J. J.; Ulbright, T. M.; Pera, M. F.; Looijenga, L. H. J. (2012). "Lessons from human teratomas to guide development of safe stem cell therapies". Nature Biotechnology. 30 (9): 849–57. doi:10.1038/nbt.2329. PMID 22965062.

92. Bellin, M.; Marchetto, M. C.; Gage, F. H.; Mummery, C. L. (2012). "Induced pluripotent stem cells: The new patient?". Nature Reviews Molecular Cell Biology. 13 (11): 713–26. doi:10.1038/nrm3448. PMID 23034453.

93. Sandoe, J.; Eggan, K. (2013). "Opportunities and challenges of pluripotent stem cell neurodegenerative disease models". Nature Neuroscience. 16 (7): 780–9. doi:10.1038/nn.3425. PMID 23799470.

94. Takahashi, K.; Yamanaka, S. (2013). "Induced pluripotent stem cells in medicine and biology". Development. 140 (12): 2457–61. doi:10.1242/dev.092551. PMID 23715538.

95. Fu, X; Xu, Y (2012). "Challenges to the clinical application of pluripotent stem cells: Towards genomic and functional stability". Genome Medicine. 4 (6): 55. doi:10.1186/gm354. PMC 3698533 . PMID 22741526.

96. Araki, R.; Uda, M.; Hoki, Y.; Sunayama, M.; Nakamura, M.; Ando, S.; Sugiura, M.; Ideno, H.; Shimada, A.; Nifuji, A.; Abe, M. (2013). "Negligible immunogenicity of terminally differentiated cells derived from induced pluripotent or embryonic stem cells". Nature. 494 (7435): 100–4. doi:10.1038/nature11807. PMID 23302801.

97. Wahlestedt, M.; Norddahl, G. L.; Sten, G.; Ugale, A.; Frisk, M. -A. M.; Mattsson, R.; Deierborg, T.; Sigvardsson, M.; Bryder, D. (2013). "An epigenetic component of hematopoietic stem cell aging amenable to reprogramming into a young state". Blood. 121 (21): 4257–64. doi:10.1182/blood-2012-11-469080. PMID 23476050.

98. Ohnishi, K.; Semi, K.; Yamamoto, T.; Shimizu, M.; Tanaka, A.; Mitsunaga, K.; Yamada, Y. (2014). "Premature Termination of Reprogramming In Vivo Leads to Cancer Development through Altered Epigenetic Regulation". Cell. 156 (4): 663–677. doi:10.1016/j.cell.2014.01.005. PMID 24529372.

99. Mfopou JK, De Groote V, Xu X, Heimberg H, Bouwens L (May 2007). "Sonic hedgehog and other soluble factors from differentiating embryoid bodies inhibit pancreas development". Stem Cells. 25 (5): 1156–65. doi:10.1634/stemcells.2006-0720. PMID 17272496.

100. Mapping out cell conversion

101. Owen, Rackham; Gough, Julian (2016). "A predictive computational framework for direct reprogramming between human cell types". Nature Genetics. 48: 331–335. doi:10.1038/ng.3487.

102. New Algorithm May Someday Enable Scientists to Regrow Limbs and Replace Damaged Organs

103. De Los, Angeles; Daley, G. Q. (2013). "A chemical logic for reprogramming to pluripotency". Cell Research. 23: 1337–1338. doi:10.1038/cr.2013.119.

104. Federation, A. J.; Bradner, J. E.; Meissner, A. (2013). "The use of small molecules in somatic-cell reprogramming". Trends in Cell Biology. 24: 179–187. doi:10.1016/j.tcb.2013.09.011. PMID 24183602.

105. Zhao, Y.; Zhao, T.; Guan, J. (2015). "A XEN-like State Bridges Somatic Cells to Pluripotency during Chemical Reprogramming". Cell. 163: 1678–1691. doi:10.1016/j.cell.2015.11.017.

106. NAKAUCHI Hiromitsu, KAMIYA Akihide, SUZUKI Nao, ITO Keiichi, YAMAZAKI Satoshi (2011) METHOD FOR PRODUCING CELLS INDUCED TO DIFFERENTIATE FROM PLURIPOTENT STEM CELLSPATENT COOPERATION TREATY APPLICATION, patno: WO2011071085 (A1) — 2011-06-16 (C12N5/07)

107. Amabile, G.; Welner, R. S.; Nombela-Arrieta, C.; d'Alise, A. M.; Di Ruscio, A.; Ebralidze, A. K.; Kraytsberg, Y.; Ye, M.; Kocher, O.; Neuberg, D. S.; Khrapko, K.; Silberstein, L. E.; Tenen, D. G. (2012). "In vivo generation of transplantable human hematopoietic cells from induced pluripotent stem cells". Blood. 121 (8): 1255–64. doi:10.1182/blood-2012-06-434407. PMID 23212524.

108. Suzuki, N.; Yamazaki, S.; Yamaguchi, T.; Okabe, M.; Masaki, H.; Takaki, S.; Otsu, M.; Nakauchi, H. (2013). "Generation of Engraftable Hematopoietic Stem Cells from Induced Pluripotent Stem Cells by Way of Teratoma Formation". Molecular Therapy. 21 (7): 1424–31. doi:10.1038/mt.2013.71. PMID 23670574.

109. Chou, B. K.; Ye, Z.; Cheng, L. (2013). "Generation and Homing of iPSC-Derived Hematopoietic Cells in Vivo". Molecular Therapy. 21 (7): 1292–3. doi:10.1038/mt.2013.129. PMID 23812546.

110. Yamauchi, T; Takenaka, K; Urata, S; Shima, T; Kikushige, Y; Tokuyama, T; Iwamoto, C; Nishihara, M; Iwasaki, H; Miyamoto, T; Honma, N; Nakao, M; Matozaki, T; Akashi, K (2013). "Polymorphic Sirpa is the genetic determinant for NOD-based mouse lines to achieve efficient human cell engraftment". Blood. 121 (8): 1316–25. doi:10.1182/blood-2012-06-440354. PMID 23293079.

111. Rong, Z.; Wang, M.; Hu, Z.; Stradner, M.; Zhu, S.; Kong, H.; Yi, H.; Goldrath, A.; Yang, Y. G.; Xu, Y.; Fu, X. (2014). "An Effective Approach to Prevent Immune Rejection of Human ESC-Derived Allografts". Cell Stem Cell. 14 (1): 121–30. doi:10.1016/j.stem.2013.11.014. PMC 4023958 . PMID 24388175.

112. Hirami, Y.; Osakada, F.; Takahashi, K.; Okita, K.; Yamanaka, S.; Ikeda, H.; Yoshimura, N.; Takahashi, M. (2009). "Generation of retinal cells from mouse and human induced pluripotent stem cells". Neuroscience Letters. 458 (3): 126–31. doi:10.1016/j.neulet.2009.04.035. PMID 19379795.

113. Buchholz, D. E.; Hikita, S. T.; Rowland, T. J.; Friedrich, A. M.; Hinman, C. R.; Johnson, L. V.; Clegg, D. O. (2009). "Derivation of Functional Retinal Pigmented Epithelium from Induced Pluripotent Stem Cells". Stem Cells. 27 (10): 2427–34. doi:10.1002/stem.189. PMID 19658190.

114. Yang, Jin; Nong, Eva; Tsang, Stephen H (2013). "Induced pluripotent stem cells and retinal degeneration treatment". Expert Rev. Ophthalmol. 8 (1): 5–8. doi:10.1586/EOP.12.75.

115. Fields,, Mark A.; Hwang,, John; Gong,, Jie; Cai,, Hui; Del Priore, Lucian (9 December 2012). Stephen Tsang, ed. The Eye as a Target Organ for Stem Cell Therapy. Springer. pp. 1–30. ISBN 978-1-4614-5493-9.

116. Li, Y; Tsai, YT; Hsu, CW; et al. (2012). "Long-term safety and efficacy of human induced pluripotent stem cell (iPS) grafts in a preclinical model of retinitis pigmentosa". Mol. Med. 18 (1): 1312–1319. doi:10.2119/molmed.2012.00242. PMC 3521789 . PMID 22895806.

117. Stem cell therapy for RP is now offered at St. Luke's Medical Center.

118. Tzouvelekis, A.; Ntolios, P.; Bouros, D. (2013). "Stem Cell Treatment for Chronic Lung Diseases". Respiration. 85 (3): 179–92. doi:10.1159/000346525. PMID 23364286.

119. Wagner, Darcy E.; Bonvillain, Ryan W.; Jensen, Todd; Girard, Eric D.; Bunnell, Bruce A.; Finck, Christine M.; Hoffman5, Andrew M.; Weiss2, Daniel J. (Jul 2013). "Can stem cells be used to generate new lungs? Ex vivo lung bioengineering with decellularized whole lung scaffolds". Respirology. 18 (6): 895–911. doi:10.1111/resp.12102. PMID 23614471.

120. Wong, A. P.; Rossant, J. (2013). "Generation of Lung Epithelium from Pluripotent Stem Cells". Current pathobiology reports. 1 (2): 137–145. doi:10.1007/s40139-013-0016-9. PMC 3646155 . PMID 23662247.

121. Mou, H.; Zhao, R.; Sherwood, R.; Ahfeldt, T.; Lapey, A.; Wain, J.; Sicilian, L.; Izvolsky, K.; Lau, F. H.; Musunuru, K.; Cowan, C.; Rajagopal, J. (2012). "Generation of Multipotent Lung and Airway Progenitors from Mouse ESCs and Patient-Specific Cystic Fibrosis iPSCs". Cell Stem Cell. 10 (4): 385–97.

doi:10.1016/j.stem.2012.01.018. PMID 22482504.

122. Ghaedi, M.; Calle, E. A.; Mendez, J. J.; Gard, A. L.; Balestrini, J.; Booth, A.; Bove, P. F.; Gui, L.; White, E. S.; Niklason, L. E. (2013). "Human iPS cell-derived alveolar epithelium repopulates lung extracellular matrix". Journal of Clinical Investigation. 123 (11): 4950–62. doi:10.1172/JCI68793. PMID 24135142.

123. Ghaedi, M.; Mendez, J. J.; Bove, P. F.; Sivarapatna, A.; Raredon, M. S. B.; Niklason, L. E. (2014). "Alveolar epithelial differentiation of human induced pluripotent stem cells in a rotating bioreactor". Biomaterials. 35 (2): 699–710. doi:10.1016/j.biomaterials.2013.10.018. PMID 24144903.

124. Huang, S. X. L.; Islam, M. N.; O'Neill, J.; Hu, Z.; Yang, Y. G.; Chen, Y. W.; Mumau, M.; Green, M. D.; Vunjak-Novakovic, G.; Bhattacharya, J.; Snoeck, H. W. (2013). "Efficient generation of lung and airway epithelial cells from human pluripotent stem cells". Nature Biotechnology. 32 (1): 84–91. doi:10.1038/nbt.2754. PMC 4101921 . PMID 24291815.

125. Niu, Z.; Hu, Y.; Chu, Z.; Yu, M.; Bai, Y.; Wang, L.; Hua, J. (2013). "Germ-like cell differentiation from induced pluripotent stem cells (iPSCs)". Cell Biochemistry and Function. 31 (1): 12–9. doi:10.1002/cbf.2924. PMID 23086862.

126. Yang, S.; Bo, J.; Hu, H.; Guo, X.; Tian, R.; Sun, C.; Zhu, Y.; Li, P.; Liu, P.; Zou, S.; Huang, Y.; Li, Z. (2012). "Derivation of male germ cells from induced pluripotent stem cells in vitro and in reconstituted seminiferous tubules". Cell Proliferation. 45 (2): 91–100. doi:10.1111/j.1365-2184.2012.00811.x. PMID 22324506.

127. Panula, S.; Medrano, J. V.; Kee, K.; Bergstrom, R.; Nguyen, H. N.; Byers, B.; Wilson, K. D.; Wu, J. C.; Simon, C.; Hovatta, O.; Reijo Pera, R. A. (2010). "Human germ cell differentiation from fetal- and adult-derived induced pluripotent stem cells". Human Molecular Genetics. 20 (4): 752–62. doi:10.1093/hmg/ddq520. PMID 21131292.

128. ^ Jump up to:a b c Qian, L.; Huang, Y.; Spencer, C. I.; Foley, A.; Vedantham, V.; Liu, L.; Conway, S. J.; Fu, J. D.; Srivastava, D. (2012). "In vivo reprogramming of murine cardiac fibroblasts into induced cardiomyocytes". Nature. 485 (7400): 593–8. doi:10.1038/nature11044. PMID 22522929.

129. Szabo, E.; Rampalli, S.; Risueño, R. M.; Schnerch, A.; Mitchell, R.; Fiebig-Comyn, A.; Levadoux-Martin, M.; Bhatia, M. (2010). "Direct conversion of human fibroblasts to multilineage blood progenitors". Nature. 468 (7323): 521–526. doi:10.1038/nature09591. PMID 21057492.

130. Efe, J. A.; Hilcove, S.; Kim, J.; Zhou, H.; Ouyang, K.; Wang, G.; Chen, J.; Ding, S. (2011). "Conversion of mouse fibroblasts into cardiomyocytes using a direct reprogramming strategy". Nature Cell Biology. 13 (3): 215–222. doi:10.1038/ncb2164. PMID 21278734.

131. ^ Jump up to:a b Lujan, E.; Chanda, S.; Ahlenius, H.; Sudhof, T. C.; Wernig, M. (2012). "Direct conversion of mouse fibroblasts to self-renewing, tripotent neural precursor cells". Proceedings of the National Academy of Sciences. 109 (7): 2527–2532. doi:10.1073/pnas.1121003109.

132. ^ Jump up to:a b Thier, M.; Wörsdörfer, P.; Lakes, Y. B.; Gorris, R.; Herms, S.; Opitz, T.; Seiferling, D.; Quandel, T.; Hoffmann, P.; Nöthen, M. M.; Brüstle, O.; Edenhofer, F. (2012). "Direct Conversion of Fibroblasts into Stably Expandable Neural Stem Cells". Cell Stem Cell. 10 (4): 473–9. doi:10.1016/j.stem.2012.03.003. PMID 22445518.

133. ^ Jump up to:a b c Han, D. W.; Tapia, N.; Hermann, A.; Hemmer, K.; Höing, S.; Araúzo-Bravo, M. J.; Zaehres, H.; Wu, G.; Frank, S.; Moritz, S. R.; Greber, B.; Yang, J. H.; Lee, H. T.; Schwamborn, J. C.; Storch, A.; Schöler, H. R. (2012). "Direct Reprogramming of Fibroblasts into Neural Stem Cells by Defined Factors". Cell Stem Cell. 10 (4): 465–72. doi:10.1016/j.stem.2012.02.021. PMID 22445517.

134. Taylor, S. M.; Jones, P. A. (1979). "Multiple new phenotypes induced in 10T1/2 and 3T3 cells treated with 5-azacytidine". Cell. 17 (4): 771–9. doi:10.1016/0092-8674(79)90317-9. PMID 90553.

135. Lassar, A. B.; Paterson, B. M.; Weintraub, H (1986). "Transfection of a DNA locus that mediates the conversion of 10T1/2 fibroblasts to myoblasts". Cell. 47 (5): 649–56. doi:10.1016/0092-8674(86)90507-6. PMID 2430720.

136. Vierbuchen, T.; Wernig, M. (2011). "Direct lineage conversions: Unnatural but useful?". Nature Biotechnology. 29 (10): 892–907. doi:10.1038/nbt.1946. PMID 21997635.

137. Chandrakanthan, Vashe; et al. (2016). "PDGF-AB and 5-Azacytidine induce conversion of somatic cells into tissue-regenerative multipotent stem cells". Proceedings of the National Academy of Sciences. 113: E2306–E2315. doi:10.1073/pnas.1518244113.

138. Scientists develop 'game changing' stem cell repair system. Stem Cells Portal

139. Could this new stem cell become the game changer for regenerative treatments?. Irish Examiner

140. Riddle, M. R.; Weintraub, A.; Nguyen, K. C. Q.; Hall, D. H.; Rothman, J. H. (2013). "Transdifferentiation and remodeling of post-embryonic C. Elegans cells by a single transcription factor". Development. 140 (24): 4844–9. doi:10.1242/dev.103010. PMID 24257624.

141. Wei, S; Zou, Q; Lai, S; et al. (2016). "Conversion of embryonic stem cells into extraembryonic lineages by CRISPR-mediated activators". Sci Rep. 6: 19648. doi:10.1038/srep19648.

142. Joshua B Black, Andrew F Adler, Hong-Gang Wang, Anthony M D'Ippolito, Hunter A Hutchinson, Timothy E Reddy, Geoffrey S Pitt, Kam W Leong, and Charles A Gersbach. (2016). Targeted Epigenetic Remodeling of Endogenous Loci by CRISPR/Cas9-Based Transcriptional Activators Directly Converts Fibroblasts to Neuronal Cells. Cell Stem Cell, doi:10.1016/j.stem.2016.07.001

143. Jung, D. W.; Williams, D. R. (2011). "Novel Chemically Defined Approach to Produce Multipotent Cells from Terminally Differentiated Tissue Syncytia". ACS Chemical Biology. 6 (6): 553–62. doi:10.1021/cb2000154. PMID 21322636.

144. "In This Issue". ACS Chemical Biology. 7 (4): 619. 2012. doi:10.1021/cb300127f.

145. Zhang, Hongkai; Wilson, Ian A.; Lerner, Richard A. (2012). "Selection of antibodies that regulate phenotype from intracellular combinatorial antibody libraries". PNAS. 109 (39): 15728–15733. doi:10.1073/pnas.1214275109. PMID 23019357.

146. Antibody that Transforms Bone Marrow Stem Cells Directly into Brain Cells

147. Liu, X.; Ory, V.; Chapman, S.; Yuan, H.; Albanese, C.; Kallakury, B.; Timofeeva, O. A.; Nealon, C.; Dakic, A.; Simic, V.; Haddad, B. R.; Rhim, J. S.; Dritschilo, A.; Riegel, A.; McBride, A.; Schlegel, R. (2012). "ROCK Inhibitor and Feeder Cells Induce the Conditional Reprogramming of Epithelial Cells". The American Journal of Pathology. 180 (2): 599–607. doi:10.1016/j.ajpath.2011.10.036. PMID 22189618.

148. Rheinwald, J. G.; Green, H (1975). "Serial cultivation of strains of human epidermal keratinocytes: The formation of keratinizing colonies from single cells". Cell. 6 (3): 331–43. doi:10.1016/S0092-8674(75)80001-8. PMID 1052771.

149. Hiew, Y.-L. (2011) Examining the biological consequences of DNA damage caused by irradiated J2-3T3 fibroblast feeder cells and HPV16: characterisation of the biological functions of Mll. Doctoral thesis, UCL (University College London)

150. Szumiel, I. (2012). "Radiation hormesis: Autophagy and other cellular mechanisms". International Journal of Radiation Biology. 88 (9): 619–28. doi: 10.3109/09553002.2012.699698. PMID 22702489.

151. Kurosawa, H. (2012). "Application of Rho-associated protein kinase (ROCK) inhibitor to human pluripotent stem cells". Journal of Bioscience and Bioengineering. 114 (6): 577–81. doi:10.1016/j.jbiosc.2012.07.013. PMID 22898436.

152. Terunuma, A.; Limgala, R. P.; Park, C. J.; Choudhary, I.; Vogel, J. C. (2010). "Efficient Procurement of Epithelial Stem Cells from Human Tissue Specimens Using a Rho-Associated Protein Kinase Inhibitor Y-27632". Tissue Engineering Part A. 16 (4): 1363–8. doi:10.1089/ten.tea.2009.0339. PMID 19912046.

153. Sandra Chapman, Xuefeng Liu, Craig Meyers, Richard Schlegel, and Alison A. McBride. (2010) Human keratinocytes are efficiently immortalized by a Rho kinase inhibitor

154. Suprynowicz, F. A.; Upadhyay, G.; Krawczyk, E.; Kramer, S. C.; Hebert, J. D.; Liu, X.; Yuan, H.; Cheluvaraju, C.; Clapp, P. W.; Boucher, R. C.; Kamonjoh, C. M.; Randell, S. H.; Schlegel, R. (2012). "Conditionally reprogrammed cells represent a stem-like state of adult epithelial cells". Proceedings of the National Academy of Sciences. 109 (49): 20035–20040. doi:10.1073/pnas.1213241109.

155. b Agarwal, S.; Rimm, D. L. (2012). "Making Every Cell Like He La". The American Journal of Pathology. 180 (2): 443–5. doi:10.1016/j.ajpath.2011.12.001. PMID 22192626.

156. Lisanti, MP; Tanowitz, HB (Apr 2012). "Translational discoveries, personalized medicine, and living biobanks of the future". The American Journal of Pathology. 180 (4): 1334–6. doi:10.1016/j.ajpath.2012.02.003. PMID 22453029.

157. Yuan, H.; Myers, S.; Wang, J.; Zhou, D.; Woo, J. A.; Kallakury, B.; Ju, A.;

Bazylewicz, M.; Carter, Y. M.; Albanese, C.; Grant, N.; Shad, A.; Dritschilo, A.; Liu, X.; Schlegel, R. (2012). "Use of Reprogrammed Cells to Identify Therapy for Respiratory Papillomatosis". New England Journal of Medicine. 367 (13): 1220–7. doi:10.1056/NEJMoa1203055. PMID 23013073.

158. Crystal, AS; Shaw, AT; Sequist, LV; Friboulet, L; Niederst, MJ; Lockerman, EL; Frias, RL; Gainor, JF; Amzallag, A; Greninger, P; Lee, D; Kalsy, A; Gomez-Caraballo, M; Elamine, L; Howe, E; Hur, W; Lifshits, E; Robinson, HE; Katayama, R; Faber, AC; Awad, MM; Ramaswamy, S; Mino-Kenudson, M; Iafrate, AJ; Benes, CH; Engelman, JA (2014). "Patient-derived models of acquired resistance can identify effective drug combinations for cancer". Science. 346 (6216): 1480–6. doi:10.1126/science.1254721. PMID 25394791.

159. Palechor-Ceron, N.; Suprynowicz, F. A.; Upadhyay, G.; Dakic, A.; Minas, T.; Simic, V.; Johnson, M.; Albanese, C.; Schlegel, R.; Liu, X. (2013). "Radiation Induces Diffusible Feeder Cell Factor(s) That Cooperate with ROCK Inhibitor to Conditionally Reprogram and Immortalize Epithelial Cells". The American Journal of Pathology. 183 (6): 1862–70. doi:10.1016/j.ajpath.2013.08.009. PMID 24096078.

160. Saenz, F. R.; Ory, V.; AlOtaiby, M.; Rosenfield, S.; Furlong, M.; Cavalli, L. R.; Johnson, M. D.; Liu, X.; Schlegel, R.; Wellstein, A.; Riegel, A. T. (2014). "Conditionally Reprogrammed Normal and Transformed Mouse Mammary Epithelial Cells Display a Progenitor-Cell–Like Phenotype". PLoS ONE. 9 (5): e97666. doi:10.1371/journal.pone.0097666. PMC 4022745 . PMID 24831228.

161. Kaur, Sukhbir; Soto-Pantoja, David R.; Stein, Erica V.; et al. (2013). "Thrombospondin-1 Signaling through CD47 Inhibits Self-renewal by Regulating c-Myc and Other Stem Cell Transcription Factors". Scientific Reports. 3: 1673. doi:10.1038/srep01673. PMC 3628113 . PMID 23591719.

162. Soto-Pantoja, D. R.; Ridnour, L. A.; Wink, D. A.; Roberts, D. D. (2013). "Blockade of CD47 increases survival of mice exposed to lethal total body irradiation". Scientific Reports. 3. doi:10.1038/srep01038.

163. Gentek, R.; Molawi, K.; Sieweke, M. H. (2014). "Tissue macrophage identity and self-renewal". Immunological Reviews. 262: 56–73. doi:10.1111/imr.12224.

164. Kurian, Leo; Sancho-Martinez, Ignacio; Nivet, Emmanuel; Juan; Izpisua Belmonte, Carlos (2012). "Conversion of human fibroblasts to angioblast-like progenitor cells". Nature Methods. 10: 77–83. doi:10.1038/nmeth.2255.

165. Morris, S. A.; Daley, G. Q. (2013). "A blueprint for engineering cell fate: current technologies to reprogram cell identity". Cell research. 23 (1): 33–48. doi:10.1038/cr.2013.1. PMID 23277278.

166. Wang, Y. C.; Nakagawa, M.; Garitaonandia, I.; Slavin, I.; Altun, G.; Lacharite, R. M.; Nazor, K. L.; Tran, H. T.; Lynch, C. L.; Leonardo, T. R.; Liu, Y.; Peterson, S. E.; Laurent, L. C.; Yamanaka, S.; Loring, J. F. (2011). "Specific lectin biomarkers for isolation of human pluripotent stem cells identified through array-based glycomic analysis". Cell Research. 21 (11): 1551–63. doi:10.1038/cr.2011.148. PMID 21894191.

167. Thomson, J. A.; Itskovitz-Eldor, J; Shapiro, S. S.; Waknitz, M. A.; Swiergiel, J. J.; Marshall, V. S.; Jones, J. M. (1998). "Embryonic Stem Cell Lines Derived from Human Blastocysts". Science. 282 (5391): 1145–7. doi:10.1126/science.282.5391.1145. PMID 9804556.
168. Suila, H.; Hirvonen, T.; Ritamo, I.; Natunen, S.; Tuimala, J.; Laitinen, S.; Anderson, H.; Nystedt, J.; Räbinä, J.; Valmu, L. (2014). "Extracellular O-Linked N-Acetylglucosamine is Enriched in Stem Cells Derived from Human Umbilical Cord Blood". BioResearch Open Access. 3 (2): 39–44. doi:10.1089/biores.2013.0050. PMID 24804163.
169. Perdigoto, C. N.; Bardin, A. J. (2013). "Sending the right signal: Notch and stem cells". Biochimica et Biophysica Acta (BBA) - General Subjects. 1830 (2): 2307–2322. doi:10.1016/j.bbagen.2012.08.009.
170. Jafar-Nejad, H.; Leonardi, J.; Fernandez-Valdivia, R. (2010). "Role of glycans and glycosyltransferases in the regulation of Notch signaling". Glycobiology. 20 (8): 931–949. doi:10.1093/glycob/cwq053. PMID 20368670.
171. Alisson-Silva, Frederico; Deivid; Rodrigues, Carvalho; Vairo, Leandro; et al. (2014). "and Adriane R Todeschini (2014). Evidences for the involvement of cell surface glycans in stem cell pluripotency and differentiation". Glycobiology. 24 (5): 458–468. doi:10.1093/glycob/cwu012. PMID 24578376.
172. Hasehira, K.; Tateno, H.; Onuma, Y.; Ito, Y.; Asashima, M.; Hirabayashi, J. (2012). "Structural and Quantitative Evidence for Dynamic Glycome Shift on Production of Induced Pluripotent Stem Cells". Molecular & Cellular Proteomics. 11 (12): 1913–1923. doi:10.1074/mcp.M112.020586.
173. Becker Kojic', Z. A. (2002). "A Novel Human Erythrocyte Glycosylphosphatidylinositol (GPI)-anchored Glycoprotein ACA. ISOLATION, PURIFICATION, PRIMARY STRUCTURE DETERMINATION, AND MOLECULAR PARAMETERS OF ITS LIPID STRUCTURE". Journal of Biological Chemistry. 277 (43): 40472–8. doi:10.1074/jbc.M202416200. PMID 12167612.
174. Becker-Kojić, Z. A.; Ureña-Peralta, J. R.; Saffrich, R; Rodriguez-Jiménez, F. J.; Rubio, M. P.; Rios, P; Romero, A; Ho, A. D.; Stojković, M (2013). "A novel human glycoprotein ACA is an upstream regulator of human hematopoiesis". Bulletin of experimental biology and medicine. 155 (4): 536–51. doi:10.1007/s10517-013-2195-0. PMID 24143385.
175. Becker-Kojič, ZA; Ureña-Peralta, JR; Zipančić, I.; Stojkovič, M. (2013). "Activation of surface glycoprotein ACA induced pluripotent hematopoietic progenitor cells" (PDF). Cell Technologies in Biology and Medicine. 9 (2): 85–101.
176. Template:Cite bok
177. Redmer, T.; Diecke, S.; Grigoryan, T.; Quiroga-Negreira, A.; Birchmeier, W.; Besser, D. (2011). "E-cadherin is crucial for embryonic stem cell pluripotency and can replace OCT4 during somatic cell reprogramming". EMBO Reports. 12 (7): 720–6. doi:10.1038/embor.2011.88. PMID 21617704.

178. Bedzhov, I.; Alotaibi, H.; Basilicata, M. F.; Ahlborn, K.; Liszewska, E.; Brabletz, T.; Stemmler, M. P. (2013). "Adhesion, but not a specific cadherin code, is indispensable for ES cell and induced pluripotency". Stem Cell Research. 11 (3): 1250–63. doi:10.1016/j.scr.2013.08.009. PMID 24036274.

179. Su, G.; Zhao, Y.; Wei, J.; Xiao, Z.; Chen, B.; Han, J.; Chen, L.; Guan, J.; Wang, R.; Dong, Q.; Dai, J. (2013). "Direct conversion of fibroblasts into neural progenitor-like cells by forced growth into 3D spheres on low attachment surfaces". Biomaterials. 34 (24): 5897–906. doi:10.1016/j.biomaterials.2013.04.040. PMID 23680365.

180. Downing, T. L.; Soto, J.; Morez, C.; Houssin, T.; Fritz, A.; Yuan, F.; Chu, J.; Patel, S.; Schaffer, D. V.; Li, S. (2013). "Biophysical regulation of epigenetic state and cell reprogramming". Nature Materials. 12 (12): 1154–62. doi:10.1038/nmat3777. PMID 24141451.

181. Sun, Yubing; Koh; Aw Yong, Meng; Villa-Diaz, Luis G.; Fu, Jianping (2014). "Hippo/YAP-mediated rigidity-dependent motor neuron differentiation of human pluripotent stem cells". Nature Materials. 13: 599–604. doi:10.1038/nmat3945.

182. Murray, P.; Prewitz, M.; Hopp, I.; Wells, N.; Zhang, H.; Cooper, A.; Parry, K. L.; Short, R.; Antoine, D. J.; Edgar, D. (2013). "The self-renewal of mouse embryonic stem cells is regulated by cell–substratum adhesion and cell spreading". The International Journal of Biochemistry & Cell Biology. 45 (11): 2698–2705. doi:10.1016/j.biocel.2013.07.001.

183. Guilak, F.; Cohen, D. M.; Estes, B. T.; et al. (2009). "Control of stem cell fate by physical interactions with the extracellular matrix". Cell stem cell. 5 (1): 17–26. doi:10.1016/j.stem.2009.06.016. PMC 2768283 . PMID 19570510.

184. Worley, K.; Certo, A.; Wan, L. Q. (2012). "Geometry–Force Control of Stem Cell Fate". BioNanoScience. 3: 43–51. doi:10.1007/s12668-012-0067-0.

185. Caiazzo, Massimiliano; Okawa, Yuya; Ranga, Adrian; Piersigilli, Alessandra; Tabata, Yoji; Lutolf, Matthias P. (2016). "Defined three-dimensional microenvironments boost induction of pluripotency". Nature Materials. 15: 344–352. doi:10.1038/nmat4536.

186. Squeezing cells into stem cells. ScienceDaily, 11 January 2016

187. Singh, A.; Suri, S.; Lee, T.; Chilton, J. M.; Cooke, M. T.; Chen, W.; Fu, J.; Stice, S. L.; Lu, H.; McDevitt, T. C.; García, A. S. J. (2013). "Adhesion strength–based, label-free isolation of human pluripotent stem cells". Nature Methods. 10 (5): 438–44. doi:10.1038/nmeth.2437. PMID 23563795.

188. Wang, Kainan; Degerny, Cindy; Xu, Minghong; Yang, Xiang-Jiao (2009). "YAP, TAZ, and Yorkie: A conserved family of signal-responsive transcriptional coregulators in animal development and human disease". Biochemistry and Cell Biology. 87 (1): 77–91. doi:10.1139/O08-114. PMID 19234525.

189. Yang, C.; Tibbitt, M.W.; Basta, L.; Anseth, K.S. (2014). "Mechanical memory and dosing influence stem cell fate". Nature Materials. 13: 645–652. doi:10.1038/nmat3889.

190. Nampe, D.; Tsutsui, H. (2013). "Engineered Micromechanical Cues Affecting

Human Pluripotent Stem Cell Regulations and Fate". Journal of laboratory automation. 18 (6): 482–493. doi:10.1177/2211068213503156. PMID 24062363.

191. Zhang, W.; Duan, S.; Li, Y.; Xu, X.; Qu, J.; Zhang, W.; Liu, G. H. (2012). "Converted neural cells: Induced to a cure?". Protein & Cell. 3 (2): 91–97. doi:10.1007/s13238-012-2029-2.

192. Yang, N.; Ng, Y. H.; Pang, Z. P.; Südhof, T. C.; Wernig, M. (2011). "Induced Neuronal Cells: How to Make and Define a Neuron". Cell Stem Cell. 9 (6): 517–25. doi:10.1016/j.stem.2011.11.015. PMID 22136927.

193. Sheng, C.; Zheng, Q.; Wu, J.; Xu, Z.; Sang, L.; Wang, L.; Guo, C.; Zhu, W.; Tong, M.; Liu, L.; Li, W.; Liu, Z. H.; Zhao, X. Y.; Wang, L.; Chen, Z.; Zhou, Q. (2012). "Generation of dopaminergic neurons directly from mouse fibroblasts and fibroblast-derived neural progenitors". Cell Research. 22 (4): 769–72. doi:10.1038/cr.2012.32. PMID 22370632.

194. Maucksch, C.; Firmin, E.; et al. (2012). "Non-viral generation of neural precursor-like cells from adult human fibroblasts". J Stem Cells Regen Med. 8 (3): 1–9.

195. Ring, K. L.; Tong, L. M.; Balestra, M. E.; Javier, R.; Andrews-Zwilling, Y.; Li, G.; Walker, D.; Zhang, W. R.; Kreitzer, A. C.; Huang, Y. (2012). "Direct Reprogramming of Mouse and Human Fibroblasts into Multipotent Neural Stem Cells with a Single Factor". Cell Stem Cell. 11 (1): 100–9. doi:10.1016/j.stem.2012.05.018. PMC 3399516 . PMID 22683203.

196. Generation of neural progenitor cells by chemical cocktails and hypoxia Cheng, L.; Hu, W.; Qiu, B.; Zhao, J.; Yu, Y.; Guan, W.; Wang, M.; Yang, W.; Pei, G. (2014). "Generation of neural progenitor cells by chemical cocktails and hypoxia". Cell Research. 24 (6): 665–79. doi:10.1038/cr.2014.32. PMID 24638034.

197. Zhang, Mingliang; Lin, Yuan-Hung; Jennifer Sun, Yujiao; Zhu, Saiyong; Zheng, Jiashun; Liu, Kai; Cao, Nan; Li, Ke; Huang, Yadong; Ding, Sheng (2016). "Pharmacological Reprogramming of Fibroblasts into Neural Stem Cells by Signaling-Directed Transcriptional Activation". Cell Stem Cell. 18: 653–667. doi:10.1016/j.stem.2016.03.020.

198. Liu, G. H.; Yi, F.; Suzuki, K.; Qu, J.; Belmonte, J. C. I. (2012). "Induced neural stem cells: A new tool for studying neural development and neurological disorders". Cell Research. 22 (7): 1087–91. doi:10.1038/cr.2012.73. PMID 22547025.

199. Torper, O.; Pfisterer, U.; Wolf, D. A.; Pereira, M.; Lau, S.; Jakobsson, J.; Bjorklund, A.; Grealish, S.; Parmar, M. (2013). "Generation of induced neurons via direct conversion in vivo". Proceedings of the National Academy of Sciences. 110 (17): 7038–7043. doi:10.1073/pnas.1303829110.

200. Niu, W.; Zang, T.; Zou, Y.; Fang, S.; Smith, D. K.; Bachoo, R.; Zhang, C. L. (2013). "In vivo reprogramming of astrocytes to neuroblasts in the adult brain". Nature Cell Biology. 15 (10): 1164–75. doi:10.1038/ncb2843. PMID 24056302.

201. Su, Z.; Niu, W.; Liu, M. L.; Zou, Y.; Zhang, C. L. (2014). "In vivo conversion of astrocytes to neurons in the injured adult spinal cord". Nature Communications. 5. doi:10.1038/ncomms4338.

202. Najm, F. J.; Lager, A. M.; Zaremba, A.; Wyatt, K.; Caprariello, A. V.; Factor, D. C.; Karl, R. T.; Maeda, T.; Miller, R. H.; Tesar, P. J. (2013). "Transcription factor–mediated reprogramming of fibroblasts to expandable, myelinogenic oligodendrocyte progenitor cells". Nature Biotechnology. 31 (5): 426–33. doi:10.1038/nbt.2561. PMID 23584611.

203. Yang, N.; Zuchero, J. B.; Ahlenius, H.; Marro, S.; Ng, Y. H.; Vierbuchen, T.; Hawkins, J. S.; Geissler, R.; Barres, B. A.; Wernig, M. (2013). "Generation of oligodendroglial cells by direct lineage conversion". Nature Biotechnology. 31 (5): 434–9. doi:10.1038/nbt.2564. PMID 23584610.

204. Xu, C. (2012). "Turning cardiac fibroblasts into cardiomyocytes in vivo". Trends in Molecular Medicine. 18 (10): 575–6. doi:10.1016/j.molmed.2012.06.009. PMID 22770847.

205. Fu, J. D.; Stone, N. R.; Liu, L.; Spencer, C. I.; Qian, L.; Hayashi, Y.; Delgado-Olguin, P.; Ding, S.; Bruneau, B. G.; Srivastava, D. (2013). "Direct Reprogramming of Human Fibroblasts toward a Cardiomyocyte-like State". Stem Cell Reports. 1 (3): 235–47. doi:10.1016/j.stemcr.2013.07.005. PMID 24319660.

206. Chen, J. X.; Krane, M.; Deutsch, M. -A.; Wang, L.; Rav-Acha, M.; Gregoire, S.; Engels, M. C.; Rajarajan, K.; Karra, R.; Abel, E. D.; Wu, J. C.; Milan, D.; Wu, S. M. (2012). "Inefficient Reprogramming of Fibroblasts into Cardiomyocytes Using Gata4, Mef2c, and Tbx5". Circulation Research. 111 (1): 50–5. doi:10.1161/CIRCRESAHA.112.270264. PMC 3390172 . PMID 22581928.

207. Burridge, P. W.; Keller, G.; Gold, J. D.; Wu, J. C. (2012). "Production of De Novo Cardiomyocytes: Human Pluripotent Stem Cell Differentiation and Direct Reprogramming". Cell Stem Cell. 10 (1): 16–28. doi:10.1016/j.stem.2011.12.013. PMC 3255078 . PMID 22226352.

208. Wang, H.; Cao, N.; Spencer, C. I.; Nie, B.; Ma, T.; Xu, T.; Zhang, Y.; Wang, X.; Srivastava, D.; Ding, S. (2014). "Small Molecules Enable Cardiac Reprogramming of Mouse Fibroblasts with a Single Factor, Oct4". Cell Reports. 6 (5): 951–60. doi:10.1016/j.celrep.2014.01.038. PMC 4004339 . PMID 24561253.

209. Carpenter, L.; Carr, C.; Yang, C. T.; Stuckey, D. J.; Clarke, K.; Watt, S. M. (2012). "Efficient Differentiation of Human Induced Pluripotent Stem Cells Generates Cardiac Cells That Provide Protection Following Myocardial Infarction in the Rat". Stem Cells and Development. 21 (6): 977–86. doi:10.1089/scd.2011.0075. PMID 22182484.

210. Nan Cao, Yu Huang, Jiashun Zheng et al & Deepak Srivastava, Sheng Ding (2016). Conversion of human fibroblasts into functional cardiomyocytes by small molecules. Science, doi:10.1126/science.aaf1502

211. Scientists Turn Skin Cells into Heart Cells and Brain Cells Using Drugs. GLADSTONE INSTITUTES. News Center

212. Yamada, S.; Nelson, T. J.; Kane, G. C.; Martinez-Fernandez, A.; Crespo-Diaz, R. J.; Ikeda, Y.; Perez-Terzic, C.; Terzic, A. (2013). "IPS Cell Intervention Rescues Wall Motion Disparity Achieving Biological Cardiac Resynchronization Post-Infarction". The Journal of Physiology. 591 (17): 4335–4349. doi:10.1113/

jphysiol.2013.252288.

213. Lian, X.; Hsiao, C.; Wilson, G.; Zhu, K.; Hazeltine, L. B.; Azarin, S. M.; Raval, K. K.; Zhang, J.; Kamp, T. J.; Palecek, S. P. (2012). "Cozzarelli Prize Winner: Robust cardiomyocyte differentiation from human pluripotent stem cells via temporal modulation of canonical Wnt signaling". Proceedings of the National Academy of Sciences. 109 (27): E1848. doi:10.1073/pnas.1200250109.

214. Willems, E.; Cabral-Teixeira, J.; Schade, D.; Cai, W.; Reeves, P.; Bushway, P. J.; Lanier, M.; Walsh, C.; Kirchhausen, T.; Izpisua Belmonte, J. C.; Cashman, J.; Mercola, M. (2012). "Small Molecule-Mediated TGF-β Type II Receptor Degradation Promotes Cardiomyogenesis in Embryonic Stem Cells". Cell Stem Cell. 11 (2): 242–52. doi:10.1016/j.stem.2012.04.025. PMID 22862949.

215. Lu, T. Y.; Lin, B.; Kim, J.; Sullivan, M.; Tobita, K.; Salama, G.; Yang, L. (2013). "Repopulation of decellularized mouse heart with human induced pluripotent stem cell-derived cardiovascular progenitor cells". Nature Communications. 4. doi:10.1038/ncomms3307.

216. Tamer M. A. Mohamed, Nicole R. Stone, Emily C. Berry, et al., & Deepak Srivastava (2016). Chemical Enhancement of In Vitro and In Vivo Direct Cardiac Reprogramming. Circulation, doi:10.1161/CIRCULATIONAHA.116.024692

217. Budniatzky, I.; Gepstein, L. (2014). "Concise Review: Reprogramming Strategies for Cardiovascular Regenerative Medicine: From Induced Pluripotent Stem Cells to Direct Reprogramming". Stem cells translational medicine. 3 (4): 448–457. doi:10.5966/sctm.2013-0163. PMID 24591731.

218. Cosgrove, B. D.; Gilbert, P. M.; Porpiglia, E.; Mourkioti, F.; Lee, S. P.; Corbel, S. Y.; Blau, H. M. (2014). "Rejuvenation of the muscle stem cell population restores strength to injured aged muscles". Nature Medicine. 20 (3): 255–264. doi:10.1038/nm.3464. PMC 3949152 . PMID 24531378.

219. Sousa-Victor, P.; Gutarra, S.; García-Prat, L.; Rodriguez-Ubreva, J.; Ortet, L.; Ruiz-Bonilla, V.; Jardí, M.; Ballestar, E.; González, S.; Serrano, A. L.; Perdiguero, E.; Muñoz-Cánoves, P. (2014). "Geriatric muscle stem cells switch reversible quiescence into senescence". Nature. 506 (7488): 316–21. doi:10.1038/nature13013. PMID 24522534.

220. Hosoyama; et al. "and Masatoshi Suzuki (March, 2014). Derivation of Myogenic Progenitors Directly From Human Pluripotent Stem Cells Using a Sphere-Based Culture". Stem Cells Trans Med. 3: 564–574. doi:10.5966/sctm.2013-0143.

221. Zhu, S.; Rezvani, M.; Harbell, J.; Mattis, A. N.; Wolfe, A. R.; Benet, L. Z.; Willenbring, H.; Ding, S. (2014). "Mouse liver repopulation with hepatocytes generated from human fibroblasts". Nature. 508 (7494): 93–7. doi:10.1038/nature13020. PMID 24572354.

222. Katsuda T, Kawamata M, Hagiwara K, Takahashi R, Yamamoto Y, Camargo FD, Ochiya T (). Conversion of Terminally Committed Hepatocytes to Culturable Bipotent Progenitor Cells with Regenerative Capacity. Cell Stem Cell, doi:10.1016/j.stem.2016.10.007 showArticle Info

223. Abdelalim, E. M.; Bonnefond, A.; Bennaceur-Griscelli, A.; Froguel, P. (2014).

"Pluripotent Stem Cells as a Potential Tool for Disease Modelling and Cell Therapy in Diabetes". Stem Cell Reviews and Reports. 10: 327–337. doi:10.1007/s12015-014-9503-6.

224. Hrvatin, S.; O'Donnell, C. W.; Deng, F.; et al. (2014). "Differentiated human stem cells resemble fetal, not adult, β cells". Proceedings of the National Academy of Sciences. 111 (8): 3038–3043. doi:10.1073/pnas.1400709111.

225. Zhu, Saiyong; Russ, Holger A.; Wang, Xiaojing; Zhang, Mingliang; Ma, Tianhua; Xu, Tao; Tang, Shibing; Hebrok, Matthias; Ding, Sheng (2016). "Human pancreatic beta-like cells converted from fibroblasts". Nature Communications. 7: 10080. doi:10.1038/ncomms10080.

226. Akinci, E; Banga, A; Tungatt, K; et al. (2013). "Reprogramming of Various Cell Types to a Beta-Like State by Pdx1, Ngn3 and MafA". PLoS ONE. 8 (11): e82424. doi:10.1371/journal.pone.0082424.

227. Chen, Y. J.; Finkbeiner, S. R.; Weinblatt, D.; Stanger, B. Z. (2014). "De Novo Formation of Insulin-Producing "Neo-β Cell Islets" from Intestinal Crypts". Cell Reports. 6: 1046–1058. doi:10.1016/j.celrep.2014.02.013.

228. Hendry, C. E.; Vanslambrouck, J. M.; Ineson, J.; Suhaimi, N.; Takasato, M.; Rae, F.; Little, M. H. (2013). "Direct Transcriptional Reprogramming of Adult Cells to Embryonic Nephron Progenitors". Journal of the American Society of Nephrology. 24 (9): 1424–34. doi:10.1681/ASN.2012121143. PMID 23766537.

229. Xinaris, C; Benedetti, V; Rizzo, P; et al. (2012). "In vivo maturation of functional renal organoids formed from embryonic cell suspensions" (PDF). J Am Soc Nephrol. 23 (11): 1857–1868. doi:10.1681/ASN.2012050505. PMC 3482737 . PMID 23085631.

230. Yin, L.; Ohanyan, V.; Fen Pung, Y.; Delucia, A.; Bailey, E.; Enrick, M.; Stevanov, K.; Kolz, C. L.; Guarini, G.; Chilian, W. M. (2011). "Induction of Vascular Progenitor Cells from Endothelial Cells Stimulates Coronary Collateral Growth". Circulation Research. 110 (2): 241–52. doi:10.1161/CIRCRESAHA.111.250126. PMID 22095729.

231. Quijada, P.; Toko, H.; Fischer, K. M.; Bailey, B.; Reilly, P.; Hunt, K. D.; Gude, N. A.; Avitabile, D.; Sussman, M. A. (2012). "Preservation of Myocardial Structure is Enhanced by Pim-1 Engineering of Bone Marrow Cells". Circulation Research. 111 (1): 77–86. doi:10.1161/CIRCRESAHA.112.265207. PMC 3398618 . PMID 22619278.

232. Mohsin, S.; Khan, M.; Toko, H.; Bailey, B.; Cottage, C. T.; Wallach, K.; Nag, D.; Lee, A.; Siddiqi, S.; Lan, F.; Fischer, K. M.; Gude, N.; Quijada, P.; Avitabile, D.; Truffa, S.; Collins, B.; Dembitsky, W.; Wu, J. C.; Sussman, M. A. (2012). "Human Cardiac Progenitor Cells Engineered with Pim-I Kinase Enhance Myocardial Repair". Journal of the American College of Cardiology. 60 (14): 1278–87. doi:10.1016/j.jacc.2012.04.047. PMID 22841153.

233. American Heart Association (2012, July 25). Adult stem cells from liposuction used to create blood vessels in the lab. ScienceDaily.

234. Wang, Z. Z.; Au, P.; Chen, T.; Shao, Y.; Daheron, L. M.; Bai, H.; Arzigian, M.; Fukumura, D.; Jain, R. K.; Scadden, D. T. (2007). "Endothelial cells derived from human embryonic stem cells form durable blood vessels in vivo". Nature Biotechnology. 25 (3): 317–8. doi:10.1038/nbt1287. PMID 17322871.

235. Samuel, R.; Daheron, L.; Liao, S.; Vardam, T.; Kamoun, W. S.; Batista, A.; Buecker, C.; Schafer, R.; Han, X.; Au, P.; Scadden, D. T.; Duda, D. G.; Fukumura, D.; Jain, R.

K. (2013). "Generation of functionally competent and durable engineered blood vessels from human induced pluripotent stem cells". Proceedings of the National Academy of Sciences. 110 (31): 12774–12779. doi:10.1073/pnas.1310675110.

236. Zangi, L.; Lui, K. O.; von Gise, A.; Ma, Q.; Ebina, W.; Ptaszek, L. M.; Später, D.; Xu, H.; Tabebordbar, M.; Gorbatov, R.; Sena, B.; Nahrendorf, M.; Briscoe, D. M.; Li, R. A.; Wagers, A. J.; Rossi, D. J.; Pu, W. T.; Chien, K. R. (2013). "Modified mRNA directs the fate of heart progenitor cells and induces vascular regeneration after myocardial infarction". Nature Biotechnology. 31 (10): 898–907. doi:10.1038/nbt.2682. PMID 24013197.

237. Zeuner, A.; Martelli, F.; Vaglio, S.; Federici, G.; Whitsett, C.; Migliaccio, A. R. (2012). "Concise Review: Stem Cell-Derived Erythrocytes as Upcoming Players in Blood Transfusion". Stem Cells. 30 (8): 1587–96. doi:10.1002/stem.1136. PMID 22644674.

238. Hirose, S. I.; Takayama, N.; Nakamura, S.; Nagasawa, K.; Ochi, K.; Hirata, S.; Yamazaki, S.; Yamaguchi, T.; Otsu, M.; Sano, S.; Takahashi, N.; Sawaguchi, A.; Ito, M.; Kato, T.; Nakauchi, H.; Eto, K. (2013). "Immortalization of Erythroblasts by c-MYC and BCL-XL Enables Large-Scale Erythrocyte Production from Human Pluripotent Stem Cells". Stem Cell Reports. 1 (6): 499–508. doi:10.1016/j.stemcr.2013.10.010. PMID 24371805.

239. Giarratana, M. -C.; Rouard, H.; Dumont, A.; Kiger, L.; Safeukui, I.; Le Pennec, P. -Y.; Francois, S.; Trugnan, G.; Peyrard, T.; Marie, T.; Jolly, S.; Hebert, N.; Mazurier, C.; Mario, N.; Harmand, L.; Lapillonne, H.; Devaux, J. -Y.; Douay, L. (2011). "Proof of principle for transfusion of in vitro-generated red blood cells". Blood. 118 (19): 5071–9. doi:10.1182/blood-2011-06-362038. PMID 21885599.

240. Kobari, L.; Yates, F.; Oudrhiri, N.; Francina, A.; Kiger, L.; Mazurier, C.; Rouzbeh, S.; El-Nemer, W.; Hebert, N.; Giarratana, M. -C.; Francois, S.; Chapel, A.; Lapillonne, H.; Luton, D.; Bennaceur-Griscelli, A.; Douay, L. (2012). "Human induced pluripotent stem cells can reach complete terminal maturation: In vivo and in vitro evidence in the erythropoietic differentiation model". Haematologica. 97 (12): 1795–803. doi:10.3324/haematol.2011.055566. PMID 22733021.

241. Keerthivasan, G.; Wickrema, A.; Crispino, J. D. (2011). "Erythroblast Enucleation". Stem Cells International. 2011: 1–9. doi:10.4061/2011/139851.

242. Smith, B. W.; Rozelle, S. S.; Leung, A.; Ubellacker, J.; Parks, A.; Nah, S. K.; French, D.; Gadue, P.; Monti, S.; Chui, D. H. K.; Steinberg, M. H.; Frelinger, A. L.; Michelson, A. D.; Theberge, R.; McComb, M. E.; Costello, C. E.; Kotton, D. N.; Mostoslavsky, G.; Sherr, D. H.; Murphy, G. J. (2013). "The aryl hydrocarbon receptor directs hematopoietic progenitor cell expansion and differentiation". Blood. 122 (3): 376–85. doi:10.1182/blood-2012-11-466722. PMID 23723449.

243. Shah, Siddharth; Huang, Xiaosong; Cheng, Linzhao (2014). "Stem Cell-Based Approaches to Red Blood Cell Production for Transfusion". Stem Cells Trans Med. 3 (3): 346–355. doi:10.5966/sctm.2013-0054.

244. Rousseau, G. F.; Mazurier, C.; Douay, L. (2016). "Culturing red blood cells from stem cells: a solution to present and future challenges of transfusion medicine?". ISBT Science Series. 11: 111–117. doi:10.1111/voxs.12235.

245. Giani, F. C.; Fiorini, C.; Wakabayashi, A.; Ludwig, L. S.; Salem, R. M.; Jobaliya, C. D.; Guo, M. H. (2016). "Targeted Application of Human Genetic Variation Can Improve Red Blood Cell Production from Stem Cells". Cell stem cell. 18 (1): 73–78. doi:10.1016/j.stem.2015.09.015.

246. Fujita, A.; Uchida, N.; Haro-Mora, J. J.; Winkler, T.; Tisdale, J. (2016). "β-Globin-

Expressing Definitive Erythroid Progenitor Cells Generated from Embryonic and Induced Pluripotent Stem Cell-Derived Sacs. STEM CELLS. doi:10.1002/stem.2335.

247. Figueiredo, C. A.; Goudeva, L.; Horn, P. A.; Eiz-Vesper, B.; Blasczyk, R.; Seltsam, A. (2010). Generation of HLA-deficient platelets from hematopoietic progenitor cells. Transfusion. 50 (8): 1690–701. doi:10.1111/j.1537-2995.2010.02644.x. PMID 20412529.

248. Nakamura, S.; Takayama, N.; Hirata, S.; Seo, H.; Endo, H.; Ochi, K.; Fujita, K. I.; Koike, T.; Harimoto, K. I.; Dohda, T.; Watanabe, A.; Okita, K.; Takahashi, N.; Sawaguchi, A.; Yamanaka, S.; Nakauchi, H.; Nishimura, S.; Eto, K. (2014). Expandable Megakaryocyte Cell Lines Enable Clinically Applicable Generation of Platelets from Human Induced Pluripotent Stem Cells. Cell Stem Cell. 14 (4): 535–48. doi:10.1016/j.stem.2014.01.011. PMID 24529595.

249. Large scale production of megakaryocytes from human pluripotent stem cells by a chemically defined forward programming approach

250. Thon JN, Medvetz DA, Karlsson SM, Italiano Jr JE. Road blocks in making platelets for transfusion. J Thromb Haemost 2015; 13 (Suppl. 1): S55–S62. doi:10.1111/jth.12942

251. Riddell, S. R.; Greenberg, P. D. (1995). Principles for Adoptive T Cell Therapy of Human Viral Diseases. Annual Review of Immunology. 13: 545–86. doi:10.1146/annurev.iy.13.040195.002553. PMID 7612234.

252. ^ Jump up to:a b Nishimura, T.; Kaneko, S.; Kawana-Tachikawa, A.; Tajima, Y.; Goto, H.; Zhu, D.; Nakayama-Hosoya, K.; Iriguchi, S.; Uemura, Y.; Shimizu, T.; Takayama, N.; Yamada, D.; Nishimura, K.; Ohtaka, M.; Watanabe, N.; Takahashi, S.; Iwamoto, A.; Koseki, H.; Nakanishi, M.; Eto, K.; Nakauchi, H. (2013). Generation of Rejuvenated Antigen-Specific T Cells by Reprogramming to Pluripotency and Redifferentiation. Cell Stem Cell. 12 (1): 114–26. doi:10.1016/j.stem.2012.11.002. PMID 23290140.

253. Vizcardo, R.; Masuda, K.; Yamada, D.; Ikawa, T.; Shimizu, K.; Fujii, S. I.; Koseki, H.; Kawamoto, H. (2013). Regeneration of Human Tumor Antigen-Specific T Cells from iPSCs Derived from Mature CD8+ T Cells. Cell Stem Cell. 12 (1): 31–6. doi:10.1016/j.stem.2012.12.006. PMID 23290135.

254. ^ Jump up to:a b Lei, F.; Haque, R.; Xiong, X.; Song, J. (2012). Directed Differentiation of Induced Pluripotent Stem Cells towards T Lymphocytes. Journal of Visualized Experiments (63). doi:10.3791/3986.

255. Sadelain, M; Brentjens, R; Rivière, I (2013). The basic principles of chimeric antigen receptor design. Cancer Discovery. 3 (4): 388–98. doi:10.1158/2159-8290.CD-12-0548. PMC 3667586 . PMID 23550147.

256. Themeli, M.; Kloss, C. C.; Ciriello, G.; Fedorov, V. D.; Perna, F.; Gonen, M.; Sadelain, M. (2013). Generation of tumor-targeted human T lymphocytes from induced pluripotent stem cells for cancer therapy. Nature Biotechnology. 31 (10): 928–33. doi:10.1038/nbt.2678. PMID 23934177.

257. Pilones, K. A.; Aryankalayil, J.; Demaria, S. (2012). Invariant NKT Cells as Novel Targets for Immunotherapy in Solid Tumors. Clinical and Developmental Immunology. 2012: 1–11. doi:10.1155/2012/720803.

258. Watarai, H.; Yamada, D.; Fujii, S. I.; Taniguchi, M.; Koseki, H. (2012). Induced pluripotency as a potential path towards iNKT cell-mediated cancer immunotherapy. International Journal of Hematology. 95 (6): 624–31. doi:10.1007/s12185-012-1091-0. PMID 22592322.

259. Haruta, M.; Tomita, Y.; Yuno, A.; Matsumura, K.; Ikeda, T.; Takamatsu, K.; Haga, E.; Koba, C.; Nishimura, Y.; Senju, S. (2012). TAP-deficient human iPS cell-derived myeloid cell lines as unlimited cell source for dendritic cell-like antigen-presenting cells. Gene Therapy. 20 (5): 504–13. doi:10.1038/gt.2012.59. PMID 22875043.

260. Xie, H.; Ye, M.; Feng, R.; Graf, T. (2004). Stepwise Reprogramming of B Cells into Macrophages. Cell. 117 (5): 663–76. doi:10.1016/S0092-8674(04)00419-2. PMID 15163413.

261. Bussmann, L. H.; Schubert, A.; Vu Manh, T. P.; De Andres, L.; Desbordes, S. C.; Parra, M.; Zimmermann, T.; Rapino, F.; Rodriguez-Ubreva, J.; Ballestar, E.; Graf, T. (2009). A Robust and Highly Efficient Immune Cell Reprogramming System. Cell Stem Cell. 5 (5): 554–66. doi:10.1016/j.stem.2009.10.004. PMID 19896445.

262. Hanna, J.; Markoulaki, S.; Schorderet, P.; Carey, B. W.; Beard, C.; Wernig, M.; Creyghton, M. P.; Steine, E. J.; Cassady, J. P.; Foreman, R.; Lengner, C. J.; Dausman, J. A.; Jaenisch, R. (2008). Direct Reprogramming of Terminally Differentiated Mature B Lymphocytes to Pluripotency. Cell. 133 (2): 250–64. doi:10.1016/j.cell.2008.03.028. PMID 18423197.

263. Di Stefano, B.; Sardina, J. L.; Van Oevelen, C.; Collombet, S.; Kallin, E. M.; Vicent, G. P.; Lu, J.; Thieffry, D.; Beato, M.; Graf, T. (2013). C/EBPα poises B cells for rapid reprogramming into induced pluripotent stem cells. Nature. 506 (7487): 235–9. doi:10.1038/nature12885. PMID 24336202.

264. Rapino, F.; Robles, E. F.; Richter-Larrea, J. A.; Kallin, E. M.; Martinez-Climent, J. A.; Graf, T. (2013). C/EBPα Induces Highly Efficient Macrophage Transdifferentiation of B Lymphoma and Leukemia Cell Lines and Impairs Their Tumorigenicity. Cell Reports. 3 (4): 1153–63. doi:10.1016/j.celrep.2013.03.003. PMID 23545498.

265. Guo, J.; Feng, Y.; Barnes, P.; Huang, F. F.; Idell, S.; Su, D. M.; Shams, H. (2012). Deletion of FoxN1 in the thymic medullary epithelium reduces peripheral T cell responses to infection and mimics changes of aging. PLoS ONE. 7 (4): e34681. doi:10.1371/journal.pone.0034681.

266. Sun, L.; Guo, J.; Brown, R.; Amagai, T.; Zhao, Y.; Su, D.-M. (2010). Declining expression of a single epithelial cell-autonomous gene accelerates age-related thymic involution. Aging Cell. 9 (3): 347–357. doi:10.1111/j.1474-9726.2010.00559.x. PMID 20156205.

267. Bredenkamp, Nicholas; Nowell, Craig S.; Blackburn, C. Clare (2014). Regeneration of the aged thymus by a single transcription factor. Development. 141 (8): 1627–1637. doi:10.1242/dev.103614. PMC 3978836 . PMID 24715454.

268. Peng, Y.; Huang, S.; Cheng, B.; Nie, X.; Enhe, J.; Feng, C.; Fu, X. (2013).

Mesenchymal stem cells: A revolution in therapeutic strategies of age-related diseases. Ageing Research Reviews. 12 (1): 103–15. doi:10.1016/j.arr.2012.04.005. PMID 22569401.

269. Bieback, K; Kern, S; Kocaömer, A; Ferlik, K; Bugert, P (2008). Comparing mesenchymal stromal cells from different human tissues: Bone marrow, adipose tissue and umbilical cord blood. Bio-medical materials and engineering. 18 (1 Suppl): S71–6. PMID 18334717.

270. Efimenko, A.; Dzhoyashvili, N.; Kalinina, N.; Kochegura, T.; Akchurin, R.; Tkachuk, V.; Parfyonova, Y. (2013). Adipose-Derived Mesenchymal Stromal Cells from Aged Patients with Coronary Artery Disease Keep Mesenchymal Stromal Cell Properties but Exhibit Characteristics of Aging and Have Impaired Angiogenic Potential. Stem Cells Translational Medicine. 3 (1): 32–41. doi:10.5966/sctm.2013-0014. PMC 3902283 . PMID 24353175.

271. Stolzing, A; Jones, E; McGonagle, D; Scutt, A (2008). Age-related changes in human bone marrow-derived mesenchymal stem cells: Consequences for cell therapies. Mechanisms of Ageing and Development. 129 (3): 163–73. doi:10.1016/j.mad.2007.12.002. PMID 18241911.

272. Irina Eberle, Mohsen Moslem, Reinhard Henschler, Tobias Cantz (2012) Engineered MSCs from Patient-Specific iPS Cells. Advances in Biochemical Engineering Biotechnology

273. Chen, Y. S.; Pelekanos, R. A.; Ellis, R. L.; Horne, R.; Wolvetang, E. J.; Fisk, N. M. (2012). Small Molecule Mesengenic Induction of Human Induced Pluripotent Stem Cells to Generate Mesenchymal Stem/Stromal Cells. Stem Cells Translational Medicine. 1 (2): 83–95. doi:10.5966/sctm.2011-0022. PMID 23197756.

274. Hynes, K; Menicanin, D; Han, J; Marino, V; Mrozik, K; Gronthos, S; Bartold, P. M. (2013). Mesenchymal stem cells from iPS cells facilitate periodontal regeneration. Journal of Dental Research. 92 (9): 833–9. doi:10.1177/0022034513498258. PMID 23884555.

275. iPSC for Dental Tissue Regeneration

276. Lai, Ruenn Chai; Yeo, Ronne Wee Yeh; Tan, Soon Sim; Zhang, Bin; Yin, Yijun; Sze, Newman Siu Kwan; Choo, Andre; Lim, Sai Kiang (2013). Mesenchymal Stem Cell Exosomes: The Future MSC-Based Therapy?. Mesenchymal Stem Cell Therapy. pp. 39–61. doi:10.1007/978-1-62703-200-1_3. ISBN 978-1-62703-199-8.

277. Lai, R. C.; Yeo, R. W. Y.; Tan, K. H.; Lim, S. K. (2013). Exosomes for drug delivery — a novel application for the mesenchymal stem cell. Biotechnology Advances. 31 (5): 543–51. doi:10.1016/j.biotechadv.2012.08.008. PMID 22959595.

278. Kosaka, N.; Takeshita, F.; Yoshioka, Y.; Hagiwara, K.; Katsuda, T.; Ono, M.; Ochiya, T. (2013). Exosomal tumor-suppressive microRNAs as novel cancer therapy. Advanced Drug Delivery Reviews. 65 (3): 376–82. doi:10.1016/j.addr.2012.07.011. PMID 22841506.

279. Jumabay, M.; Abdmaulen, R.; Ly, A.; Cubberly, M. R.; Shahmirian, L. J.; Heydarkhan-Hagvall, S.; Dumesic, D. A.; Yao, Y.; Bostrom, K. I. (2014).

Pluripotent Stem Cells Derived from Mouse and Human White Mature Adipocytes. Stem Cells Translational Medicine. 3 (2): 161–71. doi:10.5966/sctm.2013-0107. PMID 24396033.

280. Poloni, A.; Maurizi, G.; Leoni, P.; Serrani, F.; Mancini, S.; Frontini, A.; Zingaretti, M. C.; Siquini, W.; Sarzani, R.; Cinti, S. (2012). Human Dedifferentiated Adipocytes Show Similar Properties to Bone Marrow-Derived Mesenchymal Stem Cells. Stem Cells. 30 (5): 965–74. doi:10.1002/stem.1067. PMID 22367678.
281. Shen, J. F.; Sugawara, A; Yamashita, J; Ogura, H; Sato, S (2011). Dedifferentiated fat cells: An alternative source of adult multipotent cells from the adipose tissues. International Journal of Oral Science. 3 (3): 117–24. doi:10.4248/IJOS11044. PMC 3470092 . PMID 21789960.
282. Melief, S. M.; Zwaginga, J. J.; Fibbe, W. E.; Roelofs, H. (2013). Adipose Tissue-Derived Multipotent Stromal Cells Have a Higher Immunomodulatory Capacity Than Their Bone Marrow-Derived Counterparts. Stem Cells Translational Medicine. 2 (6): 455–63. doi:10.5966/sctm.2012-0184. PMID 23694810.
283. Cheng, A.; Hardingham, T. E.; Kimber, S. J. (2013). Generating Cartilage Repair from Pluripotent Stem Cells. Tissue Engineering Part B: Reviews. 20 (4): 131030093023007. doi:10.1089/ten.teb.2012.0757.
284. Outani, H.; Okada, M.; Yamashita, A.; Nakagawa, K.; Yoshikawa, H.; Tsumaki, N. (2013). Direct Induction of Chondrogenic Cells from Human Dermal Fibroblast Culture by Defined Factors. PLoS ONE. 8 (10): e77365. doi:10.1371/journal.pone.0077365. PMC 3797820 . PMID 24146984.
285. Crompton, J. G.; Rao, M.; Restifo, N. P. (2013). Memoirs of a Reincarnated T Cell. Cell Stem Cell. 12 (1): 6–8. doi:10.1016/j.stem.2012.12.009. PMID 23290132.
286. Tan, H. -K.; Toh, C. -X. D.; Ma, D.; Yang, B.; Liu, T. M.; Lu, J.; Wong, C. -W.; Tan, T. -K.; Li, H.; Syn, C.; Tan, E. -L.; Lim, B.; Lim, Y. -P.; Cook, S. A.; Loh, Y. -H. (2014). Human Finger-Prick Induced Pluripotent Stem Cells Facilitate the Development of Stem Cell Banking. Stem Cells Translational Medicine. 3 (5): 586–98. doi:10.5966/sctm.2013-0195. PMID 24646489.
287. Okita, K.; Yamakawa, T.; Matsumura, Y.; Sato, Y.; Amano, N.; Watanabe, A.; Goshima, N.; Yamanaka, S. (2013). An Efficient Nonviral Method to Generate Integration-Free Human-Induced Pluripotent Stem Cells from Cord Blood and Peripheral Blood Cells. Stem Cells. 31 (3): 458–66. doi:10.1002/stem.1293. PMID 23193063.
288. Geti, I.; Ormiston, M. L.; Rouhani, F.; Toshner, M.; Movassagh, M.; Nichols, J.; Mansfield, W.; Southwood, M.; Bradley, A.; Rana, A. A.; Vallier, L.; Morrell, N. W. (2012). A Practical and Efficient Cellular Substrate for the Generation of Induced Pluripotent Stem Cells from Adults: Blood-Derived Endothelial Progenitor Cells. Stem Cells Translational Medicine. 1 (12): 855–65. doi:10.5966/sctm.2012-0093. PMID 23283547.
289. Staerk, J.; Dawlaty, M. M.; Gao, Q.; Maetzel, D.; Hanna, J.; Sommer, C. A.; Mostoslavsky, G.; Jaenisch, R. (2010). Reprogramming of Human Peripheral

Blood Cells to Induced Pluripotent Stem Cells. Cell Stem Cell. 7 (1): 20–4. doi:10.1016/j.stem.2010.06.002. PMC 2917234 . PMID 20621045.

290. Park, T. S.; Huo, J. S.; Peters, A.; Talbot, C. C.; Verma, K.; Zimmerlin, L.; Kaplan, I. M.; Zambidis, E. T. (2012). Growth Factor-Activated Stem Cell Circuits and Stromal Signals Cooperatively Accelerate Non-Integrated iPSC Reprogramming of Human Myeloid Progenitors. PLoS ONE. 7 (8): e42838. doi:10.1371/journal.pone.0042838. PMC 3414503 . PMID 22905176.

291. Yoshikawa, K.; Naitoh, M.; Kubota, H.; Ishiko, T.; Aya, R.; Yamawaki, S.; Suzuki, S. (2013). Multipotent stem cells are effectively collected from adult human cheek skin. Biochemical and Biophysical Research Communications. 431 (1): 104–10. doi:10.1016/j.bbrc.2012.12.069. PMID 23268344.

292. Zhou, T.; Benda, C.; Duzinger, S.; Huang, Y.; Li, X.; Li, Y.; Guo, X.; Cao, G.; Chen, S.; Hao, L.; Chan, Y. -C.; Ng, K. -M.; Cy Ho, J.; Wieser, M.; Wu, J.; Redl, H.; Tse, H. -F.; Grillari, J.; Grillari-Voglauer, R.; Pei, D.; Esteban, M. A. (2011). Generation of Induced Pluripotent Stem Cells from Urine. Journal of the American Society of Nephrology. 22 (7): 1221–8. doi:10.1681/ASN.2011010106. PMID 21636641.

293. Zhou, T.; Benda, C.; Dunzinger, S.; Huang, Y.; Ho, J. C.; Yang, J.; Wang, Y.; Zhang, Y.; Zhuang, Q.; Li, Y.; Bao, X.; Tse, H. F.; Grillari, J.; Grillari-Voglauer, R.; Pei, D.; Esteban, M. A. (2012). Generation of human induced pluripotent stem cells from urine samples. Nature Protocols. 7 (12): 2080–9. doi:10.1038/nprot.2012.115. PMID 23138349.

294. Wang, L.; Wang, L.; Huang, W.; Su, H.; Xue, Y.; Su, Z.; Liao, B.; Wang, H.; Bao, X.; Qin, D.; He, J.; Wu, W.; So, K. F.; Pan, G.; Pei, D. (2012). Generation of integration-free neural progenitor cells from cells in human urine. Nature Methods. 10 (1): 84–9. doi:10.1038/nmeth.2283. PMID 23223155.

295. Cai, J; Zhang, Y; Liu, P; Chen, S; Wu, X; Sun, Y; Li, A; Huang, K; et al. (2013). Generation of tooth-like structures from integration-free human urine induced pluripotent stem cells (PDF). Cell Regeneration. 2: 6. doi:10.1186/2045-9769-2-6.

296. Bharadwaj, S.; Liu, G.; Shi, Y.; Wu, R.; Yang, B.; He, T.; Fan, Y.; Lu, X.; Zhou, X.; Liu, H.; Atala, A.; Rohozinski, J.; Zhang, Y. (2013). Multipotential differentiation of human urine-derived stem cells: Potential for therapeutic applications in urology. Stem Cells. 31 (9): 1840–56. doi:10.1002/stem.1424. PMID 23666768.

297. Wang, Y.; Liu, J.; Tan, X.; Li, G.; Gao, Y.; Liu, X.; Zhang, L.; Li, Y. (2012). Induced Pluripotent Stem Cells from Human Hair Follicle Mesenchymal Stem Cells. Stem Cell Reviews and Reports. 9 (4): 451–60. doi:10.1007/s12015-012-9420-5. PMID 23242965.

298. Schnabel, L. V.; Abratte, C. M.; Schimenti, J. C.; Southard, T. L.; Fortier, L. A. (2012). Genetic background affects induced pluripotent stem cell generation. Stem Cell Research & Therapy. 3 (4): 30. doi:10.1186/scrt121.

299. Panopoulos, A. D.; Ruiz, S.; Yi, F.; Herrerías, A. D.; Batchelder, E. M.; Belmonte, J. C. I. (2011). Rapid and Highly Efficient Generation of Induced Pluripotent

Stem Cells from Human Umbilical Vein Endothelial Cells. PLoS ONE. 6 (5): e19743. doi:10.1371/journal.pone.0019743. PMC 3095638 . PMID 21603572.

300. Polo, J. M.; Liu, S.; Figueroa, M. E.; Kulalert, W.; Eminli, S.; Tan, K. Y.; Apostolou, E.; Stadtfeld, M.; Li, Y.; Shioda, T.; Natesan, S.; Wagers, A. J.; Melnick, A.; Evans, T.; Hochedlinger, K. (2010). Cell type of origin influences the molecular and functional properties of mouse induced pluripotent stem cells. Nature Biotechnology. 28 (8): 848–55. doi:10.1038/nbt.1667. PMID 20644536.

301. Miura, K.; Okada, Y.; Aoi, T.; Okada, A.; Takahashi, K.; Okita, K.; Nakagawa, M.; Koyanagi, M.; Tanabe, K.; Ohnuki, M.; Ogawa, D.; Ikeda, E.; Okano, H.; Yamanaka, S. (2009). Variation in the safety of induced pluripotent stem cell lines. Nature Biotechnology. 27 (8): 743–5. doi:10.1038/nbt.1554. PMID 19590502.

302. Liang, Y.; Zhang, H.; Feng, Q. S.; Cai, M. B.; Deng, W.; Qin, D.; Yun, J. P.; Tsao, G. S. W.; Kang, T.; Esteban, M. A.; Pei, D.; Zeng, Y. X. (2013). The propensity for tumorigenesis in human induced pluripotent stem cells is related with genomic instability. Chinese Journal of Cancer. 32 (4): 205–12. doi:10.5732/cjc.012.10065. PMID 22704487.

303. Kim, K.; Doi, A.; Wen, B.; Ng, K.; Zhao, R.; Cahan, P.; Kim, J.; Aryee, M. J.; Ji, H.; Ehrlich, L. I. R.; Yabuuchi, A.; Takeuchi, A.; Cunniff, K. C.; Hongguang, H.; McKinney-Freeman, S.; Naveiras, O.; Yoon, T. J.; Irizarry, R. A.; Jung, N.; Seita, J.; Hanna, J.; Murakami, P.; Jaenisch, R.; Weissleder, R.; Orkin, S. H.; Weissman, I. L.; Feinberg, A. P.; Daley, G. Q. (2010). Epigenetic memory in induced pluripotent stem cells. Nature. 467 (7313): 285–90. doi:10.1038/nature09342. PMID 20644535.

304. Kim, K.; Zhao, R.; Doi, A.; Ng, K.; Unternaehrer, J.; Cahan, P.; Hongguang, H.; Loh, Y. H.; Aryee, M. J.; Lensch, M. W.; Li, H.; Collins, J. J.; Feinberg, A. P.; Daley, G. Q. (2011). Donor cell type can influence the epigenome and differentiation potential of human induced pluripotent stem cells. Nature Biotechnology. 29 (12): 1117–9. doi:10.1038/nbt.2052. PMID 22119740.

305. Bar-Nur, O.; Russ, H. A.; Efrat, S.; Benvenisty, N. (2011). Epigenetic Memory and Preferential Lineage-Specific Differentiation in Induced Pluripotent Stem Cells Derived from Human Pancreatic Islet Beta Cells. Cell Stem Cell. 9 (1): 17–23. doi:10.1016/j.stem.2011.06.007. PMID 21726830.

306. Denker, H. W. (2012). Time to Reconsider Stem Cell Induction Strategies. Cells. 1 (4): 1293–312. doi:10.3390/cells1041293. PMC 3901125 . PMID 24710555.

Stem-cell Therapy

Chapter Contents

Stem Cell Institute is one of the world's leading adult stem cell therapy and research centers. In close collaboration with universities and physicians world-wide, our comprehensive stem cell treatment protocols employ well-targeted combinations of allogeneic human umbilical cord stem cells, autologous bone marrow stem cells, and autologous adipose stem cells, and to treat the diseases listed below.

INTRODUCTION

Stem-cell therapy is the use of stem cells to treat or prevent a disease or condition.

Bone marrow transplant is the most widely used stem-cell therapy, but some therapies derived from umbilical cord blood are also in use. Research is underway to develop various sources for stem cells, and to apply stem-cell treatments for neurodegenerative diseases and conditions such as diabetes, heart disease, and other conditions.

Stem-cell therapy has become controversial following developments such as the ability of scientists to isolate and culture embryonic stem cells, to create stem cells using somatic cell nuclear transfer and their use of techniques to create induced pluripotent stem cells. This controversy is often related to abortion politics and to human cloning. Additionally, efforts to market treatments based on transplant of stored umbilical cord blood have been controversial.

MEDICAL USES

For over 30 years, bone marrow has been used to treat cancer patients with conditions such as leukaemia and lymphoma; this is the only form of stem-cell therapy that is widely practiced. During chemotherapy, most growing cells are killed by the cytotoxic agents. These agents, however, cannot discriminate between the leukaemia or neoplastic cells, and the hematopoietic stem cells within the bone marrow. It is this side effect of conventional chemotherapy strategies that the stem-cell transplant attempts to reverse; a donor's healthy bone marrow reintroduces functional stem cells to replace the cells lost in the host's body during treatment. The transplanted cells also generate an immune response that helps to kill off the cancer cells; this process can go too far, however, leading to graft vs host disease, the most serious side effect of this treatment.

Another stem-cell therapy called Prochymal, was conditionally approved in Canada in 2012 for the management of acute graft-vs-host disease in children who are unresponsive to steroids. It is an allogenic stem therapy based on mesenchymal stem cells (MSCs) derived from the bone marrow of adult donors. MSCs are purified from the marrow, cultured and packaged, with up to 10,000 doses derived from a single donor. The doses are stored frozen until needed.

The FDA has approved five hematopoietic stem-cell products derived from umbilical cord blood, for the treatment of blood and immunological diseases.

In 2014, the European Medicines Agency recommended approval of Holoclar, a treatment involving stem cells, for use in the European Union. Holoclar is used for people with severe limbal stem cell deficiency due to burns in the eye.

In March 2016 GlaxoSmithKline›s Strimvelis (GSK2696273) therapy for the treatment ADA-SCID was recommended for EU approval.

RESEARCH

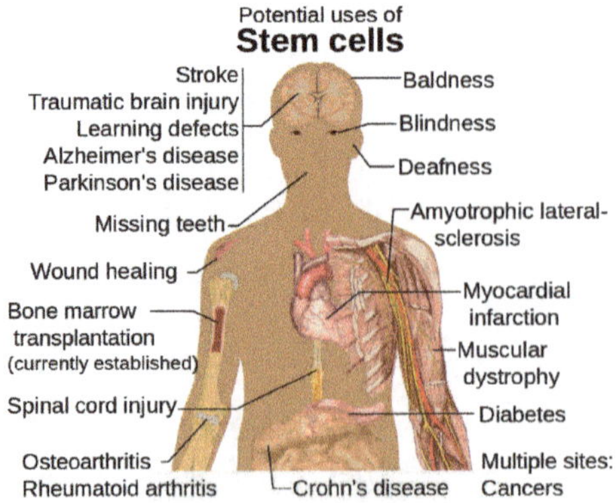

Diseases and conditions where stem cell treatment is promising or emerging.

Stem cells are being studied for a number of reasons. The molecules and exosomes released from stem cells are also being studied in an effort to make medications.

Neurodegeneration

Research has been conducted on the effects of stem cells on animal models of brain degeneration, such as in Parkinson's, Amyotrophic lateral sclerosis, and Alzheimer's disease.There have been preliminary studies related to multiple sclerosis.

Healthy adult brains contain neural stem cells which divide to maintain general stem-cell numbers, or become progenitor cells. In healthy adult laboratory animals, progenitor cells migrate within the brain and function primarily to maintain neuron populations for olfaction (the sense of smell). Pharmacological activation of endogenous neural stem cells has been reported to induce neuroprotection and behavioral recovery in adult rat models of neurological disorder.

Brain and Spinal Cord Injury

Stroke and traumatic brain injury lead to cell death, characterized by a loss of neurons and oligodendrocytes within the brain. A small clinical trial was underway in Scotland in 2013, in which stem cells were injected into the brains of stroke patients.

Clinical and animal studies have been conducted into the use of stem cells in cases of spinal cord injury.

Heart

The pioneering work by Bodo-Eckehard Strauer has now been discredited by the identification of hundreds of factual contradictions. Among several clinical trials that have reported that adult stem-cell therapy is safe and effective, powerful effects have been reported from only a few laboratories, but this has covered old and recent infarcts as well as heart failure not arising from myocardial infarction. While initial animal studies demonstrated remarkable therapeutic effects, later clinical trials achieved only modest, though statistically significant, improvements. Possible reasons for this discrepancy are patient age, timing of treatment and the recent occurrence of a myocardial infarction. It appears that these obstacles may be overcome by additional treatments which increase the effectiveness of the treatment or by optimizing the methodology although these too can be controversial. Current studies vary greatly in cell-procuring techniques, cell types, cell-administration timing and procedures, and studied parameters, making it very difficult to make comparisons. Comparative studies are therefore currently needed.

Stem-cell therapy for treatment of myocardial infarction usually makes use of autologous bone-marrow stem cells (a specific type or all), however other types of adult stem cells may be used, such as adipose-derived stem cells. Adult stem cell therapy for treating heart disease was commercially available in at least five continents as of 2007.

Possible mechanisms of recovery include:

- Generation of heart muscle cells
- Stimulation of growth of new blood vessels to repopulate damaged heart tissue
- Secretion of growth factors
- Assistance via some other mechanism

It may be possible to have adult bone-marrow cells differentiate into heart muscle cells.

The first successful integration of human embryonic stem cell derived cardiomyocytes in guinea pigs (mouse hearts beat too fast) was reported in August 2012. The contraction strength was measured four weeks after the guinea pigs underwent simulated heart attacks and cell treatment. The cells contracted synchronously with the existing cells, but it is unknown if the positive results were produced mainly from paracrine as opposed to direct electromechanical effects from the human cells. Future work will focus on how to get the cells to engraft more strongly around the scar tissue. Whether treatments from embryonic or adult bone marrow stem cells will prove more effective remains to be seen.

In 2013 the pioneering reports of powerful beneficial effects of autologous bone marrow stem cells on ventricular function were found to contain hundreds of discrepancies. Critics report that of 48 reports there seemed to be just five underlying trials, and that in many cases whether they were randomized or merely observational accepter-versus-rejecter, was contradictory between reports of the same trial. One pair of reports of identical baseline characteristics and final results, was presented in two publications as, respectively, a 578 patient randomized trial and as a 391 patient observational study. Other reports required (impossible) negative standard deviations in subsets of patients, or contained fractional patients, negative NYHA classes. Overall there were many more patients published as having receiving stem cells in trials, than the number of stem cells processed in the hospital›s laboratory during that time. A university investigation, closed in 2012 without reporting, was reopened in July 2013.

One of the most promising benefits of stem cell therapy is the potential for cardiac tissue regeneration to reverse the tissue loss underlying the development of heart failure after cardiac injury.

Initially, the observed improvements were attributed to a transdifferentiation of BM-MSCs into cardiomyocyte-like cells. Given the apparent inadequacy of unmodified stem cells for heart tissue regeneration, a more promising modern technique involves treating these cells to create cardiac progenitor cells before implantation to the injured area.

Blood-cell Formation

The specificity of the human immune-cell repertoire is what allows the human body to defend itself from rapidly adapting antigens. However, the immune system is vulnerable to degradation upon the pathogenesis of disease, and because of the critical role that it plays in overall defense, its degradation is often fatal to the organism as a whole. Diseases of hematopoietic cells are diagnosed and classified via a subspecialty of pathology known as hematopathology. The specificity of the immune cells is what allows recognition of foreign antigens, causing further challenges in the treatment of immune disease. Identical matches between donor and recipient must be made for successful transplantation treatments, but matches are uncommon, even between first-degree relatives. Research using both hematopoietic adult stem cells and embryonic stem cells has provided insight into the possible mechanisms and methods of treatment for many of these ailments.

Fully mature human red blood cells may be generated *ex vivo* by hematopoietic stem cells (HSCs), which are precursors of red blood cells. In this process, HSCs are grown together with stromal cells, creating an environment that mimics the conditions of bone marrow, the natural site of red-blood-cell growth. Erythropoietin, a growth factor, is added, coaxing the stem cells to complete terminal differentiation into red blood cells. Further research into this technique should have potential benefits to gene therapy, blood transfusion, and topical medicine.

Missing Teeth

In 2004, scientists at King's College London discovered a way to cultivate a complete tooth in miceand were able to grow bioengineered teeth stand-alone in the laboratory. Researchers are confident that the tooth regeneration technology can be used to grow live teeth in human patients.

In theory, stem cells taken from the patient could be coaxed in the lab turning into a tooth bud which, when implanted in the gums, will give rise to a new tooth, and would be expected to be grown in a time over three weeks. It will fuse with the jawbone and release chemicals that encourage nerves and blood vessels to connect with it. The process is similar to what happens when humans grow their original adult teeth. Many challenges remain, however, before stem cells could be a choice for the replacement of missing teeth in the future.

Research is ongoing in different fields, alligators which are polyphyodonts grow up to 50 times a successional tooth (a small replacement tooth) under each mature functional tooth for replacement once a year.

Cochlear hair Cell Regrowth

Heller has reported success in re-growing cochlea hair cells with the use of embryonic stem cells.

Blindness and Vision Impairment

Since 2003, researchers have successfully transplanted corneal stem cells into damaged eyes to restore vision. "Sheets of retinal cells used by the team are harvested from aborted fetuses, which some people find objectionable." When these sheets are transplanted over the damaged cornea, the stem cells stimulate renewed repair, eventually restore vision. The latest such development was in June 2005, when researchers at the Queen Victoria Hospital of Sussex, England were able to restore the sight of forty patients using the same technique. The group, led by Sheraz Daya, was able to successfully use adult stem cells obtained from the patient, a relative, or even a cadaver. Further rounds of trials are ongoing.

In April 2005, doctors in the UK transplanted corneal stem cells from an organ donor to the cornea of Deborah Catlyn, a woman who was blinded in one eye when acid was thrown in her eye at a nightclub. The cornea, which is the transparent window of the eye, is a particularly suitable site for transplants. In fact, the first successful human transplant was a cornea transplant. The absence of blood vessels within the cornea makes this area a relatively easy target for transplantation. The majority of corneal transplants carried out today are due to a degenerative disease called keratoconus.

The University Hospital of New Jersey reports that the success rate for growth of new cells from transplanted stem cells varies from 25 percent to 70 percent.

In 2014, researchers demonstrated that stem cells collected as biopsies from donor human corneas can prevent scar formation without provoking a rejection response in mice with corneal damage.

In January 2012, The Lancet published a paper by Steven Schwartz, at UCLA›s Jules Stein Eye Institute, reporting two women who had gone legally blind from macular degeneration had dramatic improvements in their vision after retinal injections of human embryonic stem cells.

In June 2015, the Stem Cell Ophthalmology Treatment Study (SCOTS), the largest adult stem cell study in ophthalmology (www.clinicaltrials.gov NCT # 01920867) published initial results on a patient with optic nerve disease who improved from 20/2000 to 20/40 following treatment with bone marrow derived stem cells.

Pancreatic Beta Cells

Diabetes patients lose the function of insulin-producing beta cells within the pancreas. In recent experiments, scientists have been able to coax embryonic stem cell to turn into beta cells in the lab. In theory if the beta cell is transplanted successfully, they will be able to replace malfunctioning ones in a diabetic patient.

Transplantation

Human embryonic stem cells may be grown in cell culture and stimulated to form insulin-producing cells that can be transplanted into the patient.

However, clinical success is highly dependent on the development of the following procedures:

- Transplanted cells should proliferate
- Transplanted cells should differentiate in a site-specific manner
- Transplanted cells should survive in the recipient (prevention of transplant rejection)
- Transplanted cells should integrate within the targeted tissue
- Transplanted cells should integrate into the host circuitry and restore function

Orthopaedics

Clinical case reports in the treatment orthopaedic conditions have been reported. To date, the focus in the literature for musculoskeletal care appears to be on mesenchymal stem cells. Centeno et al. have published MRI evidence of increased cartilage and meniscus volume in individual human subjects.The results of trials that include a large number of subjects, are yet to be published. However, a published safety study conducted in a group of 227 patients over a 3-4-year period shows adequate safety and minimal complications associated with mesenchymal cell transplantation.

Wakitani has also published a small case series of nine defects in five knees involving surgical transplantation of mesenchymal stem cells with coverage of the treated chondral defects.

Wound Healing

Stem cells can also be used to stimulate the growth of human tissues. In an adult, wounded tissue is most often replaced by scar tissue, which is characterized in the skin by disorganized collagen structure, loss of hair follicles and irregular vascular structure. In the case of wounded fetal tissue, however, wounded tissue is replaced with normal tissue through the activity of stem cells. A possible method for tissue regeneration in adults is to place adult stem cell "seeds" inside a tissue bed "soil" in a wound bed and allow the stem cells to stimulate differentiation in the tissue bed cells. This method elicits a regenerative response more similar to fetal wound-healing than adult scar tissue formation.Researchers are still investigating different aspects of the "soil" tissue that are conducive to regeneration.

Infertility

Culture of human embryonic stem cells in mitotically inactivated porcine ovarian fibroblasts (POF) causes differentiation into germ cells (precursor cells of oocytes and spermatozoa), as evidenced by gene expression analysis.

Human embryonic stem cells have been stimulated to form Spermatozoon-like cells, yet still slightly damaged or malformed. It could potentially treat azoospermia.

In 2012, oogonial stem cells were isolated from adult mouse and human ovaries and demonstrated to be capable of forming mature oocytes. These cells have the potential to treat infertility.

HIV/AIDS

Destruction of the immune system by the HIV is driven by the loss of CD4+ T cells in the peripheral blood and lymphoid tissues. Viral entry into CD4+ cells is mediated by the interaction with a cellular chemokine receptor, the most common of which are CCR5 and CXCR4. Because subsequent viral replication requires cellular gene expression processes, activated CD4+ cells are the primary targets of productive HIV infection. Recently scientists have been investigating an alternative approach to treating HIV-1/AIDS, based on the creation of a disease-resistant immune system through transplantation of autologous, gene-modified (HIV-1-resistant) hematopoietic stem and progenitor cells (GM-HSPC).

Clinical Trials

GRNOPC1

On 23 January 2009, the US Food and Drug Administration gave clearance to Geron Corporation for the initiation of the first clinical trial of an embryonic stem-cell-based therapy on humans. The trial aimed evaluate the drug GRNOPC1, embryonic stem cell-derived oligodendrocyte progenitor cells, on patients with acute spinal cord injury. The trial was discontinued in November 2011 so that the company could focus on therapies in the current environment of capital scarcity and uncertain economic conditions.In 2013 biotechnology and regenerative medicine company BioTime (NYSE MKT: BTX) acquired Geron›s stem cell assets in a stock transaction, with the aim of restarting the clinical trial.

Cryopreserved Mesenchymal Stromal Cells (MSCs)

Scientists have reported that MSCs when transfused immediately within few hours post thawing may show reduced function or show decreased efficacy in treating diseases as compared to those MSCs which are in log phase of cell growth(fresh), so cryopreserved MSCs should be brought back into log phase of cell growth in invitro culture before these are administered for clinical trials or experimental therapies, re-culturing of MSCs will help in recovering from the shock the cells get during freezing and thawing. Various clinical trials on MSCs have failed which used cryopreserved product immediately post thaw as compared to those clinical trials which used fresh MSCs.

VETERINARY MEDICINE

Research currently conducted on horses, dogs, and cats can benefit the development of stem cell treatments in veterinary medicine and can target a wide range of injuries and diseases such as myocardial infarction, stroke, tendon and ligament damage, osteoarthritis, osteochondrosis and muscular dystrophy both in large animals, as well as humans. While investigation of cell-based therapeutics generally reflects human medical needs, the high degree of frequency and severity of certain injuries in racehorses has put veterinary medicine at the forefront of this novel regenerative approach. Companion animals can serve as clinically relevant models that closely mimic human disease.

Development of Regenerative Treatment Models

Stem cells are thought to mediate repair via five primary mechanisms: 1) providing an anti-inflammatory effect, 2) homing to damaged tissues and recruiting other cells, such as endothelial progenitor cells, that are necessary for tissue growth, 3) supporting tissue remodeling over scar formation, 4) inhibiting apoptosis, and 5) differentiating into bone, cartilage, tendon, and ligament tissue.

To further enrich blood supply to the damaged areas, and consequently promote tissue regeneration, platelet-rich plasma could be used in conjunction with stem cell transplantation. The efficacy of some stem cell populations may also be affected by the method of delivery; for instance, to regenerate bone, stem cells are often introduced in a scaffold where they produce the minerals necessary for generation of functional bone.

Stem cells have also been shown to have a low immunogenicity due to the relatively low number of MHC molecules found on their surface. In addition, they have been found to secrete chemokines that alter the immune response and promote tolerance of the new tissue. This allows for allogeneic treatments to be performed without a high rejection risk.

Sources of Stem Cells

Veterinary applications of stem cell therapy as a means of tissue regeneration have been largely shaped by research that began with the use of adult-derived mesenchymal stem cells to treat animals with injuries or defects affecting bone, cartilage, ligaments and/or tendons. There are two main categories of stem cells used for treatments: allogeneic stem cells derived from a genetically different donor within the same species and autologous mesenchymal stem cells, derived from the patient prior to use in various treatments. A third category, xenogenic stem cells, or stem cells derived from different species, are used primarily for research purposes, especially for human treatments.

Most stem cells intended for regenerative therapy are generally isolated either from the patient›s bone marrow or from adipose tissue. Mesenchymal stem cells can differentiate into the cells that make up bone, cartilage, tendons, and ligaments, as well as muscle, neural and other progenitor tissues, they have been the main type of stem cells studied in the treatment of diseases affecting these tissues. The number of stem cells transplanted into damaged tissue may alter efficacy of treatment. Accordingly, stem cells derived from bone marrow aspirates, for instance, are cultured in specialized laboratories for expansion to millions of cells. Although adipose-derived tissue also requires processing prior to use, the culturing methodology for adipose-derived stem cells is not as extensive as that for bone marrow-derived cells. While it is thought that bone-marrow derived stem cells are preferred for bone, cartilage, ligament, and tendon repair, others believe that the less challenging collection techniques and the multi-cellular microenvironment already present in adipose-derived stem cell fractions make the latter the preferred source for autologous transplantation.

New sources of mesenchymal stem cells are being researched, including stem cells present in the skin and dermis which are of interest because of the ease at which they can be harvested with minimal risk to the animal. Hematopoetic stem cells have also been discovered to be travelling in the blood stream and possess equal differentiating ability as other mesenchymal stem cells, again with a very non-invasive harvesting technique.

There has been more recent interest in the use of extra embryonic mesenchymal stem cells. Research is underway to examine the differentiating capabilities of stem cells found in the umbilical cord, yolk sac and placenta of different animals. These stem cells are thought to have more differentiating ability than their adult counterparts, including the ability to more readily form tissues of endodermal and ectodermal origin.

Stem Cells and Hard-tissue Repair

Because of the general positive healing capabilities of stem cells, they have gained interest for the treatment of cutaneous wounds. This is important interest for those with reduced healing capabilities, like diabetics and those undergoing chemotherapy. In one trial, stem cells were isolated from the Wharton's jelly of the umbilical cord. These cells were injected directly into the wounds. Within a week, full re-epithelialization of the wounds had occurred, compared to minor re-epithelialization in the control wounds. This showed the capabilities of mesenchymal stem cells in the repair of epidermal tissues.

Soft-palate defects in horses are caused by a failure of the embryo to fully close at the midline during embryogenesis. These are often not found until after they have become worse because of the difficulty in visualizing the entire soft palate. This lack of visualization is thought to also contribute to the low success rate in surgical intervention to repair the defect. As a result, the horse often has to be euthanized. Recently, the use of mesenchymal stem cells has been added to the conventional treatments. After the surgeon has sutured the palate closed, autologous mesenchymal cells are injected into the soft palate. The stem cells were found to be integrated into the healing tissue especially along the border with the old tissue. There was also a large reduction in the number of inflammatory cells present, which is thought to aid in the healing process.

Stem cells and Orthopedic Repairs

Autologous stem cell-based treatments for ligament injury, tendon injury, osteoarthritis, osteochondrosis, and sub-chondral bone cysts have been commercially available to practicing veterinarians to treat horses since 2003 in the United States and since 2006 in the United Kingdom. Autologous stem cell based treatments for tendon injury, ligament injury, and osteoarthritis in dogs have been available to veterinarians in the United States since 2005. Over 3000 privately owned horses and dogs have been treated with autologous adipose-derived stem cells. The efficacy of these treatments has been shown in double-blind clinical trials for dogs with osteoarthritis of the hip and elbow and horses with tendon damage.

Tendon Repair

Race horses are especially prone to injuries of the tendon and ligaments. Conventional therapies are very unsuccessful in returning the horse to full functioning potential. Natural healing, guided by the conventional treatments, leads to the formation of fibrous scar tissue that reduces flexibility and full joint movement. Traditional treatments prevented a large number of horses from returning to full activity and also have a high incidence of re-injury due to the stiff nature of the scarred tendon. Introduction of both bone marrow and adipose derived stem cells, along with natural mechanical stimulus promoted the regeneration of tendon tissue. The natural movement promoted the alignment of the new fibers and tendocytes with the natural alignment found in uninjured tendons. Stem cell treatment not only allowed more horses to return to full duty and also greatly reduced the re-injury rate over a three-year period.

The use of embryonic stem cells has also been applied to tendon repair. The embryonic stem cells were shown to have a better survival rate in the tendon as well as better migrating capabilities to reach all areas of damaged tendon. The overall repair quality was also higher, with better tendon architecture and collagen formed. There was also no tumor formation seen during the three month experimental period. Long-term studies need to be carried out to examine the long-term efficacy and risks associated with the use of embryonic stem cells. Similar results have been found in small animals.

Joint Repair

Osteoarthritis is the main cause of joint pain both in animals and humans. Horses and dogs are most frequently affected arthritis. Natural cartilage regeneration is very limited and no current drug therapies are curative, but rather look to reduce the symptoms associated with the degeneration. Different types of mesenchymal stem cells and other additives are still being researched to find the best type of cell and method for long-term treatment.

Adipose-derived mesenchymal cells are currently the most often used because of the non-invasive harvesting. There has been a lot of success recently injecting mesenchymal stem cells directly into the joint. This is a recently developed, non-invasive technique developed for easier clinical use. Dogs receiving this treatment showed greater flexibility in their joints and less pain.

Bone Defect Repair

Bone has a unique and well documented natural healing process that normally is sufficient to repair fractures and other common injuries. Misaligned breaks due to severe trauma, as well as things like tumor resections of bone cancer, are prone to improper healing if left to the natural process alone. Scaffolds composed of natural and artificial components are seeded with mesenchymal stem cells and placed in the defect. Within four weeks of placing the scaffold, newly formed bone begins to integrate with the old bone and within 32 weeks, full union is achieved. Further studies are necessary to fully characterize the use of cell-based therapeutics for treatment of bone fractures.

Stem cells have been used to treat degenerative bone diseases. The normally recommended treatment for dogs that have Legg–Calve–Perthes disease is to remove the head of the femur after the degeneration has progressed. Recently, mesenchymal stem cells have been injected directly in to the head of the femur, with success not only in bone regeneration, but also in pain reduction.

Stem cells and Muscle Repairs

Stem cells have successfully been used to ameliorate healing in the heart after myocardial infarction in dogs. Adipose and bone marrow derived stem cells were removed and induced to a cardiac cell fate before being injected into the heart. The heart was found to have improved contractility and a reduction in the damaged area four weeks after the stem cells were applied.

A different trial is underway for a patch made of a porous substance onto which the stem cells are "seeded" in order to induce tissue regeneration in heart defects. Tissue was regenerated and the patch was well incorporated into the heart tissue. This is thought to be due, in part, to improved angiogenesis and reduction of inflammation. Although cardiomyocytes were produced from the mesenchymal stem cells, they did not appear to be contractile. Other treatments that induced a cardiac fate in the cells before transplanting had greater success at creating contractile heart tissue.

Stem cells and Nervous System Repairs

Spinal cord injuries are one of the most common traumas brought into veterinary hospitals. Spinal injuries occur in two ways after the trauma: the primary mechanical damage, and in secondary processes, like inflammation and scar formation, in the days following the trauma. These cells involved in the secondary damage response secrete factors that promote scar formation and inhibit cellular regeneration. Mesenchymal stem cells that are induced to a neural cell fate are loaded onto a porous scaffold and are then implanted at the site of injury. The cells and scaffold secrete factors that counteract those secreted by scar forming cells and promote neural regeneration. Eight weeks later, dogs treated with stem cells showed immense improvement over those treated with conventional therapies. Dogs treated with stem cells were able to occasionally support their own weight, which has not been seen in dogs undergoing conventional therapies.

Treatments are also in clinical trials to repair and regenerate peripheral nerves. Peripheral nerves are more likely to be damaged, but the effects of the damage are not as widespread as seen in injuries to the spinal cord. Treatments are currently in clinical trials to repair severed nerves, with early success. Stem cells induced to a neural fate injected in to a severed nerve. Within four weeks, regeneration of previously damaged stem cells and completely formed nerve bundles were observed.

Stem cells are also in clinical phases for treatment in ophthalmology. Hematopoietic stem cells have been used to treat corneal ulcers of different origin of several horses. These ulcers were resistant to conventional treatments available, but quickly responded positively to the stem cell treatment. Stem cells were also able to restore sight in one eye of a horse with retinal detachment, allowing the horse to return to daily activities.

Keratoconjunctivitis Sicca (KCS)

Pre-clinical models of Sjögrens syndrome have culminated in allogeneic MSCs implanted around the lacrimal glands in KSC dogs that were refractory to current therapy. Significantly improved scores in ocular discharge, conjunctival hyperaemia, corneal changes and Schirmer tear tests (STT) were seen.

Current Areas of Research

Stems Cells in the Lab

The ability to grow up functional adult tissues indefinitely in culture through Directed differentiation creates new opportunities for drug research. Researchers are able to grow up differentiated cell lines and then test new drugs on each cell type to examine possible interactions *in vitro* before performing *in vivo* studies. This is critical in the development of drugs for use in veterinary research because of the possibilities of species specific interactions. The hope is that having these cell lines available for research use will reduce the need for research animals used because effects on human tissue *in vitro* will provide insight not normally known before the animal testing phase.

With the advent of induced pluripotent stem cells (iPSC), treatments being explored and created for the used in endangered low production animals possible. Rather than needing to harvest embryos or eggs, which are limited, the researchers can remove mesenchymal stem cells with greater ease and greatly reducing the danger to the animal due to noninvasive techniques. This allows the limited eggs to be put to use for reproductive purposes only.

Stem cells and Conservation

Stem cells are being explored for use in conservation efforts. Spermatogonial stem cells have been harvested from a rat and placed into a mouse host and fully mature sperm were produced with the ability to produce viable offspring. Currently research is underway to find suitable hosts for the introduction of donor spermatogonial stem cells. If this becomes a viable option for conservationists, sperm can be produced from high genetic quality individuals who die before reaching sexual maturity, preserving a line that would otherwise be lost.

Future Clinical Uses

The use of stem cells for the treatment of liver disease in both humans and animals has been the focus of considerable interest. The liver has some natural regenerative properties, but is often insufficient to deal with the extent of some liver diseases. Hepatocytes have been formed from some sources of MSC, but they have not been applied clinically currently. There is a large effort to create stem cells differentiated along the pancreatic line as a possible cure for diabetes, but no line has been well established.

Mesenchymal stem cells are currently under clinical trials as a possible treatment for graft v. host disease and graft rejection after experiments on various animals showing that allogenic stem cell treatments were not rejected and showed no difference in healing capabilities compared with autologous stem cells. This is being further researched for creating off-the-shelf allogenic stem cell treatments for various aspects in regenerative veterinary medicine. Clinical trials are underway to explore the low immunogenic properties of stem cells and their possible use for treatment of problems with an overactive immune system seen with allergies and autoimmune disorders.

In recent years, US-based stem-cell clinics have emerged that treat patients with their own bone marrow or adipose derived adult stem cells as part of clinical trials or FDA authorized same day outpatient IRB programs, most notably for athletes to recover from osteoskeletal (bone, joint and connective tissue) related injuries. This emergence of US based human adult stem cell therapy is discussed by Rudderham in his 2012 article Adult Stem Cell US Therapy.

The long-term impact of these treatments will need to be examined outside of their contribution to medicine. Vast improvements in veterinary medicine has allowed for companion and farm animals to live longer lives. This, however, has contributed to the rise in injury and chronic illness in companion animals. Stem cell treatments, especially for the treatment of orthopedic issues in horses, allows for working animals to return to a normal state of activity at a faster rate with a reduction in the re-injury rate.

EMBRYONIC STEM-CELL CONTROVERSY

There is widespread controversy over the use of human embryonic stem cells. This controversy primarily targets the techniques used to derive new embryonic stem cell lines, which often requires the destruction of the blastocyst. Opposition to the use of human embryonic stem cells in research is often based on philosophical, moral, or religious objections. There is other stem cell research that does not involve the destruction of a human embryo, and such research involves adult stem cells, amniotic stem cells, and induced pluripotent stem cells.

AROUND THE WORLD

China

Stem-cell research and treatment was practiced in the People's Republic of China. The Ministry of Health of the People's Republic of China has permitted the use of stem-cell therapy for conditions beyond those approved of in Western countries. The Western World has scrutinized China for its failed attempts to meet international documentation standards of these trials and procedures.

Middle East

Since 2008 many universities, centers and doctors tried a diversity of methods; in Lebanon proliferation for stem cell therapy, in-vivo and in-vitro techniques were used, Thus this country is considered the launching place of the ***Regentime*** procedure. http://www.researchgate.net/publication/281712114_Treatment_of_Long_Standing_Multiple_

Sclerosis_with_Regentime_Stem_Cell_Technique The regenerative medicine also took place in Jordan and Egypt.

Mexico

Stem-cell treatment is currently being practiced at a clinical level in Mexico. An International Health Department Permit (COFEPRIS) is required. Authorized centers are found in Tijuana, Guadalajara and Cancun. Currently undergoing the approval process is Los Cabos. This permit allows the use of stem cell.

South Korea

In 2005, South Korean scientists claimed to have generated stem cells that were tailored to match the recipient. Each of the 11 new stem cell lines was developed using somatic cell nuclear transfer (SCNT) technology. The resultant cells were thought to match the genetic material of the recipient, thus suggesting minimal to no cell rejection.

Thailand

As of 2013, Thailand still considers Hematopoietic stem cell transplants as experimental. Kampon Sriwatanakul began with a clinical trial in October 2013 with 20 patients. 10 are going to receive stem-cell therapy for Type-2 diabetes and the other 10 will receive stem-cell therapy for emphysema. Chotinantakul's research is on Hematopoietic cells and their role for the hematopoietic system function in homeostasis and immune response.

Ukraine

Today, Ukraine is permitted to perform clinical trials of stem-cell treatments (Order of the MH of Ukraine № 630 "About carrying out clinical trials of stem cells", 2008) for the treatment of these pathologies: pancreatic necrosis, cirrhosis, hepatitis, burn disease, diabetes, multiple sclerosis, critical lower limb ischemia. The first medical institution granted the right to conduct clinical trials became the "Institute of Cell Therapy"(Kiev).

Other countries

Other countries where doctors did stem cells research, trials, manipulation, storage, therapy: Brazil, Cyprus, Germany, Italy, Israel, Japan, Pakistan, Philippines, Russia, Switzerland, Turkey, United Kingdom, India, and many others.

REFERENCES

1. Ian Murnaghan for Explore Stem Cells. Updated: 16 December 2013 Why Perform a Stem Cell Transplant?
2. Bone Marrow Transplantation and Peripheral Blood Stem Cell Transplantation

In National Cancer Institute Fact Sheet web site. Bethesda, MD: National Institutes of Health, U.S. Department of Health and Human Services, 2010. Cited 24 August 2010

3. Karanes C, Nelson GO, Chitphakdithai P, Agura E, Ballen KK, Bolan CD, Porter DL, Uberti JP, King RJ, Confer DL (2008). Twenty years of unrelated donor hematopoietic cell transplantation for adult recipients facilitated by the National Marrow Donor Program. Biology of Blood and Marrow Transplantation. 14 (9 Suppl): 8–15. doi:10.1016/j.bbmt.2008.06.006. PMID 18721775.
4. Malard F, Mohty M (2014). New Insight for the Diagnosis of Gastrointestinal Acute Graft-versus-Host Disease. Mediators Inflamm. 2014: 701013. doi:10.1155/2014/701013. PMID 24733964.
5. Prochymal – First Stem Cell Drug Approved. 22 May 2012.
6. A Stem-Cell-Based Drug Gets Approval in Canada. 17 May 2012.
7. Rosemann A (Dec 2014). Why regenerative stem cell medicine progresses slower than expected. J Cell Biochem. 115 (12): 2073–6. doi:10.1002/jcb.24894. PMID 25079695.
8. European Medicines Agency. First stem-cell therapy recommended for approval in EU. Retrieved 12 December 2014.
9. European Ad Comm backs Glaxo's stem cell therapy Strimvelis for rare autoimmune disorder. March 2016
10. Maguire, G (12 May 2016). Therapeutics from Adult Stem Cells and the Hype Curve.. ACS Medicinal Chemistry Letters. 7 (5): 441–3. doi:10.1021/acsmedchemlett.6b00125. PMID 27190588.
11. Cell Basics: What are the potential uses of human stem cells and the obstacles that must be overcome before these potential uses will be realized?. In Stem Cell Information World Wide Web site. Bethesda, MD: National Institutes of Health, U.S. Department of Health and Human Services, 2009. cited Sunday, 26 April 2009
12. Neural Stem Cells May Rescue Memory In Advanced Alzheimer's, Mouse Study Suggests
13. Vastag B (April 2001). Stem cells step closer to the clinic: paralysis partially reversed in rats with ALS-like disease. JAMA. 285 (13): 1691–3. doi:10.1001/jama.285.13.1691. PMID 11277806.
14. Rebeiro P, Moore J. The role of autologous haemopoietic stem cell transplantation in the treatment of autoimmune disorders. Intern Med J. 2016 Jan;46(1):17-28. PMID 26524106
15. Results Reported from Case Studies of Stem Cell Transplantation in People with Relapsing and Progressive MS. National MS Society. January 2015.
16. Androutsellis-Theotokis A, Leker RR, Soldner F, et al. (August 2006). Notch signalling regulates stem cell numbers in vitro and in vivo. Nature. 442 (7104): 823–6. doi:10.1038/nature04940. PMID 16799564.
17. Androutsellis-Theotokis A, Rueger MA, Park DM, et al. (August 2009). Targeting

neural precursors in the adult brain rescues injured dopamine neurons. Proc. Natl. Acad. Sci. U.S.A. 106 (32): 13570–5. doi:10.1073/pnas.0905125106. PMC 2714762. PMID 19628689.

18. Androutsellis-Theotokis A, Rueger MA, Mkhikian H, Korb E, McKay RD (2008). Signaling pathways controlling neural stem cells slow progressive brain disease. Cold Spring Harb. Symp. Quant. Biol. 73: 403–10. doi:10.1101/sqb.2008.73.018. PMID 19022746.
19. Ghosh, Pallab (27 May 2013) Stroke patients see signs of recovery in stem cell trial BBC News health, Retrieved 27 May 2013
20. Kang KS, Kim SW, Oh YH, et al. (2005). A 37-year-old spinal cord-injured female patient, transplanted of multipotent stem cells from human UC blood, with improved sensory perception and mobility, both functionally and morphologically: a case study. Cytotherapy. 7 (4): 368–73. doi:10.1080/14653240500238160. PMID 16162459.
21. Team co-headed by researchers at Chosun University, Seoul National University and the Seoul Cord Blood Bank (SCB) Umbilical cord cells ‹allow paralysed woman to walk› By Roger Highfield, Science Editor. Last Updated: 1:28AM GMT 30 November 2004
22. Cummings BJ, Uchida N, Tamaki SJ, et al. (September 2005). Human neural stem cells differentiate and promote locomotor recovery in spinal cord-injured mice. Proc. Natl. Acad. Sci. U.S.A. 102 (39): 14069–74. doi:10.1073/pnas.0507063102. PMC 1216836. PMID 16172374.
23. Strauer, Bodo; Steinhoff G (September 2011). 10 years of intracoronary and intramyocardial bone marrow stem cell therapy of the heart: from the methodological origin to clinical practice. J Am Coll Cardiol. 58 (11): 1095–1104. doi:10.1016/j.jacc.2011.06.016. PMID 21884944.
24. Francis, DP; Mielewczik, M; Zargaran, D; Cole, GD (26 June 2013). Autologous bone marrow-derived stem cell therapy in heart disease: Discrepancies and contradictions. International Journal of Cardiology. 168 (4): 3381–403. doi:10.1016/j.ijcard.2013.04.152. PMID 23830344. Retrieved 21 July 2013.
25. Strauer, BE; Yousef, M; Schannwell, CM (July 2010). The acute and long-term effects of intracoronary Stem cell Transplantation in 191 patients with chronic heARt failure: the STAR-heart study. European journal of heart failure. 12 (7): 721–9. doi:10.1093/eurjhf/hfq095. PMID 20576835.
26. Yousef, M; Schannwell, CM; Köstering, M; Zeus, T; Brehm, M; Strauer, BE (16 June 2009). The BALANCE Study: clinical benefit and long-term outcome after intracoronary autologous bone marrow cell transplantation in patients with acute myocardial infarction. Journal of the American College of Cardiology. 53 (24): 2262–9. doi:10.1016/j.jacc.2009.02.051. PMID 19520249.
27. Schannwell CM, Kostering M, Zeus T, Brehm M, Erdmann G, Fleissner T, Yosef M, Kogler G, Wernet P, Strauer BE (2008). Hmane autologe Stammzelltransplantation zur Myokardregeneration bei dilatativer Kardiomyopathie (NYHA Stadium II bis III)(PDF). Austrian Journal of Cardiology. 15 (1): 23–30.

28. ^ Jump up to:[a] [b] Orlic D, Kajstura J, Chimenti S, Jakoniuk I, Anderson SM, Li B, Pickel J, McKay R, Nadal-Ginard B, Bodine DM, Leri A, Anversa P (2001). Bone marrow cells regenerate infarcted myocardium. Nature. 410 (6829): 701–5. doi:10.1038/35070587. PMID 11287958.
29. Kocher A. A.; et al. Neovascularization of ischemic myocardium by human bone-marrow-derived angioblasts prevents cardiomyocyte apoptosis, reduces remodeling and improves cardiac function. Nature Medicine. 7: 430–436. doi:10.1038/86498.
30. Kuswardhani R. A.; Soejitno A. (2011). Bone marrow-derived stem cells as an adjunctive treatment for acute myocardial infarction: a systematic review and meta-analysis. Acta medica Indonesiana. 43 (3): 168–177. PMID 21979282.
31. Malliaras K.; Kreke M.; Marban E. (2011). The stuttering progress of cell therapy for heart disease. Clinical pharmacology and therapeutics. 90 (4): 532–541. doi:10.1038/clpt.2011.175. PMID 21900888.
32. Ayala-Lugo A, et al. Age-dependent availability and functionality of bone marrow stem cells in an experimental model of acute and chronic myocardial infarction. Cell transplantation. 20: 407–419. doi:10.3727/096368909X519283.
33. Zhang Y, et al. Timing of bone marrow cell therapy is more important than repeated injections after myocardial infarction. Cardiovascular Pathology. 20: 204–212. doi:10.1016/j.carpath.2010.06.007.
34. Wang X.; et al. Donor myocardial infarction impairs the therapeutic potential of bone marrow cells by an interleukin-1-mediated inflammatory response. Science Translational Medicine. 3: 100ra90. doi:10.1126/scitranslmed.3002814.
35. Krishnamurthy P, Thal M, Verma S, Hoxha E, Lambers E, Ramirez V, Qin G, Losordo D, Kishore R (2011). Interleukin-10 deficiency impairs bone marrow-derived endothelial progenitor cell survival and function in ischemic myocardium. Circ. Res. 109 (11): 1280–9. doi:10.1161/CIRCRESAHA.111.248369. PMC 3235675. PMID 21959218.
36. Paul A.; Srivastava S.; Chen G.; Shum-Tim D.; Prakash S. Functional Assessment of Adipose Stem Cells for Xenotransplantation Using Myocardial Infarction Immunocompetent Models: Comparison with Bone Marrow Stem Cells. Cell Biochemistry and Biophysics. 67: 263–273. doi:10.1007/s12013-011-9323-0.
37. Guinea pig hearts beat with human cells : Nature News & Comment
38. Francis, Darrel P (Oct 2013). Autologous bone marrow-derived stem cell therapy in heart disease: Discrepancies and contradictions. Int J Cardiol. Elsevier. 168: 3381–403. doi:10.1016/j.ijcard.2013.04.152. PMID 23830344. Retrieved 6 July 2013.
39. Berndt, Christina. A minefield of contradictions. Suddeutsche Zeitung. Retrieved 6 July 2013.
40. Haider, HKh; Ashraf, M (June 2005). Bone marrow stem cell transplantation for cardiac repair.. American Journal of Physiology. Heart and Circulatory Physiology. 288 (6): H2557–67. doi:10.1152/ajpheart.01215.2004. PMID 15897328.

41. Ptaszek LM, Mansour M, Ruskin JN, Chien KR (2012). Towards regenerative therapy for cardiac disease. The Lancet. 379 (9819): 933–942. doi:10.1016/s0140-6736(12)60075-0.

42. Giarratana MC, Kobari L, Lapillonne H, et al. (January 2005). Ex vivo generation of fully mature human red blood cells from hematopoietic stem cells. Nat. Biotechnol. 23 (1): 69–74. doi:10.1038/nbt1047. PMID 15619619.

43. Archer, Graeme. Technology. The Daily Telegraph. London. Retrieved 24 May 2010.

44. Anglin, Ian. Scientists Grow Teeth Using Stem Cells. SingularityHUB. Retrieved 31 July 2014.

45. Yen AH, Sharpe PT (January 2008). Stem cells and tooth tissue engineering. Cell Tissue Res. 331 (1): 359–72. doi:10.1007/s00441-007-0467-6. PMID 17938970.

46. Stem cell-based biological tooth repair and regeneration. Trends Cell Biol. 20: 715–22. 2010. doi:10.1016/j.tcb.2010.09.012. PMC 3000521. PMID 21035344.

47. Wu, Ping; Wu, Xiaoshan; Jiang, Ting-Xin; Elsey, Ruth M.; Temple, Bradley L.; Divers, Stephen J.; Glenn, Travis C.; Yuan, Kuo; Chen, Min-Huey; Widelitz, Randall B.; Chuon, Cheng-Ming (2013). Specialized stem cell niche enables repetitive renewal of alligator teeth (PDF). Proceedings of the National Academy of Sciences of the United States of America. 110 (22): E2009–E2018. doi:10.1073/pnas.1213202110. PMC 3670376. PMID 23671090. Archived from the original (PDF) on 4 November 2013.

48. Gene therapy is first deafness ‹cure› – health – 14 February 2005 – New Scientist

49. Fetal tissue restores lost sightMedicalNewsToday. Article Date: 28 October 2004 – 10:00 PDT

50. BBC NEWS | England | Southern Counties | Stem cells used to restore vision

51. The University Hospital of New Jersey, 2002

52. Human limbal biopsy–derived stromal stem cells prevent corneal scarring. Science Translational Medicine. 12 December 2014. Retrieved 2015-08-02.

53. Embryonic stem cells improve sight of legally blind women. CNN.com. 23 January 2012. Retrieved 2012-01-12.

54. Weiss JN, Levy S, Malkin A. Stem Cell Ophthalmology Treatment Study (SCOTS) for retinal and optic nerve diseases: a preliminary report. Neural Regen Res [serial online] 2015 [cited 2015 Sep 21];10:982-8. Available from: http://www.nrronline.org/text.asp?2015/10/6/982/158365

55. Saki N, Jalalifar MA, Soleimani M, Hajizamani S, Rahim F (2013). Adverse Effect of High Glucose Concentration on Stem Cell Therap. Int J Hematol Oncol Stem Cell Res. 7 (3): 34–40. PMC 3913149. PMID 24505533.

56. Goldstein, Ron (2007). Embryonic stem cell research is necessary to find a diabetes cure. Greenhaven Press. p. 44.

57. Centeno CJ, Busse D, Kisiday J, Keohan C, Freeman M, Karli D (December 2008). Regeneration of meniscus cartilage in a knee treated with percutaneously implanted autologous mesenchymal stem cells. Med. Hypotheses. 71 (6): 900–8.

doi:10.1016/j.mehy.2008.06.042. PMID 18786777.

58. Centeno CJ, Busse D, Kisiday J, Keohan C, Freeman M, Karli D (2008). Increased knee cartilage volume in degenerative joint disease using percutaneously implanted, autologous mesenchymal stem cells. Pain Physician. 11 (3): 343–53. PMID 18523506.

59. Centeno CJ, Schultz JR, Cheever M, Robinson B, Freeman M, Marasco W (March 2010). Safety and complications reporting on the re-implantation of culture-expanded mesenchymal stem cells using autologous platelet lysate technique. Curr Stem Cell Res Ther. 5 (1): 81–93. doi:10.2174/157488810790442796. PMID 19951252.

60. Wakitani S, Nawata M, Tensho K, Okabe T, Machida H, Ohgushi H (2007). Repair of articular cartilage defects in the patello-femoral joint with autologous bone marrow mesenchymal cell transplantation: three case reports involving nine defects in five knees. J Tissue Eng Regen Med. 1 (1): 74–9. doi:10.1002/term.8. PMID 18038395.

61. Gurtner GC, Callaghan MJ, Longaker MT (2007). Progress and potential for regenerative medicine. Annu. Rev. Med. 58 (1): 299–312. doi:10.1146/annurev.med.58.082405.095329. PMID 17076602.

62. Richards M, Fong CY, Bongso A (December 2008). Comparative evaluation of different in vitro systems that stimulate germ cell differentiation in human embryonic stem cells. Fertil. Steril. 93 (3): 986–94. doi:10.1016/j.fertnstert.2008.10.030. PMID 19064262.

63. Ledford H (7 July 2009). Sperm-like cells made from human embryonic stem cells. Nature News. doi:10.1038/news.2009.646. Archived from the original on 9 May 2011.

64. White, YAR; Woods DC; Takai Y; Ishihara O; Seki H; Tilly JL. (2012). Oocyte formation by mitotically active germ cells purified from ovaries of reproductive-age women. Nature Medicine. 18 (3): 413–421. doi:10.1038/nm.2669. PMC 3296965. PMID 22366948.

65. Allers, Kristinia; Hütter, Gero; Hofmann, Jörg; Loddenkemper, Chrtoph; Rieger, Kathrin; Thiel, Eckhard; Schneider, Thomas (14 July 2014). Evidence for the cure of HIV infection by CCR5Δ32/Δ32 stem cell transplantation. Blood. 117 (10): 2791–2799. doi:10.1182/blood-2010-09-309591. PMID 21148083.

66. DiGiusto, David; Stan, Rodica; Krishnan, Amrita; Li, Haitang; Rossi, John; Zaia, John (22 November 2013). Development of Hematopoietic Stem Cell Based Gene Therapy for HIV-1 Infection: Considerations for Proof of Concept Studies and Translation to Standard Medical Practice. Viruses. 2013 (5): 2898–2919. doi:10.3390/v5112898.

67. O›Connell, Claire (27 January 2012). Stem cells – where are we now?. The Irish Times.

68. BioTime acquires stem cell assets from Geron, raises $10 million. San Francisco Business Times. 7 January 2013.

69. Francois M et al., Cytotherapy.2012;14:147–152

70. Chen J, Li Y, Wang L, et al. (April 2001). Therapeutic benefit of intravenous administration of bone marrow stromal cells after cerebral ischemia in rats. Stroke. 32 (4): 1005–11. doi:10.1161/01.STR.32.4.1005. PMID 11283404.

71. Assmus B, Schächinger V, Teupe C, et al. (December 2002). Transplantation of Progenitor Cells and Regeneration Enhancement in Acute Myocardial Infarction (TOPCARE-AMI). Circulation. 106 (24): 3009–17. doi:10.1161/01.CIR.0000043246.74879.CD. PMID 12473544.

72. Murphy JM, Fink DJ, Hunziker EB, Barry FP (December 2003). Stem cell therapy in a caprine model of osteoarthritis. Arthritis Rheum. 48 (12): 3464–74. doi:10.1002/art.11365. PMID 14673997.

73. Sampaolesi M, Blot S, D›Antona G, et al. (November 2006). Mesoangioblast stem cells ameliorate muscle function in dystrophic dogs. Nature. 444 (7119): 574–9. doi:10.1038/nature05282. PMID 17108972.

74. Taylor SE, Smith RK, Clegg PD (March 2007). Mesenchymal stem cell therapy in equine musculoskeletal disease: scientific fact or clinical fiction?. Equine Vet. J. 39 (2): 172–80. doi:10.2746/042516407X180868. PMID 17378447.

75. Tecirlioglu RT, Trounson AO (2007). Embryonic stem cells in companion animals (horses, dogs and cats): present status and future prospects. Reprod. Fertil. Dev. 19 (6): 740–7. doi:10.1071/RD07039. PMID 17714628.

76. Koch TG, Betts DH (November 2007). Stem cell therapy for joint problems using the horse as a clinically relevant animal model. Expert Opin Biol Ther. 7 (11): 1621–6. doi:10.1517/14712598.7.11.1621. PMID 17961087.

77. Richardson LE, Dudhia J, Clegg PD, Smith R (September 2007). Stem cells in veterinary medicine—attempts at regenerating equine tendon after injury. Trends Biotechnol. 25 (9): 409–16. doi:10.1016/j.tibtech.2007.07.009. PMID 17692415.

78. Csaki C, Matis U, Mobasheri A, Ye H, Shakibaei M (December 2007). Chondrogenesis, osteogenesis and adipogenesis of canine mesenchymal stem cells: a biochemical, morphological and ultrastructural study. Histochem. Cell Biol. 128 (6): 507–20. doi:10.1007/s00418-007-0337-z. PMID 17922135.

79. Kane, Ed (May 2008). Stem-cell therapy shows promise for soft-tissue injury, disease. DVM Newsmagazine. 6E-10E.

80. Yamada Y, Ueda M, Naiki T, Takahashi M, Hata K, Nagasaka T (2004). "Autogenous injectable bone for regeneration with mesenchymal stem cells and platelet-rich plasma: tissue-engineered bone regeneration". Tissue Eng. 10 (5–6): 955–64. doi:10.1089/1076327041348284. PMID 15265313.

81. Singec I, Jandial R, Crain A, Nikkhah G, Snyder EY (2007). The leading edge of stem cell therapeutics. Annu. Rev. Med. 58 (1): 313–28. doi:10.1146/annurev.med.58.070605.115252. PMID 17100553.

82. Zachos TA, Smith TJ (September 2008). Use of adult stem cells in clinical orthopedics. DVM Newsmagazine. 36–39.

83. Brehm W, Burk J, Delling U, Gittel C, Ribitsch I (2012). Stem cell-based tissue engineering in veterinary orthopaedics. Cell Tissue Res. 347 (3): 677–688.

doi:10.1007/s00441-011-1316-1. PMID 22287044.

84. Young RG, Butler DL, Weber W, Caplan AI, Gordon SL, Fink DJ (July 1998). Use of mesenchymal stem cells in a collagen matrix for Achilles tendon repair. J. Orthop. Res. 16 (4): 406–13. doi:10.1002/jor.1100160403. PMID 9747780.

85. Awad HA, Butler DL, Boivin GP, et al. (June 1999). Autologous mesenchymal stem cell-mediated repair of tendon. Tissue Eng. 5 (3): 267–77. doi:10.1089/ten.1999.5.267. PMID 10434073.

86. Bruder SP, Kraus KH, Goldberg VM, Kadiyala S (July 1998). The effect of implants loaded with autologous mesenchymal stem cells on the healing of canine segmental bone defects. J Bone Joint Surg Am. 80 (7): 985–96. PMID 9698003.

87. Kraus KH, Kirker-Head C (April 2006). Mesenchymal stem cells and bone regeneration. Vet Surg. 35 (3): 232–42. doi:10.1111/j.1532-950X.2006.00142.x. PMID 16635002.

88. Gattegno-Ho D, Argyle SA, Argyle DJ (2012). Stem cells and veterinary medicine: tools to understand diseases and enable tissue regeneration and drug discovery. Vet. J. 191 (1): 19–27. doi:10.1016/j.tvjl.2011.08.007. PMID 21958722.

89. Nathan S, Das De S, Thambyah A, Fen C, Goh J, Lee EH (August 2003). Cell-based therapy in the repair of osteochondral defects: a novel use for adipose tissue. Tissue Eng. 9 (4): 733–44. doi:10.1089/107632703768247412. PMID 13678450.

90. Fraser JK, Wulur I, Alfonso Z, Hedrick MH (April 2006). Fat tissue: an underappreciated source of stem cells for biotechnology. Trends Biotechnol. 24 (4): 150–4. doi:10.1016/j.tibtech.2006.01.010. PMID 16488036.

91. Nakagami H, Morishita R, Maeda K, Kikuchi Y, Ogihara T, Kaneda Y (April 2006). Adipose tissue-derived stromal cells as a novel option for regenerative cell therapy. J. Atheroscler. Thromb. 13 (2): 77–81. doi:10.5551/jat.13.77. PMID 16733294.

92. Park BW, Kang DH, Kang EJ, Byun JH, Lee JS, Maeng GH, Rho GJ (2012). "Peripheral nerve regeneration using autologous porcine skin-derived mesenchymal stem cells". J Tissue Eng Regen Med. 6 (2): 113–24. doi:10.1002/term.404. PMID 21337707.

93. Marfe G, Massaro-Giordano M, Ranalli M, Cozzoli E, Di Stefano C, Malafoglia V, Polettini M, Gambacurta A (2012). Blood derived stem cells: an ameliorative therapy in veterinary ophthalmology. J. Cell. Physiol. 227 (3): 1250–6. doi:10.1002/jcp.22953. PMID 21792938.

94. Azari O, Babaei H, Derakhshanfar A, Nematollahi-Mahani SN, Poursahebi R, Moshrefi M (2011). Effects of transplanted mesenchymal stem cells isolated from Wharton›s jelly of caprine umbilical cord on cutaneous wound healing; histopathological evaluation. Vet. Res. Commun. 35 (4): 211–22. doi:10.1007/s11259-011-9464-z. PMID 21340694.

95. Carstanjen B, Desbois C, Hekmati M, Behr L (2006). Successful engraftment of cultured autologous mesenchymal stem cells in a surgically repaired soft

palate defect in an adult horse. The Canadian Journal of Veterinary Research. 70 (2): 143–147. PMC 1410720. PMID 16639947.

96. Black LL, Gaynor J, Adams C, et al. (2008). Effect of intraarticular injection of autologous adipose-derived mesenchymal stem and regenerative cells on clinical signs of chronic osteoarthritis of the elbow joint in dogs. Vet. Ther. 9 (3): 192–200. PMID 19003780.

97. Nixon AJ, Dahlgren LA, Haupt JL, Yeager AE, Ward DL (July 2008). Effect of adipose-derived nucleated cell fractions on tendon repair in horses with collagenase-induced tendinitis. Am. J. Vet. Res. 69 (7): 928–37. doi:10.2460/ajvr.69.7.928. PMID 18593247.

98. Guercio A, Di Marco P, Casella S, Cannella V, Russotto L, Purpari G, Di Bella S, Piccione G (2012). Production of canine mesenchymal stem cells from adipose tissue and their application in dogs with chronic osteoarthritis of the humeroradial joints. Cell Biol. Int. 36 (2): 189–94. doi:10.1042/CBI20110304. PMID 21936851.

99. Ribitsch I, Burk J, Delling U, Geißler C, Gittel C, Jülke H, Brehm W (2010). Basic Science and Clinical Application of Stem Cells in Veterinary Medicine: 219–263. doi:10.1007/10_2010_66.

100. Kim U, Shin DG, Park JS, Kim YJ, Park SI, Moon YM, Jeong KS (2011). Homing of adipose-derived stem cells to radiofrequency catheter ablated canine atrium and differentiation into cardiomyocyte-like cells. Int. J. Cardiol. 146 (3): 371–8. doi:10.1016/j.ijcard.2009.07.016. PMID 19683815.

101. Chang Y, Lai PH, Wei HJ, Lin WW, Chen CH, Hwang SM, Chen SC, Sung HW (2007). Tissue regeneration observed in a basic fibroblast growth factor–loaded porous acellular bovine pericardium populated with mesenchymal stem cells. The Journal of Thoracic and Cardiovascular Surgery. 134 (1): 65–73.e4. doi:10.1016/j.jtcvs.2007.02.019. ISSN 0022-5223.

102. Sung Su Park; et al. (2012). Functional recovery after spinal cord injury in dogs treated with a combination of Matrigel and neural-induced adipose-derived mesenchymal Stem cells. Cytotherapy. 14 (5): 584–597. doi:10.3109/14653249.2012.658913. PMID 22348702.

103. Ryu HH, Lim JH, Byeon YE, Park JR, Seo MS, Lee YW, Kim WH, Kang KS, Kweon OK (2009). Functional recovery and neural differentiation after transplantation of allogenic adipose-derived stem cells in a canine model of acute spinal cord injury. J. Vet. Sci. 10 (4): 273–84. doi:10.4142/jvs.2009.10.4.273. PMC 2807262. PMID 19934591.

104. Nishida H, Nakayama M, Tanaka H, Kitamura M, Hatoya S, Sugiura K, Harada Y, Suzuki Y, Ide C, Inaba T (2012). Safety of Autologous Bone Marrow Stromal Cell Transplantation in Dogs with Acute Spinal Cord Injury. Veterinary Surgery. 41 (4): 437–442. doi:10.1111/j.1532-950X.2011.00959.x. ISSN 0161-3499.

105. Xu, J., Wang, D., Liu, D., Fan, Z., Zhang, H., Liu, O., et al. (2012). Allogeneic mesenchymal stem cell treatment alleviates experimental and clinical Sjogren syndrome. Blood, 120(15), 3142–3151.

106. Beyazyıldız, E., Pınarlı, F. A., Beyazyıldız, Ö., Hekimoğlu, E. R., Acar, U., Demir, M. N., et al. (2014). Efficacy of Topical Mesenchymal Stem Cell Therapy in the Treatment of Experimental Dry Eye Syndrome Model. Stem Cells International, 2014(3), 250230–9

107. Villatoro, A. J., Fernández, V., Claros, S., Rico-Llanos, G. A., Becerra, J., & Andrades, J. A. (2015). Use of adipose-derived mesenchymal stem cells in keratoconjunctivitis sicca in a canine model. BioMed Research International, 2015(3), 527926–10. http://doi.org/10.1155/2015/527926

108. I. Dobrinski; A.J. Travis (2007). Germ cell transplantation for the propagation of companion animals, non-domestic and endangered species. Reproduction, Fertility, and Development. 19: 732–739. doi:10.1071/RD07036.

109. Health, Wellness, Nutrition and Anti-Aging Integrative Medicine Experts & Information – Superior Raw Super Food Supplements – Online Wellness Community

110. Mlsna, Lucas J. (2010). Stem Cell Based Treatments and Novel Considerations for Conscience Clause Legislation. Indiana Health Law Review. United States: Indiana University Robert H. McKinney School of Law. 8 (2): 471–496. ISSN:1549–3199. LCCN:2004212209. OCLC:OCLC 54703225.

111. Dobkin BH, Curt A, Guest J (2006). Cellular transplants in China: observational study from the largest human experiment in chronic spinal cord injury. Neurorehabil Neural Repair. 20 (1): 5–13. doi:10.1177/1545968305284675. PMC 4169140. PMID 16467274.

112. http://www.regentime.com

113. Stem cells tailored to patients. BBC News. 20 May 2005. Retrieved 24 May 2010.

114. Chotinantakul K, Leeanansaksiri W (June 2012). Hematopoietic stem cell development, niches, and signaling pathways. Bone Marrow Research. 2012: 12–16. doi:10.1155/2012/270425. PMC 3413998. PMID 22900188.

CHAPTER 4

Cell Potency

Chapter Contents

INTRODUCTION

Cell potency is a cell's ability to differentiate into other cell types. The more cell types a cell can differentiate into, the greater its potency. Potency is also described as the gene activation potential within a cell which like a continuum begins with totipotency to designate a cell with the most differentiation potential, pluripotency, multipotency, oligopotency and finally unipotency. Potency is taken from the Latin term potens which means having power.

TOTIPOTENCY

Totipotency is the ability of a single cell to divide and produce all of the differentiated cells in an organism. Spores and zygotes are examples of totipotent cells. In the spectrum of cell potency, totipotency represents the cell with the greatest differentiation potential. *Toti* comes from the Latin *totus* which means "entirely".

It is possible for a fully differentiated cell to return to a state of totipotency. This conversion to totipotency is complex, not fully understood and the subject of recent research. Research in 2011 has shown that cells may differentiate not into a fully totipotent cell, but instead into a complex cellular variation of totipotency. Stem cells resembling totipotent blastomeres from 2-cell stage embryos can arise spontaneously in the embryonic stem cell cultures and also can be induced to arise more frequently in vitro through down-regulation of the chromatin assembly activity of CAF-1.

The human development model is one which can be used to describe how totipotent cells arise. Human development begins when a sperm fertilizes an egg and the resulting fertilized egg creates a single totipotent cell, a zygote. In the first hours after fertilization, this zygote divides into identical totipotent cells, which can later develop into any of the three germ layers of a human (endoderm, mesoderm, or ectoderm), into cells of the cytotrophoblast layer or syncytiotrophoblast layer of the placenta. After reaching a 16-cell stage, the totipotent cells of the morula differentiate into cells that will eventually become either the blastocyst's Inner cell mass or the outer trophoblasts. Approximately four days after fertilization and after several cycles of cell division, these totipotent cells begin to specialize. The inner cell mass, the source of embryonic stem cells, becomes pluripotent.

Research on *Caenorhabditis elegans* suggests that multiple mechanisms including RNA regulation may play a role in maintaining totipotency at different stages of development in some species. Work with zebrafish and mammals suggest a further interplay between miRNA and RNA binding proteins (RBPs) in determining development differences.

In September 2013, a team from the Spanish national Cancer Research Centre was able for the first time to make adult cells from mice retreat to the characteristics of embryonic stem cells, thereby achieving totipotency.

PLURIPOTENCY

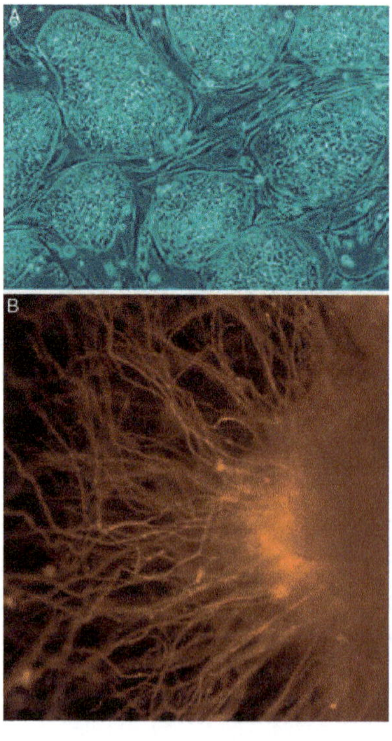

A: Human embryonic stem cells (cell colonies that are not yet differentiated).B: Nerve cells.

In cell biology, pluripotency (from the Latin plurimus, meaning *very many*, and potens, meaning *having power*) refers to a stem cell that has the potential to differentiate into any of the three germ layers: endoderm (interior stomach lining, gastrointestinal tract, the lungs), mesoderm (muscle, bone, blood, urogenital), or ectoderm (epidermal tissues and nervous system). However, cell pluripotency is a continuum, ranging from the completely pluripotent cell that can form every cell of the embryo proper, e.g., embryonic stem cells and iPSCs (see below), to the incompletely or partially pluripotent cell that can form cells of all three germ layers but that may not exhibit all the characteristics of completely pluripotent cells.

Induced Pluripotency

Induced pluripotent stem cells, commonly abbreviated as iPS cells or iPSCs are a type of pluripotent stem cell artificially derived from a non-pluripotent cell, typically an adult somatic cell, by inducing a forced expression of certain genes and transcription factors. These transcription factors play a key role in determining the state of these cells and also highlights the fact that these somatic cells do preserve the same genetic information as early embryonic cells. The ability to induce cells into a pluripotent state was initially pioneered in 2006 using mouse fibroblasts and four transcription factors, Oct4, Sox2, Klf4 and c-Myc; this technique, called reprogramming, earned Shinya Yamanaka and John Gurdon the Nobel Prize in Physiology or Medicine 2012. This was then followed in 2007 by the successful induction of human iPSCs derived from human dermal fibroblasts using methods similar to those used for the induction of mouse cells. These induced cells exhibit similar traits to those of embryonic stem cells (ESCs) but do not require the use of embryos. Some of the similarities between ESCs and iPSCs include pluripotency, morphology, self-renewal ability, a trait that implies that they can divide and replicate indefinitely, and gene expression.

Epigenetic factors are also thought to be involved in the actual reprogramming of somatic cells in order to induce pluripotency. It has been theorized that certain epigenetic factors might actually work to clear the original somatic epigenetic marks in order to acquire the new epigenetic marks that are part of achieving a pluripotent state. Chromatin is also reorganized in iPSCs and becomes like that found in ESCs in that it is less condensed and therefore more accessible. Euchromatin modifications are also common which is also consistent with the state of euchromatin found in ESCs.

Due to their great similarity to ESCs, iPSCs have been of great interest to the medical and research community. iPSCs could potentially have the same therapeutic implications and applications as ESCs but without the controversial use of embryos in the process, a topic of great bioethical debate. In fact, the induced pluripotency of somatic cells into undifferentiated iPS cells was originally hailed as the end of the controversial use of embryonic stem cells. However, iPSCs were found to be potentially tumorigenic, and, despite advances, were never approved for clinical stage research in the United States. Setbacks such as low replication rates and early senescence have also been encountered when making iPSCs, hindering their use as ESCs replacements.

Additionally, it has been determined that the somatic expression of combined transcription factors can directly induce other defined somatic cell fates (transdifferentiation); researchers identified three neural-lineage-specific transcription factors that could directly convert mouse fibroblasts (skin cells) into fully functional neurons. This result challenges the terminal nature of cellular differentiation and the integrity of lineage commitment; and implies that with the proper tools, *all* cells are totipotent and may form all kinds of tissue.

Some of the possible medical and therapeutic uses for iPSCs derived from patients include their use in cell and tissue transplants without the risk of rejection that is commonly encountered. iPSCs can potentially replace animal models unsuitable as well as in-vitro models used for disease research.

MULTIPOTENCY

Multipotency describes progenitor cells which have the gene activation potential to differentiate into discrete cell types. For example, a multipotent blood stem cell is a hematopoietic cell — and this cell type can differentiate itself into several types of blood cell types like lymphocytes, monocytes, neutrophils, etc., but cannot differentiate into brain cells, bone cells or other non-blood cell types.

New research related to multipotent cells suggests that multipotent cells may be capable of conversion into unrelated cell types. In another case, human umbilical cord blood stem cells were converted into human neurons. Research is also focusing on converting multipotent cells into pluripotent cells.

Multipotent cells are found in many, but not all human cell types. Multipotent cells have been found in cord blood, adipose tissue, cardiac cells, bone marrow, and mesenchymal stem cells (MSCs) which are found in the third molar.

MSCs may prove to be a valuable source for stem cells from molars at 8–10 years of age, before adult dental calcification. MSCs can differentiate into osteoblasts, chondrocytes, and adipocytes.

OLIGOPOTENCY

In biology, oligopotency is the ability of progenitor cells to differentiate into a few cell types. It is a degree of potency. Examples of oligopotent stem cells are the lymphoid or myeloid stem cells. A lymphoid cell specifically, can give rise to various blood cells such as B and T cells, however, not to a different blood cell type like a red blood cell. Examples of progenitor cells are vascular stem cells that have the capacity to become both endothelial or smooth muscle cells.

UNIPOTENCY

Further information: Precursor cell

In cell biology, a unipotent cell is the concept that one stem cell has the capacity to differentiate into only one cell type. It is currently unclear if true unipotent stem cells exist. Hepatoblasts, which differentiate into hepatocytes (which constitute most of the liver) or cholangiocytes (epithelial cells of the bile duct), are bipotent. A close synonym for *unipotent cell* is *precursor cell.*

CELLULAR DIFFERENTIATION

In developmental biology, **cellular differentiation** is the process where a cell changes from one cell type to another. Most commonly the cell changes to a more specialized type. Differentiation occurs numerous times during the development of a multicellular organism as it changes from a simple zygote to a complex system of tissues and cell types. Differentiation continues in adulthood as adult stem cells divide and create fully differentiated daughter cells during tissue repair and during normal cell turnover. Some differentiation occurs in response to antigen exposure. Differentiation dramatically changes a cell's size, shape, membrane potential, metabolic activity, and responsiveness to signals. These changes are largely due to highly controlled modifications in gene expression and are the study of epigenetics. With a few exceptions, cellular differentiation almost never involves a change in the DNA sequence itself. Thus, different cells can have very different physical characteristics despite having the same genome.

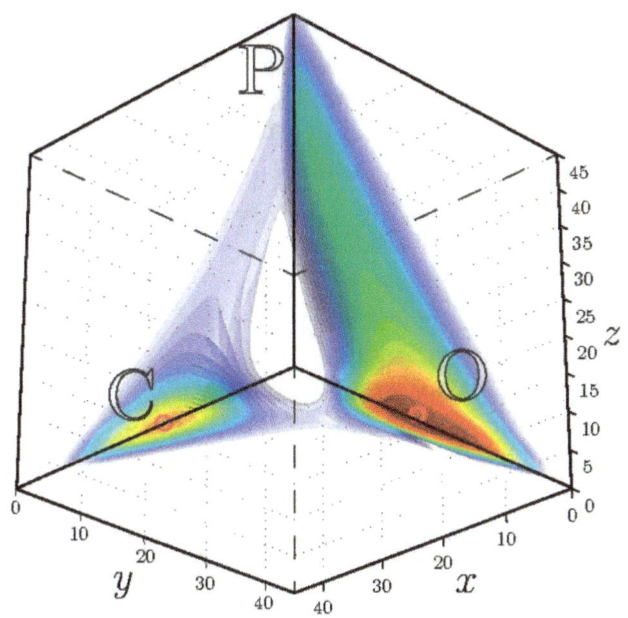

Cell-count distribution featuring cellular differentiation for three types of cells z, osteoblast y, and chondrocyte x exposed to pro-osteoblast stimulus.

There are multiple levels of cell potency, the cell's ability to differentiate into other cell types. A greater potency indicates a larger number of cells that can be derived. A cell that can differentiate into all cell types, including the placental tissue, is known as *totipotent*. In mammals, only the zygote and subsequent blastomeres are totipotent, while in plants many differentiated cells can become totipotent with simple laboratory techniques. A cell that can differentiate into all cell types of the adult organism is known as *pluripotent*. Such cells are called meristematic cells in higher plants and embryonic stem cells in animals, though some groups report the presence of adult pluripotent cells. Virally induced expression of four transcription factors Oct4, Sox2, c-Myc, and Kfl4 (Yamanaka factors) is sufficient to create pluripotent (iPS) cells from adult fibroblasts. A multipotent cell is one that can differentiate into multiple different, but closely related cell types. Oligopotent cells are more restricted than multipotent, but can still differentiate into a few closely related cell types. Finally, unipotent cells can differentiate into only one cell type, but are capable of self-renewal. In cytopathology, the level of cellular differentiation is used as a measure of cancer progression. "Grade is a marker of how differentiated a cell in a tumor is.

Mammalian Cell Types

Three basic categories of cells make up the mammalian body: germ cells, somatic cells, and stem cells. Each of the approximately 100 trillion (10^{14}) cells in an adult human has its own copy or copies of the genome except certain cell types, such as red blood cells, that lack nuclei in their fully differentiated state. Most cells are diploid; they have two copies of each chromosome. Such cells, called somatic cells, make up most of the human body, such as skin and muscle cells. Cells differentiate to specialize for different functions.

Germ line cells are any line of cells that give rise to gametes—eggs and sperm—and thus are continuous through the generations. Stem cells, on the other hand, have the ability to divide for indefinite periods and to give rise to specialized cells. They are best described in the context of normal human development.

Development begins when a sperm fertilizes an egg and creates a single cell that has the potential to form an entire organism. In the first hours after fertilization, this cell divides into identical cells. In humans, approximately four days after fertilization and after several cycles of cell division, these cells begin to specialize, forming a hollow sphere of cells, called a blastocyst. The blastocyst has an outer layer of cells, and inside this hollow sphere, there is a cluster of cells called the inner cell mass. The cells of the inner cell mass go on to form virtually all of the tissues of the human body. Although the cells of the inner cell mass can form virtually every type of cell found in the human body, they cannot form an organism. These cells are referred to as pluripotent.

Pluripotent stem cells undergo further specialization into multipotent progenitor cells that then give rise to functional cells. Examples of stem and progenitor cells include:

- *Radial glial cells* (embryonic neural stem cells) that give rise to excitatory neurons in the fetal brain through the process of neurogenesis.
- *Hematopoietic stem cells* (adult stem cells) from the bone marrow that give rise to red blood cells, white blood cells, and platelets
- *Mesenchymal stem cells* (adult stem cells) from the bone marrow that give rise to stromal cells, fat cells, and types of bone cells
- *Epithelial stem cells* (progenitor cells) that give rise to the various types of skin cells

- *Muscle satellite cells* (progenitor cells) that contribute to differentiated muscle tissue.

A pathway that is guided by the cell adhesion molecules consisting of four amino acids, arginine, glycine, asparagine, and serine, is created as the cellular blastomere differentiates from the single-layered blastula to the three primary layers of germ cells in mammals, namely the ectoderm, mesoderm and endoderm (listed from most distal (exterior) to proximal (interior)). The ectoderm ends up forming the skin and the nervous system, the mesoderm forms the bones and muscular tissue, and the endoderm forms the internal organ tissues.

Dedifferentiation

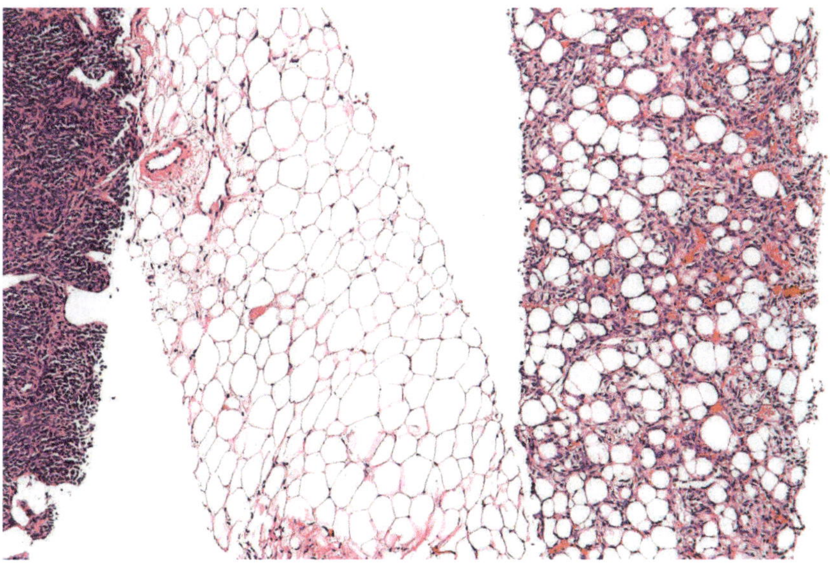

Micrograph of a liposarcoma with some dedifferentiation, that is not identifiable as a liposarcoma, (left edge of image) and a differentiated component (with lipoblasts and increased vascularity (right of image)). Fully differentiated (morphologically benign) adipose tissue (center of the image) has few blood vessels. H&E stain.

Dedifferentiation, or integration is a cellular process often seen in more basal life forms such as worms and amphibians in which a partially or terminally differentiated cell reverts to an earlier developmental stage, usually as part of a regenerative process. Dedifferentiation also occurs in plants. Cells in cell culture can lose properties they originally had, such as protein expression, or change shape. This process is also termed dedifferentiation.

Some believe dedifferentiation is an aberration of the normal development cycle that results in cancer,whereas others believe it to be a natural part of the immune response lost by humans at some point as a result of evolution.

A small molecule dubbed reversine, a purine analog, has been discovered that has proven to induce dedifferentiation in myotubes. These dedifferentiated cells could then redifferentiate into osteoblasts and adipocytes.

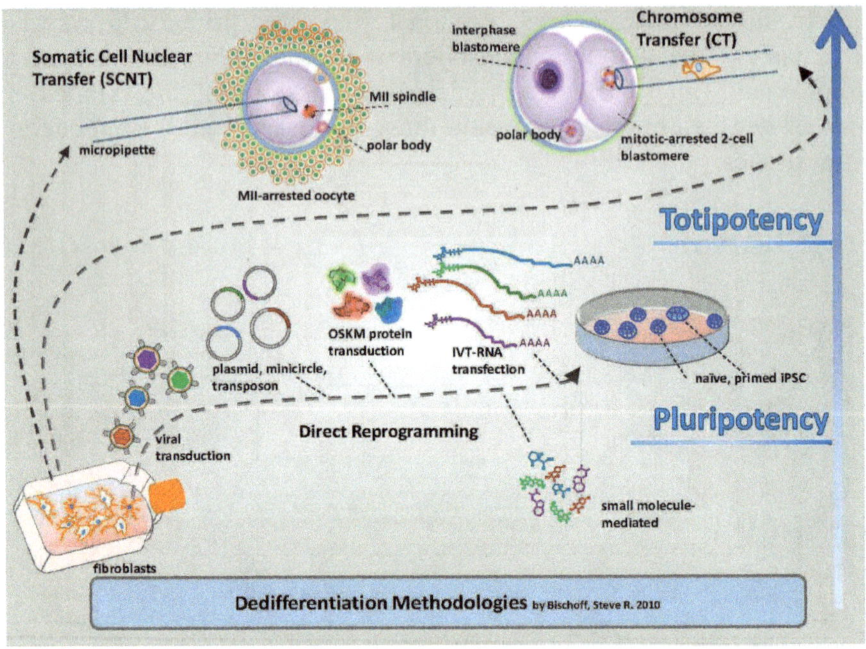

Diagram exposing several methods used to revert adult somatic cells to totipotency or pluripotency.

Mechanisms

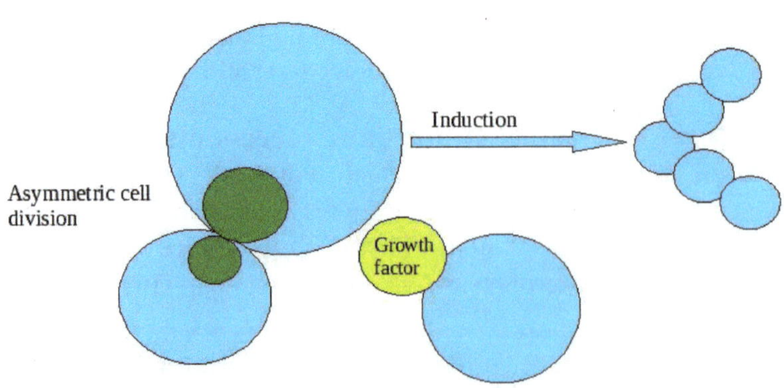

Mechanisms of Cellular Differentiation.

Each specialized cell type in an organism expresses a subset of all the genes that constitute the genome of that species. Each cell type is defined by its particular pattern of regulated gene expression. Cell differentiation is thus a transition of a cell from one cell type to another and it involves a switch from one pattern of gene expression to another. Cellular differentiation during development can be understood as the result of a gene regulatory network. A regulatory gene and its cis-regulatory modules are nodes in a gene regulatory network; they receive input and create output elsewhere in the network. The systems biology approach to developmental biology emphasizes the importance of investigating how developmental mechanisms interact to produce predictable patterns (morphogenesis). (However, an alternative view has been proposed recently. Based on stochastic gene expression, cellular differentiation is the result of a Darwinian selective process occurring among cells. In this frame, protein and gene networks are the result of cellular processes and not their cause. See: Cellular Darwinism)

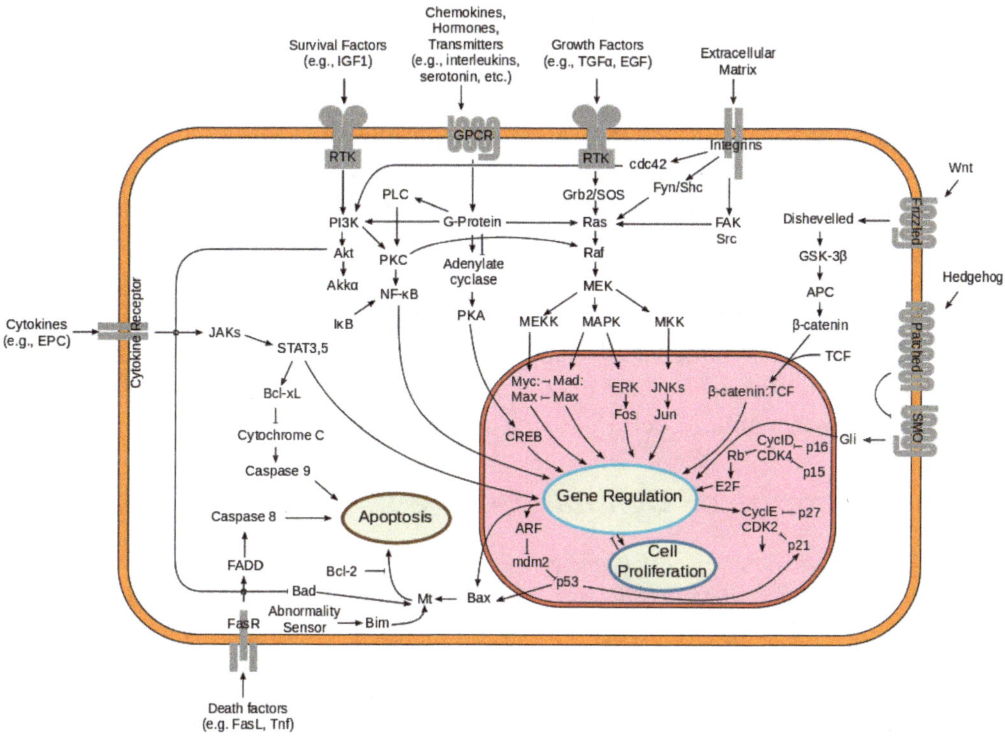

An overview of major signal transduction pathways.

A few evolutionarily conserved types of molecular processes are often involved in the cellular mechanisms that control these switches. The major types of molecular processes that control cellular differentiation involve cell signaling. Many of the signal molecules that convey information from cell to cell during the control of cellular differentiation are called growth factors. Although the details of specific signal transduction pathways vary, these pathways often share the following general steps. A ligand produced by one cell binds to a receptor in the extracellular region of another cell, inducing a conformational change in the receptor. The shape of the cytoplasmic domain of the receptor changes, and the receptor acquires enzymatic activity. The receptor then catalyzes reactions that phosphorylate other proteins, activating them. A cascade of phosphorylation reactions eventually activates a dormant transcription factor or cytoskeletal protein, thus contributing to the differentiation process in the target cell. Cells and tissues can vary in competence, their ability to respond to external signals.

Signal induction refers to cascades of signaling events, during which a cell or tissue signals to another cell or tissue to influence its developmental fate. Yamamoto and Jeffery investigated the role of the lens in eye formation in cave- and surface-dwelling fish, a striking example of induction. Through reciprocal transplants, Yamamoto and Jeffery found that the lens vesicle of surface fish can induce other parts of the eye to develop in cave- and surface-dwelling fish, while the lens vesicle of the cave-dwelling fish cannot.

Other important mechanisms fall under the category of asymmetric cell divisions, divisions that give rise to daughter cells with distinct developmental fates. Asymmetric cell divisions can occur because of asymmetrically expressed maternal cytoplasmic determinants or because of signaling. In the former mechanism, distinct daughter cells are created during cytokinesis because of an uneven distribution of regulatory molecules in the parent cell; the distinct cytoplasm that each daughter cell inherits results in a distinct pattern of differentiation for each daughter cell. A well-studied example of pattern formation by asymmetric divisions is body axis patterning in Drosophila. RNA molecules are an important type of intracellular differentiation control signal. The molecular and genetic basis of asymmetric cell divisions has also been studied in green algae of the genus *Volvox*, a model system for studying how unicellular organisms can evolve into multicellular organisms. In *Volvox carteri*, the 16 cells in the anterior hemisphere of a 32-cell embryo divide asymmetrically, each producing one large and one small daughter cell. The size of the cell at the end of all cell divisions determines whether it becomes a specialized germ or somatic cell.

Epigenetic control of Cellular Differentiation

Since each cell, regardless of cell type, possesses the same genome, determination of cell type must occur at the level of gene expression. While the regulation of gene expression can occur through cis- and trans-regulatory elements including a gene's promoter and enhancers, the problem arises as to how this expression pattern is maintained over numerous generations of cell division. As it turns out, epigenetic processes play a crucial role in regulating the decision to adopt a stem, progenitor, or mature cell fate. This section will focus primarily on mammalian stem cells.

In systems biology and mathematical modeling of gene regulatory networks, cell-fate determination is predicted to exhibit certain dynamics, such as attractor-convergence (the attractor can be an equilibrium point, limit cycle or strange attractor) or oscillatory.

Importance of Epigenetic Control

The first question that can be asked is the extent and complexity of the role of epigenetic processes in the determination of cell fate. A clear answer to this question can be seen in the 2011 paper by Lister R, *et al.* on aberrant epigenomic programming in human induced pluripotent stem cells. As induced pluripotent stem cells (iPSCs) are thought to mimic embryonic stem cells in their pluripotent properties, few epigenetic differences should exist between them. To test this prediction, the authors conducted whole-genome profiling of DNA methylation patterns in several human embryonic stem cell (ESC), iPSC, and progenitor cell lines.

Female adipose cells, lung fibroblasts, and foreskin fibroblasts were reprogrammed into induced pluripotent state with the OCT4, SOX2, KLF4, and MYC genes. Patterns of DNA methylation in ESCs, iPSCs, somatic cells were compared. Lister R, *et al.* observed significant resemblance in methylation levels between embryonic and induced pluripotent cells. Around 80% of CG dinucleotides in ESCs and iPSCs were methylated, the same was true of only 60% of CG dinucleotides in somatic cells. In addition, somatic cells possessed minimal levels of cytosine methylation in non-CG dinucleotides, while induced pluripotent cells possessed similar levels of methylation as embryonic stem cells, between 0.5 and 1.5%. Thus, consistent with their respective transcriptional activities, DNA methylation patterns, at least on the genomic level, are similar between ESCs and iPSCs.

However, upon examining methylation patterns more closely, the authors discovered 1175 regions of differential CG dinucleotide methylation between at least one ES or iPS cell line. By comparing these regions of differential methylation with regions of cytosine methylation in the original somatic cells, 44-49% of differentially methylated regions reflected methylation patterns of the respective progenitor somatic cells, while 51-56% of these regions were dissimilar to both the progenitor and embryonic cell lines. In vitro-induced differentiation of iPSC lines saw transmission of 88% and 46% of hyper and hypo-methylated differentially methylated regions, respectively.

Two conclusions are readily apparent from this study. First, epigenetic processes are heavily involved in cell fate determination, as seen from the similar levels of cytosine methylation between induced pluripotent and embryonic stem cells, consistent with their respective patterns of transcription. Second, the mechanisms of de-differentiation (and by extension, differentiation) are very complex and cannot be easily duplicated, as seen by the significant number of differentially methylated regions between ES and iPS cell lines. Now that these two points have been established, we can examine some of the epigenetic mechanisms that are thought to regulate cellular differentiation.

Mechanisms of Epigenetic Regulation

Pioneering factors **(Oct4, Sox2, Nanog)**

Three transcription factors, OCT4, SOX2, and NANOG – the first two of which are used in induced pluripotent stem cell (iPSC) reprogramming, along with Klf4 and c-Myc – are highly expressed in undifferentiated embryonic stem cells and are necessary for the maintenance of their pluripotency. It is thought that they achieve this through alterations in chromatin structure, such as histone modification and DNA methylation, to restrict or permit the transcription of target genes. While highly expressed, their levels require a precise balance to maintain pluripotency, perturbation of which will promote differentiation towards different lineages based on how the gene expression levels change. Differential regulation of Oct-4 and SOX2 levels have been shown to precede germ layer fate selection. Increased levels of Oct4 and decreased levels of Sox2 promote a mesendodermal fate, with Oct4 actively suppressing genes associated with a neural ectodermal fate. Similarly, Increased levels of Sox2 and decreased levels of Oct4 promote differentiation towards a neural ectodermal fate, with Sox2 inhibiting differentiation towards a mesendodermal fate. Regardless of the lineage cells differentiate down, suppression of NANOG has been identified as a necessary prerequisite for differentiation.

Polycomb Repressive Complex (PRC2)

In the realm of gene silencing, Polycomb repressive complex 2, one of two classes of the Polycomb group (PcG) family of proteins, catalyzes the di- and tri-methylation of histone H3 lysine 27 (H3K27me2/me3). By binding to the H3K27me2/3-tagged nucleosome, PRC1 (also a complex of PcG family proteins) catalyzes the mono-ubiquitinylation of histone H2A at lysine 119 (H2AK119Ub1), blocking RNA polymerase II activity and resulting in transcriptional suppression. PcG knockout ES cells do not differentiate efficiently into the three germ layers, and deletion of the PRC1 and PRC2 genes leads to increased expression of lineage-affiliated genes and unscheduled differentiation. Presumably, PcG complexes are responsible for transcriptionally repressing differentiation and development-promoting genes.

Trithorax Group Proteins (TrxG)

Alternately, upon receiving differentiation signals, PcG proteins are recruited to promoters of pluripotency transcription factors. PcG-deficient ES cells can begin differentiation but cannot maintain the differentiated phenotype. Simultaneously, differentiation and development-promoting genes are activated by Trithorax group (TrxG) chromatin regulators and lose their repression. TrxG proteins are recruited at regions of high transcriptional activity, where they catalyze the trimethylation of histone H3 lysine 4 (H3K4me3) and promote gene activation through histone acetylation. PcG and TrxG complexes engage in direct competition and are thought to be functionally antagonistic, creating at differentiation and development-promoting loci what is termed a “bivalent domain” and rendering these genes sensitive to rapid induction or repression.

DNA Methylation

Regulation of gene expression is further achieved through DNA methylation, in which the DNA methyltransferase-mediated methylation of cytosine residues in CpG dinucleotides maintains heritable repression by controlling DNA accessibility. The majority of CpG sites in embryonic stem cells are unmethylated and appear to be associated with H3K4me3-carrying nucleosomes. Upon differentiation, a small number of genes, including OCT4 and NANOG, are methylated and their promoters repressed to prevent their further expression. Consistently, DNA methylation-deficient embryonic stem cells rapidly enter apoptosis upon in vitro differentiation.

Nucleosome Positioning

While the DNA sequence of most cells of an organism is the same, the binding patterns of transcription factors and the corresponding gene expression patterns are different. To a large extent, differences in transcription factor binding are determined by the chromatin accessibility of their binding sites through histone modification and/or pioneer factors. In particular, it is important to know whether a nucleosome is covering a given genomic binding site or not. This can be determined using a chromatin immunoprecipitation (ChIP) assay. ChIP Overview.

Histone Acetylation and Methylation

DNA-nucleosome interactions are characterized by two states: either tightly bound by nucleosomes and transcriptionally inactive, called heterochromatin, or loosely bound and usually, but not always, transcriptionally active, called euchromatin. The epigenetic processes of histone methylation and acetylation, and their inverses demethylation and deacetylation primarily account for these changes. The effects of acetylation and deacetylation are more predictable. An acetyl group is either added to or removed from the positively charged Lysine residues in histones by enzymes called histone acetyltransferases or histone deacteylases, respectively. The acetyl group prevents Lysine's association with the negatively charged DNA backbone. Methylation is not as straightforward, as neither methylation nor demethylation consistently correlate with either gene activation or repression. However, certain methylations have been repeatedly shown to either activate or repress genes. The trimethylation of lysine 4 on histone 3 (H3K4Me3) is associated with gene activation, whereas trimethylation of lysine 27 on histone 3 represses genes

In Stem Cells

During differentiation, stem cells change their gene expression profiles. Recent studies have implicated a role for nucleosome positioning and histone modifications during this process. There are two components of this process: turning off the expression of embryonic stem cell (ESC) genes, and the activation of cell fate genes. Lysine specific demethylase 1 (KDM1A) is thought to prevent the use of enhancer (genetics) regions of pluripotency genes, thereby inhibiting their transcription. It interacts with Mi-2/NuRD complex (nucleosome remodelling and histone deacetylase) complex, giving an instance where methylation and acetylation are not discrete and mutually exclusive, but intertwined processes.

Role of Signaling in Epigenetic Control

A final question to ask concerns the role of cell signaling in influencing the epigenetic processes governing differentiation. Such a role should exist, as it would be reasonable to think that extrinsic signaling can lead to epigenetic remodeling, just as it can lead to changes in gene expression through the activation or repression of different transcription factors. Interestingly, little direct data is available concerning the specific signals that influence the epigenome, and the majority of current knowledge consist of speculations on plausible candidate regulators of epigenetic remodeling. We will first discuss several major candidates thought to be involved in the induction and maintenance of both embryonic stem cells and their differentiated progeny, and then turn to one example of specific signaling pathways in which more direct evidence exists for its role in epigenetic change.

The first major candidate is Wnt signaling pathway. The Wnt pathway is involved in all stages of differentiation, and the ligand Wnt3a can substitute for the overexpression of c-Myc in the generation of induced pluripotent stem cells. On the other hand, disruption of ß-catenin, a component of the Wnt signaling pathway, leads to decreased proliferation of neural progenitors.

Growth factors comprise the second major set of candidates of epigenetic regulators of cellular differentiation. These morphogens are crucial for development, and include bone morphogenetic proteins, transforming growth factors (TGFs), and fibroblast growth factors (FGFs). TGFs and FGFs have been shown to sustain expression of OCT4, SOX2, and NANOG by downstream signaling to Smad proteins. Depletion of growth factors promotes the differentiation of ESCs, while genes with bivalent chromatin can become either more restrictive or permissive in their transcription.

Several other signaling pathways are also considered to be primary candidates. Cytokine leukemia inhibitory factors are associated with the maintenance of mouse ESCs in an undifferentiated state. This is achieved through its activation of the Jak-STAT3 pathway, which has been shown to be necessary and sufficient towards maintaining mouse ESC pluripotency. Retinoic acid can induce differentiation of human and mouse ESCs, and Notch signaling is involved in the proliferation and self-renewal of stem cells. Finally, Sonic hedgehog, in addition to its role as a morphogen, promotes embryonic stem cell differentiation and the self-renewal of somatic stem cells.

The problem, of course, is that the candidacy of these signaling pathways was inferred primarily on the basis of their role in development and cellular differentiation. While epigenetic regulation is necessary for driving cellular differentiation, they are certainly not sufficient for this process. Direct modulation of gene expression through modification of transcription factors plays a key role that must be distinguished from heritable epigenetic changes that can persist even in the absence of the original environmental signals. Only a few examples of signaling pathways leading to epigenetic changes that alter cell fate currently exist, and we will focus on one of them.

Expression of Shh (Sonic hedgehog) upregulates the production of BMI1, a component of the PcG complex that recognizes H3K27me3. This occurs in a Gli-dependent manner, as Gli1 and Gli2 are downstream effectors of the Hedgehog signaling pathway. In culture, Bmi1 mediates the Hedgehog pathway's ability to promote human mammary stem cell self-renewal. In both humans and mice, researchers showed Bmi1 to be highly expressed in proliferating immature cerebellar granule cell precursors. When Bmi1 was knocked out in mice, impaired cerebellar development resulted, leading to significant reductions in postnatal brain mass along with abnormalities in motor control and behavior. A separate study showed a significant decrease in neural stem cell proliferation along with increased astrocyte proliferation in Bmi null mice.

In summary, the role of signaling in the epigenetic control of cell fate in mammals is largely unknown, but distinct examples exist that indicate the likely existence of further such mechanisms.

Effect of Matrix Elasticity on Differentiation

In order to fulfill the purpose of regenerating a variety of tissues, adult stems are known to migrate from their niches, adhere to new extracellular matrices (ECM) and differentiate. The ductility of these microenvironments are unique to different tissue types. The ECM surrounding brain, muscle and bone tissues range from soft to stiff. The transduction of the stem cells into these cells types is not directed solely by chemokine cues and cell to cell signaling. The elasticity of the microenvironment can also affect the differentiation of mesenchymal stem cells (MSCs which originate in bone marrow.) When MSCs are placed on substrates of the same stiffness as brain, muscle and bone ECM, the MSCs take on properties of those respective cell types. Matrix sensing requires the cell to pull against the matrix at focal adhesions, which triggers a cellular mechano-transducer to generate a signal to be informed what force is needed to deform the matrix. To determine the key players in matrix-elasticity-driven lineage specification in MSCs, different matrix microenvironments were mimicked. From these experiments, it was concluded that focal adhesions of the MSCs were the cellular mechano-transducer sensing the differences of the matrix elasticity. The non-muscle myosin IIa-c isoforms generates the forces in the cell that lead to signaling of early commitment markers. Nonmuslce myosin IIa generates the least force increasing to non-muscle myosin IIc. There are also factors in the cell that inhibit non-muscle myosin II, such as blebbistatin. This makes the cell effectively blind to the surrounding matrix. Researchers have obtained some success in inducing stem cell-like properties in HEK 239 cells by providing a soft matrix without the use of diffusing factors. The stem-cell properties appear to be linked to tension in the cells' actin network. One identified mechanism for matrix-induced differentiation is tension-induced proteins, which remodel chromatin in response to mechanical stretch. The RhoA pathway is also implicated in this process.

PROGENITOR CELL

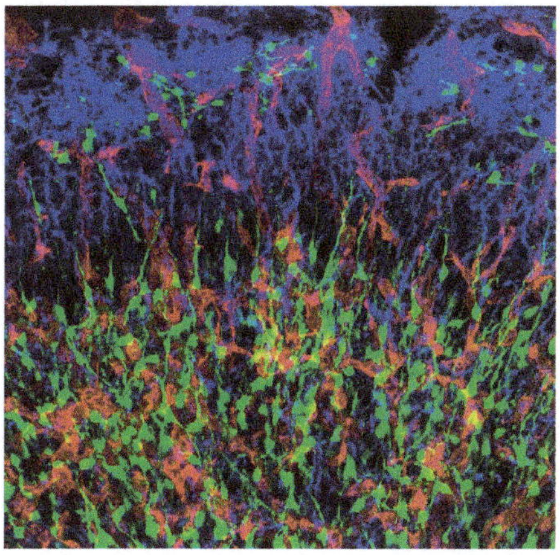

Neural progenitors (green) in olfactory bulb with astrocytes (blue).

A **progenitor cell** is a biological cell that, like a stem cell, has a tendency to differentiate into a specific type of cell, but is already more specific than a stem cell and is pushed to differentiate into its target cell. The most important difference between stem cells and progenitor cells is that stem cells can replicate indefinitely, whereas progenitor cells can divide only a limited number of times. Controversy about the exact definition remains and the concept is still evolving.

The terms progenitor cell and stem cell are sometimes equated.

Properties

Most progenitors are described as oligopotent. In this point of view, they may be compared to adult stem cells. But progenitors are said to be in a further stage of cell differentiation. They are in the "center" between stem cells and fully differentiated cells. The kind of potency they have depends on the type of their "parent" stem cell and also on their niche. Some progenitor cells were found during research, and were isolated. After their marker was found, it was proven that these progenitor could move through the body and migrate towards the tissue where they are needed. Many properties are shared by adult stem cells and progenitor cells.

Progenitor cells are found in adult organisms and they act as a repair system for the body. They replenish special cells, but also maintain the blood, skin and intestinal tissues. They can also be found in developing embryonic pancreatic tissue.

	Stem Cell	**Progenitor Cell**
Self-renewal in vitro	Unlimited	Limited
Potentiality	Multipotent	Unipotent, sometimes oligopotent
Maintenance of self-renewal	Yes	No
Population	Reaches maximum number of cells before differentiating	Does not reach maximum population

Function

The majority of progenitor cells lie dormant or possess little activity in the tissue in which they reside. They exhibit slow growth and their main role is to replace cells lost by normal attrition. In case of tissue injury, damaged or dead cells, progenitor cells can be activated. Growth factors or cytokines are two substances that trigger the progenitors to mobilize toward the damaged tissue. At the same time, they start to differentiate into the target cells. Not all progenitors are mobile and are situated near the tissue of their target differentiation. When the cytokines, growth factors and other cell division enhancing stimulators take on the progenitors, a higher rate of cell division is introduced. It leads to the recovery of the tissue.

Examples

The characterization or the defining principle of progenitor cells, in order to separate them from others, is based on the different cell markers rather than their morphological appearance.

- Satellite cells found in muscles. They play a major role in muscle cell differentiation and injury recoveries.
- Intermediate progenitor cells formed in the subventricular zone. Some of these transit amplifying neural progenitors migrate via rostral migratory stream to the olfactory bulb and differentiate further into specific types of neural cells.
- Bone marrow stromal cells, basal cell of epidermis have 10% of progenitor cell, although they are often classed as stem cells due to their high plasticity and potential for unlimited capacity for self-renewal.
- Periosteum contains progenitor cells that develop into osteoblasts and chondroblasts.
- Pancreatic progenitor cells are among the most studied progenitors. They are used in research to develop a cure against diabetes type-1.
- Angioblasts or endothelial progenitor cells (EPC). These are very important for research on fracture and wounds healing.
- Blast cells are involved in generation of B- and T-lymphocytes, which participate in immune responses.

Development of the Human Cerebral Cortices

Before embryonic day 40 (E40), progenitor cells generate other progenitor cells; after that period, progenitor cells produce only dissimilar mesenchymal stem cell daughters. The cells from a single progenitor cell form a proliferative unit that creates one cortical column; these columns contain a variety of neurons with different shapes.

ENDOTHELIAL STEM CELL

Endothelial stem cells (ESCs) are one of three types of stem cells found in bone marrow. They are multipotent, which describes the ability to give rise to many cell types, whereas a pluripotent stem cell can give rise to all types. ESCs have the characteristic properties of a stem cell: self-renewal and differentiation. These parent stem cells, ESCs, give rise to progenitor cells, which are intermediate stem cells that lose potency. Progenitor stem cells are committed to differentiating along a particular cell developmental pathway. ESCs will eventually produce endothelial cells (ECs), which create the thin-walled endothelium that lines the inner surface of blood vessels and lymphatic vessels.

ECs were first thought to arise from extraembryonic tissues because blood vessels were observed in the avian and mammalian embryos. However, after histological analysis, it was seen that ECs were in the embryo. This meant that blood vessels come from an intraembryonic source, the mesoderm.

Properties

Self-renewal and differentiation

Stem cells have the unique ability make identical copies of themselves. This property maintains unspecialized and undifferentiated cells within the body. Differentiation is the process by which a cell becomes more specialized. For stem cells, this usually occurs through several stages, where a cell proliferates giving rise to daughter cells that are further specialized. For example, an endothelial progenitor cell (EPC) is more specialized than an ESC, and an EC is more specialized than an EPC. The further specialized a cell is, the more differentiated it is and as a result it is considered to be more committed to a certain cellular lineage.

Blood vessel formation

Blood vessels are made of a thin layer of ECs. As part of the circulatory system, blood vessels play a critical role in transporting blood throughout the body. Consequently, ECs have unique functions such as fluid filtration, homeostasis and hormone trafficking. ECs are the most differentiated form of an ESC. Formation of new blood vessels occurs by two different processes: vasculogenesis and angiogenesis.The former requires differentiation of endothelial cells from hemangioblasts and then the further organization into a primary capillary network. The latter occurs when new vessels are built from preexisting blood vessels.

Markers

The vascular system is made up of two parts: 1) Blood vasculature 2) Lymphatic vessels

Both parts consist of ECs that show differential expression of various genes. A study showed that ectopic expression of Prox-1 in blood vascular ECs (BECs) induced one-third of LEC specific gene expression. Prox-1is a homeobox transcription factor found in lymphatic ECs (LECs). For example, specific mRNAs such as VEGFR-3 and p57Kip2 were expressed by the BEC that was induced to express Prox-1.

Lymphatic-specific vascular endothelial growth factors VEGF-C and VEGF-D function as ligands for the vascular endothelial growth factor receptor 3 (VEGFR-3). The ligand-receptor interaction is essential for normal development of lymphatic tissues.

Tal1 gene is specifically found in the vascular endothelium and developing brain. This gene encodes the basic helix-loop-helix structure and functions as a transcription factor. Embryos lacking *Tal1* fail to develop past embryonic day 9.5. However, the study found that *Tal1* is actually required for vascular remodeling of the capillary network, rather than early endothelial development itself.

Fetal liver kinase-1 (Flk-1) is a cell surface receptor protein that is commonly used as a marker for ESCs and EPCs.

CD34 is another marker that can be found on the surface of ESCs and EPCs. It is characteristic of hematopoietic stem cells, as well as muscle stem cells.

Role in Formation of Vascular System

The two lineages arising from the EPC and the hematopoietic progenitor cell (HPC) form the blood circulatory system. Hematopoietic stem cells can of course undergo self-renewal, and are multipotent cells that give rise to erythrocytes (red blood cells), megakaryocytes/platelets, mast cells, T-lymphocytes, B-lymphocytes, dendritic cells, natural killer cells, monocyte/macrophage, and granulocytes. A study found that in the beginning stages of mouse embryogenesis, commencing at embryonic day 7.5, HPCs are produced close to the emerging vascular system. In the yolk sac's blood islands, HPCs and EC lineages emerge from the extraembryonic mesoderm in near unison. This creates a formation in which early erythrocytes are enveloped by angioblasts, and together they give rise to mature ECs. This observation gave rise to the hypothesis that the two lineages come from the same precursor, termed hemangioblast. Even though there is evidence that corroborates a hemangioblast, the isolation and exact location in the embryo has been difficult to pinpoint. Some researchers have found that cells with hemangioblast properties have been located in the posterior end of the primitive streak during gastrulation.

In 1917, Florence Sabin first observer of blood vessels and red blood cells in the yolk sac of chick embryos occur in close proximity and time. Then, in 1932, Murray detected the same event and created the term hemangioblast for what Sabin had seen.

Further evidence to corroborate hemangioblasts come from the expression of various genes such as CD34 and Tie2 by both lineages. The fact that this expression was seen in both EC and HPC lineages led researchers to propose a common origin. However, endothelial markers like Flk1/VEGFR-2 are exclusive to ECs but stop HPCs from progressing into an EC. It is accepted that VEGFR-2+ cells are a common precursor for HPCs and ECs. If the *Vegfr3* gene is deleted then both HPC and EC differentiation comes to a halt in embryos. VEGF promotes angioblast differentiation; whereas, VEGFR-1 stops the hemangioblast from becoming an EC. In addition, basic fibroblast growth factor FGF-2 is also involved in promoting angioblasts from the mesoderm. After angioblasts commit to becoming an EC, the angioblasts gather and rearrange to assemble in a tube similar to a capillary. Angioblasts can travel during the formation of the circulatory system to configure the branches to allow for directional blood flow. Pericytes and smooth muscle cells encircle ECs when they are differentiating into arterial or venous arrangements. Surrounding the ECs creates a brace to help stabilize the vessels known as the pericellular basal lamina. It is suggested pericytes and smooth muscle cells come from neural crest cells and the surrounding mesenchyme.

Role of insulin-like Growth factors in Endothelium Differentiation

ECs derived from stem cells are the beginning of vasculogenesis. Vasculogenesis is the new production of a vascular network from mesodermal progenitor cells. This can be distinguished from angiogenesis, which is the creation of new capillaries from vessels that already exist through the process of splitting or sprouting. This can occur "in vitro" in embryoid bodies (EB) derived from embryonic stem cells; this process in EB is similar to "in vivo" vasculogenesis. Important signaling factors for vasculogenesis are TGF-β, BMP4, and VEGF, all of which promote pluripotent stem cells to differentiate into mesoderm, endothelial progenitor cells, and then into mature endothelium.

It is well established that insulin-like growth factor (IGF) signaling is important for cell responses such as mitogenesis, cell growth, proliferation, angiogenesis, and differentiation. IGF1 and IGF2 increase the production of ECs in EB. A method that IGF employs to increase vasculogenesis is upregulation of VEGF. Not only is VEGF critical for mesoderm cells to become an EC, but also for EPCs to differentiate into mature endothelium. Understanding this process can lead to further research in vascular regeneration.

Animal models of vasculogenesis

There are a number of models used to study vasculogenesis. Avian embryos, Xenopus laevis embryos, are both fair models. However, zebrafish and mouse embryos have widespread use for easily observed development of vascular systems, and the recognition of key parts of molecular regulation when ECs differentiate.

Role in Recovery

ESCs and EPCs eventually differentiate into ECs. The endothelium secretes soluble factors to regulate vasodilatation and to preserve homeostasis. When there is any dysfunction in the endothelium, the body aims to repair the damage. Resident ESCs can generate mature ECs that replace the damaged ones. However, the intermediate progenitor cell cannot always generate functional ECs. This is because some of the differentiated cells may just have angiogenic properties.

Studies have shown that when vascular trauma occurs, EPCs and circulating endothelial progenitors (CEPs) are attracted to the site due to the release of specific chemokines. CEPs are derived from EPCs within the bone marrow, and the bone marrow is a reservoir of stem and progenitor cells. These cell types accelerate the healing process and prevent further complications such as hypoxia by gathering the cellular materials to reconstruct the endothelium.

Endothelium dysfunction is a prototypical characteristic of vascular disease, common in patients with autoimmune diseases such as systemic lupus erythematosus. Further, there is an inverse relationship between age and levels of EPCs. With a decline in EPCs the body loses its ability to repair the endothelium.

The use of stem cells for treatment has become a growing interest in the scientific community. Distinguishing between an ESC and its intermediate progenitor is nearly impossible, so research is now being done broadly on EPCs. One study showed that brief exposure to sevoflurane promoted growth and proliferation of EPCs. Sevoflurane is used in general anesthesia, but this finding shows the potential to induce endothelial progenitors. Using stem cells for cell replacement therapies is known as "regenerative medicine, which is a booming field that is now working on transplanting cells as opposed to bigger tissues or organs.

Role in Cancer

Understanding more about ESCs is important in cancer research. Tumours induce angiogenesis, which is the formation of new blood vessels. These cancerous cells do this by secreting factors such as VEGF and by reducing the amount of PGK, an anti-VEGF enzyme. The result is an uncontrolled production of beta-catenin, which regulates cell growth and cell mobility. With uncontrolled beta-catenin, the cell loses its adhesive properties. As ECs get packed together to create the lining for a new blood vessel, a single cancer cell is able to travel through the vessel to a distant site. If that cancer cell implants itself and begins forming a new tumour, the cancer has metastasized.

Future Efforts

Stem cells have always been a huge interest for scientists due to their unique properties that make them unlike any other cell in the body. Generally, the idea boils down to harnessing the power of plasticity and the ability to go from an unspecialized cell to a highly specialized differentiated cell. ESCs play an incredibly important role in establishing the vascular network that is vital for a functional circulatory system. Consequently, EPCs are under study to determine the potential for treatment of ischemic heart disease. Scientists are still trying to find a way to definitely distinguish the stem cell from the progenitor. In the case of endothelial cells, it is even difficult to distinguish a mature EC from an EPC. However, because of the multipotency of the ESC, the discoveries made about EPCs will parallel or understate the powers of the ESC.

MESENCHYMAL STEM CELL

Mesenchymal stem cells, or **MSCs**, are multipotentstromal cells that can differentiate into a variety of cell types, including: osteoblasts (bone cells),chondrocytes (cartilage cells), myocytes (muscle cells)and adipocytes (fat cells). This phenomenon has been documented in specific cells and tissues in living animals and their counterparts growing in tissue culture.

While the terms *mesenchymal stem cell* and *marrow stromal cell* have been used interchangeably, neither term is sufficiently descriptive:

- Mesenchyme is embryonic connective tissue that is derived from the mesoderm and that differentiates into hematopoietic and connective tissue, whereas MSCs do not differentiate into hematopoietic cells.
- Stromal cells are connective tissue cells that form the supportive structure in which the functional cells of the tissue reside. While this is an accurate description for one function of MSCs, the term fails to convey the relatively recently discovered roles of MSCs in the repair of tissue.
- The cells can encompass multipotent cells derived from other non-marrow tissues, such as placenta, umbilical cord blood, adipose tissue, adult muscle, corneal stroma or the dental pulp of deciduous baby teeth, but do not have the capacity to reconstitute an entire organ. The term multipotent stromal cell has been proposed as a replacement.

In 1924, Russian-born morphologist Alexander A. Maximow used extensive histological findings to identify a singular type of precursor cell within mesenchyme that develops into different types of blood cells.

Scientists Ernest A. McCulloch and James E. Till first revealed the clonal nature of marrow cells in the 1960s. An *ex vivo* assay for examining the clonogenic potential of multipotent marrow cells was later reported in the 1970s by Friedenstein and colleagues. In this assay system, stromal cells were referred to as colony-forming unit-fibroblasts (CFU-f).

The first clinical trials of MSCs were completed in 1995 when a group of 15 patients were injected with cultured MSCs to test the safety of the treatment. Since then, over 200 clinical trials have been started. However, most are still in the safety stage of testing.

Subsequent experimentation revealed the plasticity of marrow cells and how their fate could be determined by environmental cues. Culturing marrow stromal cells in the presence of osteogenic stimuli such as *ascorbic acid*, *inorganic phosphate* and *dexamethasone* could promote their differentiation into osteoblasts. In contrast, the addition of *transforming growth factor-beta* (TGF-b) could induce chondrogenic markers.

Sources

Bone Marrow

Bone marrow was the first source of MSCs ever used and still is the most important source of them. These non-hematopoietic bone marrow stem cells are not expressing hematopoietic stem cells marker CD34 are also known as bone marrow stromal stem cells.

Cord Cells

The youngest, most primitive MSCs can be obtained from umbilical cord tissue, namely Wharton's jelly and the umbilical cord blood. However MSCs are found in much higher concentration in the Wharton's jelly compared to cord blood, which is a rich source of hematopoietic stem cells. The umbilical cord is easily obtained after a birth. It is normally thrown away and poses no risk for collection. The cord MSCs have more primitive properties than other adult MSCs obtained later in life, which might make them a useful source of MSCs for clinical applications.

Adipose Tissue

Adipose tissue is a ritch source of MSCs (or adipose-derived mesenchymal stem cells, AdMSCs).

Molar Cells

A rich source for mesenchymal stem cells is the developing tooth bud of the mandibular third molar. While considered multipotent, they may prove to be pluripotent. They eventually form enamel, dentin, blood vessels, dental pulp and nervous tissues, a minimum of 24 other different unique end organs. Because of ease in collection at 8–10 years of age before calcification and minimal-to-no-morbidity, they probably constitute a major source for research and multiple therapies. These stem cells have been shown capable of producing hepatocytes.

Additionally, amniotic fluid has been shown to be a rich source of stem cells. As many as 1 in 100 cells collected during amniocentesis has been shown to be a pluripotent mesenchymal stem cell.

Adipose tissue is one of the richest sources of MSCs. There are more than 500 times more stem cells in 1 gram of fat than in 1 gram of aspirated bone marrow. Adipose stem cells are actively being researched in clinical trials for treatment of a variety of diseases.

The presence of MSCs in peripheral blood has been controversial. A few groups have successfully isolated MSCs from human peripheral blood and been able to expand them in culture. Australian company Cynata claims the ability to mass-produce MSCs from induced pluripotent stem cells obtained from blood cells.

Characteristics

Morphology

Mesenchymal stem cells are characterized morphologically by a small cell body with a few cell processes that are long and thin. The cell body contains a large, round nucleus with a prominent nucleolus, which is surrounded by finely dispersed chromatin particles, giving the nucleus a clear appearance. The remainder of the cell body contains a small amount of Golgi apparatus, rough endoplasmic reticulum, mitochondria and polyribosomes. The cells, which are long and thin, are widely dispersed and the adjacent extracellular matrix is populated by a few reticular fibrils but is devoid of the other types of collagen fibrils.

Detection

The International Society for Cellular Therapy (ISCT) has proposed a set of standards to define MSCs. A cell can be classified as an MSC if it shows plastic adherent properties under normal culture conditions and has a fibroblast-like morphology. In fact, some argue that MSCs and fibroblasts are functionally identical. Furthermore, MSCs can undergo osteogenic, adipogenic and chondrogenic differentiation ex-vivo. The cultured MSCs also express on their surface CD73, CD90 and CD105, while lacking the expression of CD11b, CD14, CD19, CD34, CD45, CD79a and HLA-DR surface markers.

Differentiation Capacity

MSCs have a great capacity for self-renewal while maintaining their multipotency. Beyond that, there is little that can be definitively said. The standard test to confirm multipotency is differentiation of the cells into osteoblasts, adipocytes and chondrocytes as well as myocytes and neurons. MSCs have been seen to even differentiate into neuron-like cells, but there is lingering doubt whether the MSC-derived neurons are functional. The degree to which the culture will differentiate varies among individuals and how differentiation is induced, e.g., chemical vs. mechanical; and it is not clear whether this variation is due to a different amount of "true" progenitor cells in the culture or variable differentiation capacities of individuals' progenitors. The capacity of cells to proliferate and differentiate is known to decrease with the age of the donor, as well as the time in culture. Likewise, whether this is due to a decrease in the number of MSCs or a change to the existing MSCs is not known.

Immunomodulatory effects

Numerous studies have demonstrated that human MSCs avoid allorecognition, interfere with dendritic cell and T-cell function and generate a local immunosuppressive microenvironment by secreting cytokines. It has also been shown that the immunomodulatory function of human MSC is enhanced when the cells are exposed to an inflammatory environment characterised by the presence of elevated local interferon-gamma levels. Other studies contradict some of these findings, reflecting both the highly heterogeneous nature of MSC isolates and the considerable differences between isolates generated by the many different methods under development.

Culturing

The majority of modern culture techniques still take a colony-forming unit-fibroblasts (CFU-F) approach, where raw unpurified bone marrow or ficoll-purified bone marrow Mononuclear cell are plated directly into cell culture plates or flasks. Mesenchymal stem cells, but not red blood cells or haematopoetic progenitors, are adherent to tissue culture plastic within 24 to 48 hours. However, at least one publication has identified a population of non-adherent MSCs that are not obtained by the direct-plating technique.

Other flow cytometry-based methods allow the sorting of bone marrow cells for specific surface markers, such as STRO-1. STRO-1+ cells are generally more homogenous and have higher rates of adherence and higher rates of proliferation, but the exact differences between STRO-1+ cells and MSCs are not clear.

Methods of immunodepletion using such techniques as MACS have also been used in the negative selection of MSCs.

The supplementation of basal media with fetal bovine serum or human platelet lysate is common in MSC culture. Prior to the use of platelet lysates for MSC culture, the pathogen inactivation process is recommended to prevent pathogen transmission.

Applications

Typical gross appearance of a tubular cartilaginous construct engineered from amniotic mesenchymal stem cells Mesenchymal stem cells in the body can be activated and mobilized if needed. However, the efficiency is low. For instance, damage to muscles heals very slowly but further study into mechanisms of MSC action may provide avenues for increasing their capacity for tissue repair.

Osteo-Diseases

A statistical-based analysis of MSC therapy for osteo-diseases (e.g., osteoarthritis) noted that most studies are still underway. Wakitani published a small case series of nine defects in five knees involving surgical transplantation of MSCs with coverage of the treated chondral defects.

Autoimmune Disease

At least 218 clinical trials investigating the efficacy of mesenchymal stem cells in treating diseases have been initiated - many of which study autoimmune diseases. Promising results have been shown in conditions such as graft versus host disease, Crohn's disease, multiple sclerosis, systemic lupus erythematosus and systemic sclerosis. While their anti-inflammatory/immunomodulatory effects appear to greatly ameliorate autoimmune disease severity, the durability of these effects are unclear.

However, it is becoming more accepted that diseases involving peripheral tissues, such as inflammatory bowel disease, may be better treated with methods that increase the local concentration of cells.

Other Diseases

Many of the early clinical successes using intravenous transplantation came in systemic diseases such as graft versus host disease and sepsis. Direct injection or placement of cells into a site in need of repair may be the preferred method of treatment, as vascular delivery suffers from a pulmonary first pass effect where intravenous injected cells are sequestered in the lungs. Clinical case reports in orthopedic applications have been published, though the number of patients treated is small and these methods still lack demonstrated effectiveness.

Clinical trials of cryopreserved MSCs

Scientists have reported that MSCs when transfused immediately a few hours post thawing may show reduced function or show decreased efficacy in treating diseases as compared to those MSCs which are in log phase of cell growth, so cryopreserved MSCs should be brought back into log phase of cell growth in *in vitro* culture before these are administered for clinical trials or experimental therapies, re-culturing of MSCs will help in recovering from the shock the cells get during freezing and thawing. Various clinical trials on MSCs have failed which used cryopreserved product immediately post thaw as compared to those clinical trials which used fresh MSCs.

Cancer

Mesenchymal stem cells have been shown to contribute to cancer progression in a number of different cancers, particularly the hematological malignancies because they contact the transformed blood cells in the bone marrow.

NEURAL STEM CELL

Neural stem cells (**NSCs**) are self-renewing, multipotent cells that generate the neurons and glia of the nervous system of all animals during embryonic development. Some neural stem cells persist in the adult vertebrate brain and continue to produce neurons throughout life. Stem cells are characterized by their capacity to differentiate into multiple cell types. They undergo symmetric or asymmetric cell division into two daughter cells. In symmetric cell division, both daughter cells are also stem cells. In asymmetric division, a stem cells produces one stem cell and one specialized cell. NSCs primarily differentiate into neurons, astrocytes, and oligodendrocytes.

In 1989, Sally Temple described multipotent, self-renewing progenitor and stem cells in the subventricular zone (SVZ) of the mouse brain. In 1992, Brent A. Reynolds and Samuel Weiss were the first to isolate neural progenitor and stem cells from the adult striatal tissue, including the SVZ — one of the neurogenic areas — of adult mice brain tissue. In the same year the team of Constance Cepko and Evan Y. Snyder were the first to isolate multipotent cells from the mouse cerebellum and stably transfected them with the oncogene v-myc. Interestingly, this molecule is one of the genes widely used now to reprogram adult non-stem cells into pluripotent stem cells. Since then, neural progenitor and stem cells have been isolated from various areas of the adult brain, including non-neurogenic areas, such as the spinal cord, and from various species including humans.

Aging and Development

In vivo origin

There are two basic types of stem cell: adult stem cells, which are limited in their ability to differentiate, and embryonic stem cells (ESCs), which are pluripotent. ESCs are not limited to a particular cell fate; rather they have the capability to differentiate into any cell type.

Neural stem cells are more specialized than ESCs because they generate only neural cells (neurons or glial cells). During embryonic development of vertebrates, NSCs of the central nervous system (CNS) are called radial glial cells (RGCs), and reside in a transient zone called the ventricular zone (VZ).Neurons are generated in large numbers by NSCs during a specific period of embryonic development through the process of neurogenesis, and continue to be generated in adult life in restricted regions of the adult brain. Adult NSCs differentiate into new neurons within the adult subventricular zone (SVZ), a remnant of the embryonic germinal neuroepithelium, as well as the dentate gyrus of the hippocampus.

In vitro origin

Adult NSCs were first isolated from mouse striatum in the early 1990s. They are capable of forming multipotent neurospheres when cultured *in vitro*. Neurospheres can produce self-renewing and proliferating specialized cells. These neurospheres can differentiate to form the specified neurons, glial cells, and oligodendrocytes. In previous studies, cultured neurospheres have been transplanted into the brains of immunodeficient neonatal mice and have shown engraftment, proliferation, and neural differentiation.

Communication and Migration

NSCs are stimulated to begin differentiation via exogenous cues from the microenvironment, or stem cell niche. Some neural cells are migrated from the SVZ along the rostral migratory stream which contains a marrow-like structure with ependymal cells and astrocytes when stimulated. The ependymal cells and astrocytes form glial tubes used by migrating neuroblasts. The astrocytes in the tubes provide support for the migrating cells as well as insulation from electrical and chemical signals released from surrounding cells. The astrocytes are the primary precursors for rapid cell amplification. The neuroblasts form tight chains and migrate towards the specified site of cell damage to repair or replace neural cells. One example is a neuroblast migrating towards the olfactory bulb to differentiate into periglomercular or granule neurons which have a radial migration pattern rather than a tangential one.

Aging

Neural stem cell proliferation declines as a consequence of aging. Various approaches have been taken to counteract this age-related decline. Because FOXO proteins regulate neural stem cell homeostasis, FOXO proteins have been used to protect neural stem cells by inhibiting Wnt signaling.

Functions during differentiation and disease

Epidermal growth factor (EGF) and fibroblast growth factor (FGF) are mitogens that promote neural progenitor and stem cell growth *in vitro*, though other factors synthesized by the neural progenitor and stem cell populations are also required for optimal growth. It is hypothesized that neurogenesis in the adult brain originates from NSCs. The origin and identity of NSCs in the adult brain remain to be defined.

During Differentiation

The most widely accepted model of an adult NSC is a radial, astrocytes-like, GFAP-positive cell. Quiescent stem cells are Type B that are able to remain in the quiescent state due to the renewable tissue provided by the specific niches composed of blood vessels, astrocytes, microglia, ependymal cells, and extracellular matrix present within the brain. These niches provide nourishment, structural support, and protection for the stem cells until they are activated by external stimuli. Once activated, the Type B cells develop into Type C cells, active proliferating intermediate cells, which then divide into neuroblasts consisting of Type A cells. The undifferentiated neuroblasts form chains that migrate and develop into mature neurons. In the olfactory bulb, they mature into GABAergic granule neurons, while in the hippocampus they mature into dentate granule cells.

During Disease

NSCs have an important role during development producing the enormous diversity of neurons, astrocytes and oligodendrocytes in the developing CNS. They also have important role in adult animals, for instance in learning and hippocampal plasticity in the adult mice in addition to supplying neurons to the olfactory bulb in mice.

Notably the role of NSCs during diseases is now being elucidated by several research groups around the world. The responses during stroke, multiple sclerosis, and Parkinson's disease in animal models and humans is part of the current investigation. The results of this ongoing investigation may have future applications to treat human neurological diseases.

Neural stem cells have been shown to engage in migration and replacement of dying neurons in classical experiments performed by Sanjay Magavi and Jeffrey Macklis. Using a laser-induced damage of cortical layers, Magavi showed that SVZ neural progenitors expressing Doublecortin, a critical molecule for migration of neuroblasts, migrated long distances to the area of damage and differentiated into mature neurons expressing NeuN marker. In addition Masato Nakafuku's group from Japan showed for the first time the role of hippocampal stem cells during stroke in mice. These results demonstrated that NSCs can engage in the adult brain as a result of injury. Furthermore, in 2004 Evan Y. Snyder's group showed that NSCs migrate to brain tumors in a directed fashion. Jaime Imitola, M.D and colleagues from Harvard demonstrated for the first time, a molecular mechanism for the responses of NSCs to injury. They showed that chemokines released during injury such as SDF-1a were responsible for the directed migration of human and mouse NSCs to areas of injury in mice. Since then other molecules have been found to participate in the responses of NSCs to injury. All these results have been widely reproduced and expanded by other investigators joining the classical work of Richard L. Sidman in autoradiography to visualize neurogenesis during development, and neurogenesis in the adult by Joseph Altman in the 1960s, as evidence of the responses of adult NSCs activities and neurogenesis during homeostasis and injury.

The search for additional mechanisms that operate in the injury environment and how they influence the responses of NSCs during acute and chronic disease is matter of intense research.

Potential Clinical Applications

Regenerative Therapy of the CNS

Cell death is a characteristic of acute CNS disorders as well as neurodegenerative disease. The loss of cells is amplified by the lack of regenerative abilities for cell replacement and repair in the CNS. One way to circumvent this is to use cell replacement therapy via regenerative NSCs. NSCs can be cultured *in vitro* as neurospheres. These neurospheres are composed of neural stem cells and progenitors (NSPCs) with growth factors such as EGF and FGF. The withdrawal of these growth factors activate differentiation into neurons, astrocytes, or oligodendrocytes which can be transplanted within the brain at the site of injury. The benefits of this therapeutic approach have been examined in

Parkinson's disease, Huntington's disease, and multiple sclerosis. NSPCs induce neural repair via intrinsic properties of neuroprotection and immunomodulation. Some possible routes of transplantation include intracerebral transplantation and xenotransplantation.

An alternative therapeutic approach to the transplantation of NSPCs is the pharmacological activation of endogenous NSPCs (eNSPCs). Activated eNSPCs produce neurotrophic factors,several treatments that activate a pathway that involves the phosphorylation of STAT3 on the serine residue and subsequent elevation of Hes3 expression (STAT3-Ser/Hes3 Signaling Axis) oppose neuronal death and disease progression in models of neurological disorder.

Basic laboratory studies

Generation of 3D in vitro Models of the Human CNS

Human midbrain-derived neural progenitor cells (hmNPCs) have the ability to differentiate down multiple neural cell lineages that lead to neurospheres as well as multiple neural phenotypes. The hmNPC can be used to develop a 3D *in vitro* model of the human CNS. There are two ways to culture the hmNPCs, the adherent monolayer and the neurosphere culture systems. The neurosphere culture system has previously been used to isolate and expand CNS stem cells by its ability to aggregate and proliferate hmNPCs under serum-free media conditions as well as with the presence of epidermal growth factor (EGF) and fibroblast growth factor-2 (FGF2). Initially, the hmNPCs were isolated and expanded before performing a 2D differentiation which was used to produce a single-cell suspension. This single-cell suspension helped achieve a homogenous 3D structure of uniform aggregate size. The 3D aggregation formed neurospheres which was used to form an *in vitro* 3D CNS model.

Bioactive Scaffolds as Traumatic Brain Injury Treatment

Traumatic brain injury (TBI) can deform the brain tissue, leading to necrosis primary damage which can then cascade and activate secondary damage such as excitotoxicity, inflammation, ischemia, and the breakdown of the blood-brain-barrier. Damage can escalate and eventually lead to apoptosis or cell death. Current treatments focus on preventing further damage by stabilizing bleeding, decreasing intracranial pressure and inflammation, and inhibiting pro-apoptoic cascades. In order to repair TBI damage, an upcoming therapeutic option involves the use of NSCs derived from the embryonic periventricular region. Stem cells can be cultured in a favorable 3-dimensional, low cytotoxic environment, a hydrogel, that will increase NSC survival when injected into TBI patients. The intracerebrally injected, primed NSCs were seen to migrate to damaged tissue and differentiate into oligodendrocytes or neuronal cells that secreted neuroprotective factors.

Galectin-1 in Neural Stem Cells

Galectin-1 is expressed in adult NSCs and has been shown to have a physiological role in the treatment of neurological disorders in animal models. There are two approaches to using NSCs as a therapeutic treatment: (1) stimulate intrinsic NSCs to promote proliferation in order to replace injured tissue, and (2) transplant NSCs into the damaged brain area in order to allow the NSCs to restore the tissue. Lentivirus vectors were used to infect human NSCs (hNSCs) with Galectin-1 which were later transplanted into the damaged tissue. The hGal-1-hNSCs induced better and faster brain recovery of the injured tissue as well as a reduction in motor and sensory deficits as compared to only hNSC transplantation.

Assays

Neural stem cells are routinely studied *in vitro* using a method referred to as the Neurosphere Assay (or Neurosphere culture system), first developed by Reynolds and Weiss. Neurospheres are intrinsically heterogeneous cellular entities almost entirely formed by a small fraction (1 to 5%) of slowly dividing neural stem cells and by their progeny, a population of fast-dividing nestin-positive progenitor cells. The total number of these progenitors determines the size of a neurosphere and, as a result, disparities in sphere size within different neurosphere populations may reflect alterations in the proliferation, survival and/or differentiation status of their neural progenitors. Indeed, it has been reported that loss of β1-integrin in a neurosphere culture does not significantly affect the capacity of β1-integrin deficient stem cells to form new neurospheres, but it influences the size of the neurosphere: β1-integrin deficient neurospheres were overall smaller due to increased cell death and reduced proliferation.

While the Neurosphere Assay has been the method of choice for isolation, expansion and even the enumeration of neural stem and progenitor cells, several recent publications have highlighted some of the limitations of the neurosphere culture system as a method for determining neural stem cell frequencies. In collaboration with Reynolds, STEMCELL Technologies has developed a collagen-based assay, called the Neural Colony-Forming Cell (NCFC) Assay, for the quantification of neural stem cells. Importantly, this assay allows discrimination between neural stem and progenitor cells.

Neural Stem Cell Institute

The damaged CNS tissue has very limited regenerative and repair capacity so that loss of neurological function is often chronic and progressive. Cell replacement from stem cells is being actively pursued as a therapeutic option. In 2009, a research institute dedicated solely to translating neural stem research into therapies for patients was created outside of Albany, New York, The Neural Stem Cell Institute.

HEMATOPOIETIC STEM CELL

Hematopoietic stem cells (HSCs) or **hemocytoblasts** are the stem cells that give rise to all the other blood cells through the process of haematopoiesis. They are derived from mesoderm and located in the red bone marrow, which is contained in the core of most bones.

HSCs give rise to both the myeloid and lymphoid lineages of blood cells. (Myeloid cells include monocytes, macrophages, neutrophils, basophils, eosinophils, erythrocytes, dendritic cells, and megakaryocytes or platelets. Lymphoid cells include T cells, B cells, and natural killer cells.) The definition of hematopoietic stem cells has evolved since

HSCs were first discovered in 1961. The hematopoietic tissue contains cells with long-term and short-term regeneration capacities and committed multipotent, oligopotent, and unipotent progenitors. HSCs constitute 1:10.000 of cells in myeloid tissue.

HSC studies through much of the past half century have led to a much deeper understanding. More recent advances have resulted in the use of HSC transplants in the treatment of cancers and other immune system disorders.

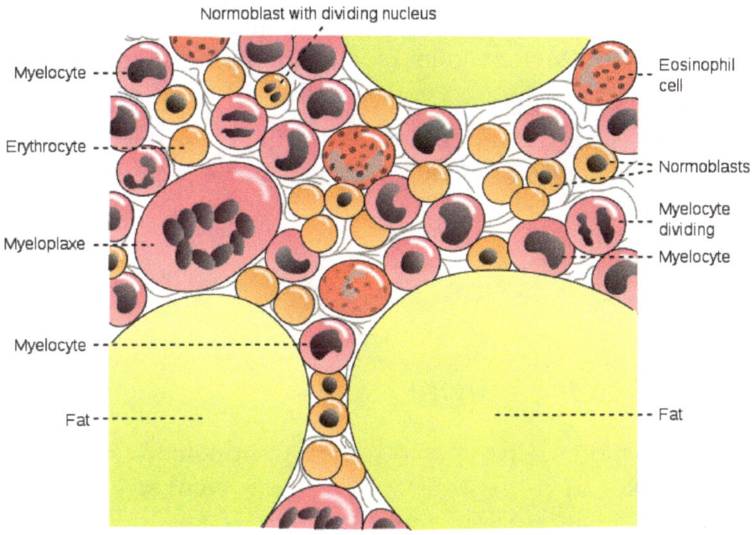

Sketch of bone marrow and its cells.

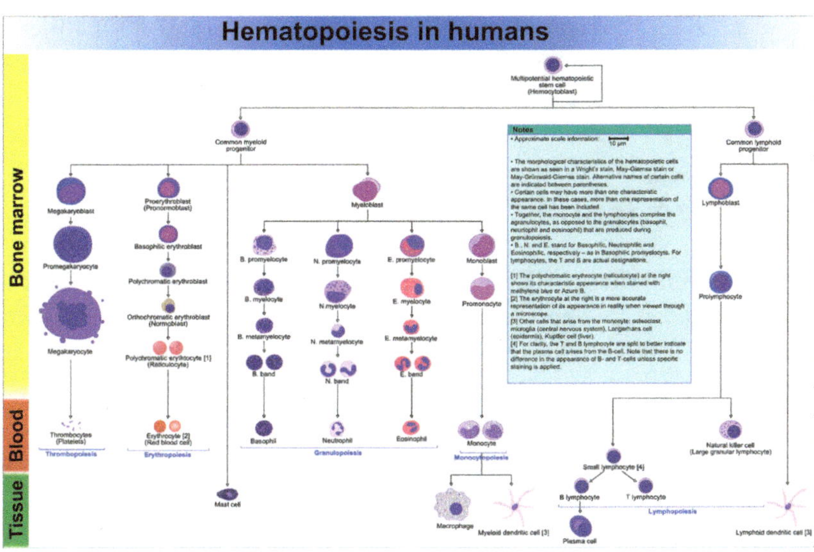

Hematopoiesis.

HSCs are found in the bone marrow of adults, specially in the pelvis, femur, and sternum. They are also found in umbilical cord blood and, in small numbers, in peripheral blood.

Stem and progenitor cells can be taken from the pelvis, at the iliac crest, using a needle and syringe. The cells can be removed as liquid (to perform a smear to look at the cell morphology) or they can be removed via a core biopsy (to maintain the architecture or relationship of the cells to each other and to the bone).

In order to harvest stem cells from the circulating peripheral blood, blood donors are injected with a cytokine, such as granulocyte-colony stimulating factor (G-CSF), that induces cells to leave the bone marrow and circulate in the blood vessels.

In mammalian embryology, the first definitive HSCs are detected in the AGM (aorta-gonad-mesonephros), and then massively expanded in the fetal liver prior to colonising the bone marrow before birth.

Functional Characteristics

Multipotency and self-renewal

HSCs can replenish all blood cell types (i.e., are multipotent) and self-renew. A small number of HSCs can expand to generate a very large number of daughter HSCs. This phenomenon is used in bone marrow transplantation, when a small number of HSCs reconstitute the hematopoietic system. This process indicates that, subsequent to bone marrow transplantation, symmetrical cell divisions into two daughter HSCs must occur.

Stem cell self-renewal is thought to occur in the stem cell niche in the bone marrow, and it is reasonable to assume that key signals present in this niche will be important in self-renewal. There is much interest in the environmental and molecular requirements for HSC self-renewal, as understanding the ability of HSC to replenish themselves will eventually allow the generation of expanded populations of HSC *in vitro* that can be used therapeutically.

Stem Cell Heterogeneity

It was originally believed that all HSCs were alike in their self-renewal and differentiation abilities. This view was first challenged by the 2002 discovery by the Muller-Sieburg group in San Diego, who illustrated that different stem cells can show distinct repopulation patterns that are epigenetically predetermined intrinsic properties of clonal Thy-1^{lo} Sca-1^{+} lin^{-} c-kit^{+} HSC. The results of these clonal studies led to the notion of **lineage bias**. Using the ratio $\rho = L/M$ of lymphoid (L) to myeloid (M) cells in blood as a quantitative marker, the stem cell compartment can be split into three categories of HSC. **Balanced (Bala) HSCs** repopulate peripheral white blood cells in the same ratio of myeloid to lymphoid cells as seen in unmanipulated mice (on average about 15% myeloid and 85% lymphoid cells, or $3 \leq \rho \leq 10$). **Myeloid-biased (My-bi) HSCs** give rise to very few lymphocytes resulting in ratios $0 < \rho < 3$, while **lymphoid-biased (Ly-bi) HSCs** generate very few myeloid cells, which results in lymphoid-to-myeloid ratios of $\rho > 10$. All three types are normal types of HSC, and they do not represent stages of differentiation. Rather, these are three classes of HSC, each with an epigenetically fixed differentiation program. These studies also showed that lineage bias is not stochastically regulated or dependent on differences in environmental influence. My-bi HSC self-renew longer than balanced or Ly-bi HSC. The myeloid bias results from reduced responsiveness to the lymphopoetin interleukin 7 (IL-7).

Subsequently, other groups confirmed and highlighted the original findings. For example, the Eaves group confirmed in 2007 that repopulation kinetics, long-term self-renewal capacity, and My-bi and Ly-bi are stably inherited intrinsic HSC properties. In 2010, the Goodell group provided additional insights about the molecular basis of lineage bias in side population (SP) SCA-1^+ lin^- c-kit^+ HSC. As previously shown for IL-7 signaling, it was found that a member of the transforming growth factor family (TGF-beta) induces and inhibits the proliferation of My-bi and Ly-bi HSC, respectively.

Behavior in Culture

A *cobblestone area-forming cell (CAFC)* assay is a cell culture-based empirical assay. When plated onto a confluent culture of stromal feeder layer, a fraction of HSCs creep between the gaps (even though the stromal cells are touching each other) and eventually settle between the stromal cells and the substratum (here the dish surface) or trapped in the cellular processes between the stromal cells. Emperipolesis is the *in vivo* phenomenon in which one cell is completely engulfed into another (e.g. thymocytes into thymic nurse cells); on the other hand, when *in vitro*, lymphoid lineage cells creep beneath nurse-like cells, the process is called pseudoemperipolesis. This similar phenomenon is more commonly known in the HSC field by the cell culture terminology *cobble stone area-forming cells (CAFC)*, which means areas or clusters of cells look dull cobblestone-like under phase contrast microscopy, compared to the other HSCs, which are refractile. This happens because the cells that are floating loosely on top of the stromal cells are spherical and thus refractile. However, the cells that creep beneath the stromal cells are flattened and, thus, not refractile. The mechanism of pseudoemperipolesis is only recently coming to light. It may be mediated by interaction through CXCR4 (CD184) the receptor for CXC Chemokines (e.g., SDF1) and $\alpha4\beta1$ integrins.

Mobility

HSCs have a higher potential than other immature blood cells to pass the bone marrow barrier, and, thus, may travel in the blood from the bone marrow in one bone to another bone. If they settle in the thymus, they may develop into T cells. In the case of fetuses and other extramedullary hematopoiesis, HSCs may also settle in the liver or spleen and develop.

This enables HSCs to be harvested directly from the blood.

Physical Characteristics

With regard to morphology, hematopoietic stem cells resemble lymphocytes. They are non-adherent, and rounded, with a rounded nucleus and low cytoplasm-to-nucleus ratio. Since HSCs cannot be isolated as a pure population, it is not possible to identify them in a microscope.

Markers

HSCs can be identified or isolated by the use of flow cytometry where the combination of several different cell surface markers are used to separate the rare HSCs from the surrounding blood cells. HSCs lack expression of mature blood cell markers and are thus, called Lin-. Lack of expression of lineage markers is used in combination with detection of several positive cell-surface markers to isolate HSCs. In addition, HSCs are characterised by their small size and low staining with vital dyes such as rhodamine 123 (rhodamine ^{lo}) or Hoechst 33342 (side population).

Cluster of Differentiation and other Markers

The classical marker of human HSC is CD34 first described independently by Civin et al. and Tindle et al. It is used to isolate HSC for reconstitution of patients who are haematologically incompetent as a result of chemotherapy or disease.

Many markers belong to the cluster of differentiation series, like: CD34, CD38, CD90, CD133, CD105, CD45, and also c-kit, - the receptor for stem cell factor.

There are many differences between the human and mice hematopoietic cell markers for the commonly accepted type of hematopoietic stem cells.

- **Mouse HSC**: $CD34^{lo/-}$, $SCA\text{-}1^{+}$, $Thy1.1^{+/lo}$, $CD38^{+}$, $C\text{-}kit^{+}$, lin^{-}
- **Human HSC**: $CD34^{+}$, $CD59^{+}$, $Thy1/CD90^{+}$, $CD38^{lo/-}$, $C\text{-}kit/CD117^{+}$, lin^{-}

However, not all stem cells are covered by these combinations that, nonetheless, have become popular. In fact, even in humans, there are hematopoietic stem cells that are $CD34^{-}/CD38^{-}$. Also some later studies suggested that earliest stem cells may lack c-kit on the cell surface. For human HSCs use of CD133 was one step ahead as both $CD34^{+}$ and $CD34^{-}$ HSCs were $CD133^{+}$.

Traditional purification method used to yield a reasonable purity level of mouse hematopoietic stem cells, in general, requires a large(~10-12) battery of markers, most of which were surrogate markers with little functional significance, and thus partial overlap with the stem cell populations and sometimes other closely related cells that are not stem cells. Also, some of these markers (e.g., Thy1) are not conserved across mouse species, and use of markers like $CD34^{-}$ for HSC purification requires mice to be at least 8 weeks old.

SLAM code

Alternative methods that could give rise to a similar or better harvest of stem cells is an active area of research, and are presently emerging. One such method uses a signature of *SLAM* family of cell surface molecules. The SLAM (Signaling lymphocyte activation molecule) family is a group of more than 10 molecules whose genes are located mostly tandemly in a single locus on chromosome 1 (mouse), all belonging to a subset of the immunoglobulin gene superfamily, and originally thought to be involved in T-cell stimulation. This family includes CD48, CD150, CD244, etc., CD150 being the founding member, and, thus, also known as slamF1, i.e., SLAM family member 1.

The signature **SLAM codes** for the hemopoietic hierarchy are:

- Hematopoietic stem cells (HSC): $CD150^{+}CD48^{-}CD244^{-}$
- Multipotent progenitor cells (MPPs): $CD150^{-}CD48^{-}CD244^{+}$
- Lineage-restricted progenitor cells (LRPs): $CD150^{-}CD48^{+}CD244^{+}$
- Common myeloid progenitor (CMP): $lin^{-}SCA\text{-}1^{-}c\text{-}kit^{+}CD34^{+}CD16/32^{mid}$
- Granulocyte-macrophage progenitor (GMP): $lin^{-}SCA\text{-}1^{-}c\text{-}kit^{+}CD34^{+}CD16/32^{hi}$
- Megakaryocyte-erythroid progenitor (MEP): $lin^{-}SCA\text{-}1^{-}c\text{-}kit^{+}CD34^{-}CD16/32^{low}$

For HSCs, $CD150^{+}CD48^{-}$ was sufficient instead of $CD150^{+}CD48^{-}CD244^{-}$ because CD48 is a ligand for CD244, and both would be positive only in the activated lineage-restricted progenitors. It seems that this code was more efficient than the more tedious earlier set of the large number of markers, and are also conserved across the mouse strains; however, recent work has shown that this method excludes a large number of HSCs and includes an equally large number of non-stem cells. $CD150^{+}CD48^{-}$ gave stem cell purity comparable to $Thy1^{lo}SCA\text{-}1^{+}lin^{-}c\text{-}kit^{+}$ in mice.

LT-HSC/ST-HSC/early MPP/late MPP

Irving Weissman's group at Stanford University was the first to isolate mouse hematopoietic stem cells in 1988 and was also the first to work out the markers to distinguish the mouse long-term (LT-HSC) and short-term (ST-HSC) hematopoietic stem cells (self-renew-capable), and the Multipotent progenitors (MPP, low or no self-renew capability — the later the developmental stage of MPP, the lesser the self-renewal ability and the more of some of the markers like CD4 and CD135):

- **LT-HSC**: $CD34^{-}$, $CD38^{-}$, $SCA\text{-}1^{+}$, $Thy1.1^{+/lo}$, $C\text{-}kit^{+}$, lin^{-}, $CD135^{-}$, $Slamf1/CD150^{+}$
- **ST-HSC**: $CD34^{+}$, $CD38^{+}$, $SCA\text{-}1^{+}$, $Thy1.1^{+/lo}$, $C\text{-}kit^{+}$, lin^{-}, $CD135^{-}$, $Slamf1/CD150^{+}$, Mac-1 $(CD11b)^{lo}$
- **Early MPP**: $CD34^{+}$, $SCA\text{-}1^{+}$, $Thy1.1^{-}$, $C\text{-}kit^{+}$, lin^{-}, $CD135^{+}$, $Slamf1/CD150^{-}$, Mac-1 $(CD11b)^{lo}$, $CD4^{lo}$
- **Late MPP**: $CD34^{+}$, $SCA\text{-}1^{+}$, $Thy1.1^{-}$, $C\text{-}kit^{+}$, lin^{-}, $CD135^{high}$, $Slamf1/CD150^{-}$, Mac-1 $(CD11b)^{lo}$, $CD4^{lo}$

Nomenclature of Hematopoietic Colonies and Lineages

Between 1948 and 1950, the Committee for Clarification of the Nomenclature of Cells and Diseases of the Blood and Blood-forming Organs issued reports on the nomenclature of blood cells. An overview of the terminology is shown below, from earliest to final stage of development:

- [root]blast
- pro[root]cyte
- [root]cyte
- meta[root]cyte
- mature cell name

The root for erythrocyte colony-forming units (CFU-E) is "rubri", for granulocyte-monocyte colony-forming units (CFU-GM) is "granulo" or "myelo" and "mono", for lympocyte colony-forming units (CFU-L) is "lympho" and for megakaryocyte colony-forming units (CFU-Meg) is "megakaryo". According to this terminology, the stages of red blood cell formation would be: rubriblast, prorubricyte, rubricyte, metarubricyte, and erythrocyte. However, the following nomenclature seems to be, at present, the most prevalent:

Committee	**"lympho"**	**"rubri"**	**"granulo" or "myelo"**	**"mono"**	**"megakaryo"**
Lineage	Lymphoid	Myeloid	Myeloid	Myeloid	Myeloid
CFU	CFU-L	CFU-GEMM→CFU-E	CFU-GEMM→CFU-GM→CFU-G	CFU-GEMM→CFU-GM→CFU-M	CFU-GEMM→CFU-Meg
Process	lymphocytopoiesis	erythropoiesis	granulocytopoiesis	monocytopoiesis	thrombocytopoiesis
[root]blast	Lymphoblast	Proerythroblast	Myeloblast	Monoblast	Megakaryoblast
pro[root]cyte	Prolymphocyte	Polychromatophilic erythrocyte	Promyelocyte	Promonocyte	Promegakaryocyte
[root]cyte	-	Normoblast	Eosino/neutro/basophilic myelocyte		Megakaryocyte
meta[root]cyte	Large lymphocyte	Reticulocyte	Eosinophilic/neutrophilic/ basophilic metamyelocyte, Eosinophilic/neutrophilic/ basophilic band cell	Early monocyte	-
mature cell name	Small lymphocyte	Erythrocyte	granulocytes (Eosino/neutro/ basophil)	Monocyte	thrombocytes (Platelets)

Osteoclasts also arise from hemopoietic cells of the monocyte/neutrophil lineage, specifically CFU-GM.

Colony-forming units

In the context of hematopoietic stem cells, a colony-forming unit is a subtype of HSC. (This sense of the term is different from colony-forming units of microbes, which is a cell counting unit.) There are various kinds of HSC colony-forming units:

- Colony-forming unit–granulocyte-erythrocyte-monocyte-megakaryocyte (CFU-GEMM)
- Colony-forming unit–lymphocyte (CFU-L)

- Colony-forming unit–erythrocyte (CFU-E)
- Colony-forming unit–granulocyte-macrophage (CFU-GM)
- Colony-forming unit–megakaryocyte (CFU-Meg)
- Colony-forming unit–basophil (CFU-B)
- Colony-forming unit–eosinophil (CFU-Eos)

The above CFUs are based on the lineage. Another CFU, the colony-forming unit–spleen (CFU-S), was the basis of an *in vivo* clonal colony formation, which depends on the ability of infused bone marrow cells to give rise to clones of maturing hematopoietic cells in the spleens of irradiated mice after 8 to 12 days. It was used extensively in early studies, but is now considered to measure more mature progenitor or **transit-amplifying cells** rather than stem cells.

HSC Repopulation Kinetics

Hematopoietic stem cells (HSC) cannot be easily observed directly, and, therefore, their behaviors need to be inferred indirectly. Clonal studies are likely the closest technique for single cell in vivo studies of HSC. Here, sophisticated experimental and statistical methods are used to ascertain that, with a high probability, a single HSC is contained in a transplant administered to a lethally irradiated host. The clonal expansion of this stem cell can then be observed over time by monitoring the percent donor-type cells in blood as the host is reconstituted. The resulting time series is defined as the repopulation kinetic of the HSC.

The reconstitution kinetics are very heterogeneous. However, using symbolic dynamics, one can show that they fall into a limited number of classes. To prove this, several hundred experimental repopulation kinetics from clonal Thy-1^{lo} SCA-1^{+} lin^{-} c-kit^{+} HSC were translated into symbolic sequences by assigning the symbols "+", "-", "~" whenever two successive measurements of the percent donor-type cells have a positive, negative, or unchanged slope, respectively. By using the Hamming distance, the repopulation patterns were subjected to cluster analysis yielding 16 distinct groups of kinetics. To finish the empirical proof, the Laplace add-one approach was used to determine that the probability of finding kinetics not contained in these 16 groups is very small. By corollary, this result shows that the hematopoietic stem cell compartment is also heterogeneous by dynamical criteria.

DNA Damage and Aging

DNA strand breaks accumulate in long term HSCs during aging. This accumulation is associated with a broad attenuation of DNA repair and response pathways that depends on HSC quiescence. Non-homologous end joining (NHEJ) is a pathway that repairs double-strand breaks in DNA. NHEJ is referred to as "non-homologous" because the break ends are directly ligated without the need for a homologous template. The NHEJ pathway depends on several proteins including ligase 4, DNA polymerase mu and NHEJ factor 1 (NHEJ1, also known as Cernunnos or XLF).

DNA ligase 4 (Lig4) has a highly specific role in the repair of double-strand breaks by NHEJ. Lig4 deficiency in the mouse causes a progressive loss of HSCs during aging. Deficiency of lig4 in pluripotent stem cells results in accumulation of DNA double-strand breaks and enhanced apoptosis.

In polymerase mu mutant mice, hematopoietic cell development is defective in several peripheral and bone marrow cell populations with about a 40% decrease in bone marrow cell number that includes several hematopoietic lineages. Expansion potential of hematopoietic progenitor cells is also reduced. These characteristics correlate with reduced ability to repair double-strand breaks in hematopoietic tissue.

Deficiency of NHEJ factor 1 in mice leads to premature aging of hematopoietic stem cells as indicated by several lines of evidence including evidence that long-term repopulation is defective and worsens over time. Using a human induced pluripotent stem cell model of NHEJ1 deficiency, it was shown that NHEJ1 has an important role in promoting survival of the primitive hematopoietic progenitors. These NHEJ1 deficient cells possess a weak NHEJ1-mediated repair capacity that is apparently incapable of coping with DNA damages induced by physiological stress, normal metabolism, and ionizing radiation.

The sensitivity of haematopoietic stem cells to Lig4, DNA polymerase mu and NHEJ1 deficiency suggests that NHEJ is a key determinant of the ability of stem cells to maintain themselves against physiological stress over time. Rossi et al. found that endogenous DNA damage accumulates with age even in wild type HSCs, and suggested that DNA damage accrual may be an important physiological mechanism of stem cell aging.

REFERENCES

1. Kryven, I.; Röblitz, S.; Schütte, Ch. (2015). Solution of the chemical master equation by radial basis functions approximation with interface tracking. BMC systems biology. **9** *(9.1). doi:10.1186/s12918-015-0210-y.*
2. Slack, J.M.W. (2013) Essential Developmental Biology. Wiley-Blackwell, Oxford.
3. Slack, J.M.W. (2007). Metaplasia and transdifferentiation: from pure biology to the clinic. Nature Reviews Molecular Cell Biology. **8** *(5): 369–378. doi:10.1038/nrm2146.*
4. Takahashi, K; Yamanaka, S (2006). Induction of pluripotent stem cells from mouse embryonic and adult fibroblast cultures by defined factors. Cell. **126** *(4): 663–76. doi:10.1016/j.cell.2006.07.024. PMID 16904174.*
5. Schöler, Hans R. (2007). The Potential of Stem Cells: An Inventory. In Nikolaus Knoepffler; Dagmar Schipanski; Stefan Lorenz Sorgner. Humanbiotechnology as Social Challenge. Ashgate Publishing. p. 28. ISBN 978-0-7546-5755-2.
6. NCI Dictionary of Cancer Terms. National Cancer Institute. Retrieved 1 November 2013.
7. Lodish, Harvey (2000). Molecular Cell Biology (4th ed.). New York: W. H. Freeman. Section 14.2. ISBN 0-7167-3136-3.

8. Kumar, Rani (2008). Textbook of Human Embryology. I.K. International Publishing House. p. 22. ISBN 9788190675710.

9. D. Binder, Marc; Hirokawa, Nobutaka; Windhorst, Uwe (2009). Encyclopedia of Neuroscience. Springer. ISBN 3540237356.

10. Rakic, P (October 2009). Evolution of the neocortex: a perspective from developmental biology. Nature reviews. Neuroscience. **10** *(10): 724–35. doi:10.1038/nrn2719. PMC 2913577. PMID 19763105.*

11. Lui, JH; Hansen, DV; Kriegstein, AR (8 July 2011). Development and evolution of the human neocortex.. Cell. **146** *(1): 18–36. PMID 21729779.*

12. Rash, BG; Ackman, JB; Rakic, P (February 2016). Bidirectional radial Ca(2+) activity regulates neurogenesis and migration during early cortical column formation.. Science advances. **2** *(2): e1501733. PMID 26933693.*

13. Stocum DL (2004). Amphibian regeneration and stem cells. Curr. Top. Microbiol. Immunol. Current Topics in Microbiology and Immunology. **280**: 1–70. doi:10.1007/978-3-642-18846-6_1. ISBN 978-3-540-02238-1. PMID 14594207.

14. Casimir CM, Gates PB, Patient RK, Brockes JP (1988-12-01). Evidence for dedifferentiation and metaplasia in amphibian limb regeneration from inheritance of DNA methylation. Development. **104** *(4): 657–668. PMID 3268408.*

15. Giles KL (1971). Dedifferentiation and Regeneration in Bryophytes: A Selective Review. New Zealand Journal of Botany. **9** *(4): 689–94. doi:10.1080/0028825x.1971.10430231.*

16. Schnabel M, Marlovits S, Eckhoff G, et al. (January 2002). Dedifferentiation-associated changes in morphology and gene expression in primary human articular chondrocytes in cell culture. Osteoarthr. Cartil. **10** *(1): 62–70. doi:10.1053/joca.2001.0482. PMID 11795984.*

17. Sell S (December 1993). Cellular origin of cancer: dedifferentiation or stem cell maturation arrest?. Environ. Health Perspect. **101** *(Suppl 5): 15–26. doi:10.2307/3431838. JSTOR 3431838. PMC 1519468. PMID 7516873.*

18. Tsonis PA (April 2004). Stem cells from differentiated cells. Mol. Interv. **4** *(2): 81–3. doi:10.1124/mi.4.2.4. PMID 15087480.*

19. Ben-Tabou de-Leon S, Davidson EH (2007). Gene regulation: gene control network in development.. Annu Rev Biophys Biomol Struct. **36** *(191): 191–212. doi:10.1146/annurev.biophys.35.040405.102002. PMID 17291181.*

20. Knisely, Karen; Gilbert, Scott F. (2009). Developmental Biology (8th ed.). Sunderland, Mass: Sinauer Associates. p. 147. ISBN 0-87893-371-9.

21. Rudel and Sommer; The evolution of developmental mechanisms. Developmental Biology 264, 15-37, 2003 Rudel, D.; Sommer, R. J. (2003). The evolution of developmental mechanisms. Developmental Biology. **264** *(1): 15–37. doi:10.1016/S0012-1606(03)00353-1. PMID 14623229.*

22. Yamamoto Y and WR Jeffery; Central role for the lens in cave fish eye degeneration. Science 289 (5479), 631-633, 2000 Yamamoto, Y.; Jeffery, W. R. (2000). Central Role for the Lens in Cave Fish Eye Degeneration. Science. **289**

(5479): 631–633. Bibcode:2000Sci...289..631Y. doi:10.1126/science.289.5479.631. PMID 10915628.

23. Kirk MM, A Ransick, SE Mcrae, DL Kirk; The relationship between cell size and cell fate in Volvox carteri. Journal of Cell Biology 123, 191-208, 1993 Kirk, M. M.; Ransick, A.; McRae, S. E.; Kirk, D. L. (1993). The relationship between cell size and cell fate in Volvox carteri. Journal of Cell Biology. **123** *(1): 191–208. doi:10.1083/jcb.123.1.191. PMC 2119814. PMID 8408198.*
24. Rabajante JF, Babierra AL (January 30, 2015). Branching and oscillations in the epigenetic landscape of cell-fate determination. Progress in Biophysics and Molecular Biology. **117** *(2–3): 240–9. doi:10.1016/j.pbiomolbio.2015.01.006. PMID 25641423.*
25. Lister R; et al. (2011). Hotspots of aberrant epigenomic reprogramming in human induced pluripotent stem cells. Nature. **471** *(7336): 68–73. Bibcode:2011Natur.471...68L. doi:10.1038/nature09798. PMC 3100360. PMID 21289626.*
26. Christophersen NS, Helin K (2010). Epigenetic control of embryonic stem cell fate. J Exp Med. **207** *(11): 2287–95. doi:10.1084/jem.20101438. PMC 2964577. PMID 20975044.*
27. Thomson, M; Liu, S. J.; Zou, L. N.; Smith, Z; Meissner, A; Ramanathan, S (2011). Pluripotency factors in embryonic stem cells regulate differentiation into germ layers. Cell. **145** *(6): 875–89. doi:10.1016/j.cell.2011.05.017. PMID 21663792.*
28. Thomson, M; Liu, S. J.; Zou, L. N.; Smith, Z; Meissner, A; Ramanathan, S (2011). Pluripotency factors in embryonic stem cells regulate differentiation into germ layers. Cell. **145** *(6): 875–89. doi:10.1016/j.cell.2011.05.017. PMID 21663792.*
29. Zhu, J.; et al. (2013). Genome-wide chromatin state transitions associated with developmental and environmental cues. Cell. **152** *(3): 642–654. doi:10.1016/j.cell.2012.12.033. PMC 3563935. PMID 23333102.*
30. Guenther MG, Young RA (2010). Repressive Transcription. Science. **329** *(5988): 150–1. Bibcode:2010Sci...329..150G. doi:10.1126/science.1193995. PMC 3006433. PMID 20616255.*
31. Meissner A (2010). Epigenetic modifications in pluripotent and differentiated cells. Nat Biotechnol. **28** *(10): 1079–88. doi:10.1038/nbt.1684. PMID 20944600.*
32. Krogan NJ, Dover J, Wood A, Schneider J, Heidt J, Boateng MA, Dean K, Ryan OW, Golshani A, Johnston M, Greenblatt JF, Shilatifard A (Mar 2003). The Paf1 complex is required for histone H3 methylation by COMPASS and Dot1p: linking transcriptional elongation to histone methylation. Molecular Cell. **11** *(3): 721–9. doi:10.1016/S1097-2765(03)00091-1. PMID 12667454.*
33. Ng HH, Robert F, Young RA, Struhl K (Mar 2003). Targeted recruitment of Set1 histone methylase by elongating Pol II provides a localized mark and memory of recent transcriptional activity. Molecular Cell. **11** *(3): 709–19. doi:10.1016/S1097-2765(03)00092-3. PMID 12667453.*

34. Bernstein BE, Kamal M, Lindblad-Toh K, Bekiranov S, Bailey DK, Huebert DJ, McMahon S, Karlsson EK, Kulbokas EJ, Gingeras TR, Schreiber SL, Lander ES (Jan 2005). Genomic maps and comparative analysis of histone modifications in human and mouse. Cell. **120** *(2): 169–81. doi:10.1016/j.cell.2005.01.001. PMID 15680324.*

35. Teif VB, Vainshtein Y, Caudron-Herger M, Mallm JP, Marth C, Höfer T, Rippe K (2012). Genome-wide nucleosome positioning during embryonic stem cell development. Nat Struct Mol Biol. **19** *(11): 1185–92. doi:10.1038/nsmb.2419. PMID 23085715.*

36. Whyte, W. A.; Bilodeau, S; Orlando, D. A.; Hoke, H. A.; Frampton, G. M.; Foster, C. T.; Cowley, S. M.; Young, R. A. (2012). Enhancer decommissioning by LSD1 during embryonic stem cell differentiation. Nature. **482** *(7384): 221–5. doi:10.1038/nature10805. PMC 4144424. PMID 22297846.*

37. Whyte, W. A.; Bilodeau, S; Orlando, D. A.; Hoke, H. A.; Frampton, G. M.; Foster, C. T.; Cowley, S. M.; Young, R. A. (2012). Enhancer decommissioning by LSD1 during embryonic stem cell differentiation. Nature. **482** *(7384): 221–5. doi:10.1038/nature10805. PMC 4144424. PMID 22297846.*

38. Mohammad HP, Baylin SB (2010). Linking cell signaling and the epigenetic machinery. Nat Biotechnol. **28** *(10): 1033–8. doi:10.1038/nbt1010-1033. PMID 20944593.*

39. Niwa H, Burdon T, Chambers I, Smith A (1998). Self-renewal of pluripotent embryonic stem cells is mediated via activation of STAT3. Genes Dev. **12** *(13): 2048–60. doi:10.1101/gad.12.13.2048. PMC 316954. PMID 9649508.*

40. Liu S; et al. (2006). Hedgehog Signaling and Bmi-1 Regulate Self-renewal of Normal and Malignant Human Mammary Stem Cells. Cancer Res. **66** *(12): 6063–71. doi:10.1158/0008-5472.CAN-06-0054. PMC 4386278. PMID 16778178.*

41. Leung C; et al. (2004). Bmi1 is essential for cerebellar development and is overexpressed in human medulloblastomas. Nature. **428** *(6980): 337–41. Bibcode:2004Natur.428..337L. doi:10.1038/nature02385. PMID 15029199.*

42. Zencak D; et al. (2005). Bmi1 loss produces an increase in astroglial cells and a decrease in neural stem cell population and proliferation. J Neurosci. **25** *(24): 5774–83. doi:10.1523/JNEUROSCI.3452-04.2005. PMID 15958744.*

43. Engler, AJ; Sen, S; Sweeney, HL; Discher, DE (August 2006). Matrix Elasticity Directs Stem Cell Lineage Specification. Cell. **126** *(4): 677–689. doi:10.1016/j.cell.2006.06.044. PMID 16923388. Retrieved 2016-04-22.*

44. Guo, Jun; Wang, Yuexiu; Sachs, Frederick; Meng, Fanjie (2014-12-09). Actin stress in cell reprogramming. Proceedings of the National Academy of Sciences. **111** *(49): E5252–E5261. doi:10.1073/pnas.1411683111. ISSN 0027-8424. PMC 4267376. PMID 25422450.*

45. Guilak, Farshid; Cohen, Daniel M.; Estes, Bradley T.; Gimble, Jeffrey M.; Liedtke, Wolfgang; Chen, Christopher S. (2009-07-02). Control of Stem Cell Fate by Physical Interactions with the Extracellular Matrix. Cell Stem Cell. **5** *(1): 17–26. doi:10.1016/j.stem.2009.06.016. PMC 2768283. PMID 19570510.*

Stem Cell Laws and Policy

Chapter Contents

This is an interactive map that provides information on human ES cell policies throughout the world. Colored maps indicate if countries or states have permissive legislation, place restrictions on or prohibit human ES cell research. The site also contains excerpts from countries with written policy statements. The site was created by the Hinxton Group, an international consortium of human ES cell researchers, ethicists and policy experts.

INTRODUCTRION

Stem cell laws and policy in the United States have had a complicated legal and political history.

SCIENCE BACKGROUND

Stem cells are cells found in all multi-cellular organisms. They were isolated in mice in 1981, and in humans in 1998. In humans there are many types of stem cells, each with varying levels of potency. Potency is a measure of a cell's differentiation potential, or the number of other cell types that can be made from that stem cell. Embryonic stem cells are pluripotent stem cells derived from the inner cell mass of the blastocyst. These stem cells can differentiate into all other cells in the human body and are the subject of much scientific research. However, since they must be derived from early human embryos their production and use in research has been a hotly debated topic as the embryo most likely is destroyed in the process.

Stem cell treatments are a type of cell therapy that introduce new cells into adult bodies for possible treatment of cancer, diabetes, neurological disorders and other medical conditions. Stem cells have been used to repair tissue damaged by disease or age. Cloning also might be done with stem cells. Pluripotent stem cells can also be derived from Somatic cell nuclear transfer which is a laboratory technique where a clone embryo is created from a donor nucleus. Somatic cell nuclear transfer is also tightly regulated amongst various countries.

Until recently, the principal source of human embryonic stem cells has been donated embryos from fertility clinics. In January 2007, researchers at Wake Forest University reported that "stem cells drawn from amniotic fluid donated by pregnant women hold much of the same promise as embryonic stem cells."

In 2000, the NIH, under the administration of President Bill Clinton, issued guidelines that allow federal funding of embryonic stem-cell research.

POLITICAL BEGINNINGS

In 1973, Roe v. Wade legalized abortion in the United States. Five years later, the first successful human *in vitro* fertilization resulted in the birth of Louise Brown in England. These developments prompted the federal government to create regulations barring the use of federal funds for research that experimented on human embryos. In 1995, the NIH Human Embryo Research Panel advised the administration of President Bill Clinton to permit federal funding for research on embryos left over from *in vitro* fertility treatments and also recommended federal funding of research on embryos specifically created for experimentation. In response to the panel's recommendations, the Clinton administration, citing moral and ethical concerns, declined to fund research on embryos created solely for research purposes, but did agree to fund research on left-over embryos created by *in vitro* fertility treatments. At this point, the Congress intervened and passed the Dickey-Wicker Amendment in 1995 (the final bill, which included the Dickey Amendment, was signed into law by Bill Clinton) which prohibited any federal funding for the Department of Health and Human Services be used for research that resulted in the destruction of an embryo regardless of the source of that embryo. In 1998, privately funded research led to the breakthrough discovery of human Embryonic stem cells (hESC).

FEDERAL LAW

No federal law ever did ban stem cell research in the United States, but only placed restrictions on funding and use, under Congress's power to spend.

In February 2001, George W. Bush requested a review of the NIH's guidelines, and after a policy discussion within his circle of supporters, implemented a policy in August of that year to limit the number of embryonic stem cell lines that could be used for research. (While he claimed that 78 lines would qualify for federal funding, only 19 lines were actually available.)

In April 2004, 206 members of Congress, including many moderate Republicans, signed a letter urging President Bush to expand federal funding of embryonic stem cell research beyond what Bush had already supported.

In May 2005, the House of Representatives voted 238-194 to loosen the limitations on federally funded embryonic stem-cell research — by allowing government-funded research on surplus frozen embryos from in vitro fertilization clinics to be used for stem cell research with the permission of donors — despite Bush's promise to veto if passed. On July 29, 2005, Senate Majority Leader William H. Frist (R-TN), announced that he too favored loosening restrictions on federal funding of embryonic stem cell research. On July 18, 2006, the Senate passed three different bills concerning stem cell research. The Senate passed the first bill, 63-37, which would have made it legal for the Federal government to spend Federal money on embryonic stem cell research that uses embryos left over from *in vitro* fertilization procedures. On July 19, 2006 President Bush vetoed this bill. The second bill makes it illegal to create, grow, and abort fetuses for research purposes. The third bill would encourage research that would isolate pluripotent, i.e., embryonic-like, stem cells without the destruction of human embryos.

The National Institutes of Health has hundreds of funding opportunities for researchers interested in hESC. In 2005 the NIH funded $607 million worth of stem cell research, of which $39 million was specifically used for hESC.

During Bush›s second term, in July 2006, he used his first Presidential veto on the Stem Cell Research Enhancement Act. The Stem Cell Research Enhancement Act was the name of two similar bills, and both were vetoed by President George W. Bush and were not enacted into law. New Jersey congressman Chris Smith wrote a Stem Cell Therapeutic and Research Act of 2005, which was signed into law by President Bush. It provided $265 million for adult stem cell therapy, umbilical cord blood and bone marrow treatment, and authorized $79 million for the collection of cord blood stem cells.

By executive order on March 9, 2009, President Barack Obama removed certain restrictions on federal funding for research involving new lines of human embryonic stem cells. Prior to President Obama's executive order, federal funding was limited to non-embryonic stem cell research and embryonic stem cell research based upon embryonic stem cell lines in existence prior to August 9, 2001. Federal funding originating from current appropriations to the Department of Health and Human Services (including the National Institutes of Health) under the Omnibus Appropriations Act of 2009, remains prohibited under the Dickey Amendment for (1) the creation of a human embryo for research purposes; or (2) research in which a human embryo or embryos are destroyed, discarded, or knowingly subjected to risk of injury or death greater than that allowed for research on fetuses in utero.

In a speech before signing the executive order, Mr. Obama noted the following:

In 2011, a United States District Court "threw out a lawsuit that challenged the use of federal funds for embryonic stem cell research." The decision was a case on remand from the United States Court of Appeals for the District of Columbia Circuit.

STATE LAW

Legalization and Funding

S1909/A2840 is a bill that was passed by the New Jersey legislature in December 2003, and signed into law by Governor James McGreevey on January 4, 2004, that permits human cloning for the purpose of developing and harvesting human stem cells. Specifically, it legalizes the process of cloning a human embryo, and implanting the clone into a womb, provided that the clone is then aborted and used for medical research. Missouri Constitutional Amendment 2 (2006) (Missouri Amendment Two) was a 2006 law that legalized certain forms of embryonic stem cell research in the state.

California voters in November 2004 approved Proposition 71, creating a US$3 billion state taxpayer-funded institute for stem cell research, the California Institute for Regenerative Medicine. It hopes to provide $300 million a year. However, as of June 6, 2006, there were delays in the implementation of the California program and it is believed that the delays will continue for the significant future. On July 21, 2006, Governor Arnold Schwarzenegger (R-Calif.) authorized $150 million in loans to the Institute in an attempt to jump start the process of funding research.

Several states, in what was initially believed to be a national migration of biotech researchers to California, have shown interest in providing their own funding support of embryonic and adult stem cell research. These states include Connecticut , Florida, Illinois, Massachusetts , Missouri, New Hampshire, New York, Pennsylvania, Texas , Washington, and Wisconsin.

Bans and Restrictions

Other states have, or have shown interest in, additional restrictions or even complete bans on embryonic stem cell research. These states include Arkansas, Iowa, Kansas, Louisiana, Nebraska, North Dakota, South Dakota, and Virginia. (*States play catch-up on stem cells*, *USA Today*, December 2004) Arkansas, Indiana, Louisiana, Michigan, North Dakota and South Dakota have passed laws to "prohibit the creation or destruction of human embryos for medical research."

Bans and Restrictions on Relevant Stem Cell/Cloning Controversies

States with Statutes specifically Banning Human Reproductive and Therapeutic Cloning

- Arkansas, [2003 SB 185]; Ark. Code § 20- 16-1001 et. seq. (2004)
- Indiana, Ind. Code § 1 6-18-2-5.5. -56.5, -128.5, -183.5 (2005)
- Michigan, Mich. Comp. Laws §§ 333.26401-06, 333.16274, 16275, 20197, 750.430a (2004), reversed by constitutional amendment in proposal 2008-02.
- North Dakota, [2003 HB 1424]; N.D. Cent. Code §§ 12.1-39-01, 12.1-39-02 (2004)
- South Dakota, 2004 SB 184
- Virginia, Va. Code Ann. §§ 32.1-162.21- .22 (2004) (unclear whether therapeutic cloning is included in the ban)

States with statutes specifically banning Human Reproductive Cloning

- Iowa, Iowa Code §§ 707C (2007)
- Maryland, 2006 SB 144

States banning the use of Public Monies for Reproductive and/or Therapeutic Cloning

- Arizona, HB 2221 (2005) (human reproductive and therapeutic cloning)
- Missouri, Mo. Rev. Stat. § 1.217 (2004) (human reproductive cloning)

States with Statutes Specifically Allowing therapeutic Cloning

- California, Cal. Bus. & Prof. §§ 16004, 16105; Cal. Health & Safety §§24185-24187 (2004)
- Missouri, Mo. Rev. Stat. § 1.217 (2004)
- New Jersey, [2003 SB 1909/2003 AB 2840]; N.J. Stat. § 2C:11A-1 (2004)
- Rhode Island, R.I. Gen. Laws §§ 23-16.4-1 - .4-4 (2004) (Sunset provision: July 7, 2010)
- Connecticut, Public Act 05-149 (2005)

POLICY STANCES OF POLITICAL PARTIES AND POLITICIANS

Policy stances on stem cell research of various political leaders in the United States have not always been predictable.

As a rule, most Democratic Party leaders and high profile supporters and even rank and file members have pushed for laws and policies almost exclusively favoring embryonic stem cell research.President Bill Clinton supported the NIH›s guidelines in 2000. Both the major candidates in 2008 had supported the 2005 and 2007 bills, in particular Hillary Rodham Clinton, Bill Clinton›s First Lady, then U. S. Senator for New York, and Barack Obama, then U.S. Senator for Illinois, who promised to sign the EFCA into law, and was a cosponsor of such bills. Massachusetts governor Deval Patrick is also a proponent of embryonic stem cell research. There have been some Democrats who have asked for boundaries be placed on human embryo use. For example, Carolyn McCarthy has publicly stated she only supports using human embryos "that would be discarded".

The Republicans largely oppose embryonic stem cell research in favor of adult stem cell research which has already produced cures and treatments for cancer and paralysis for example, but there are some high profile exceptions who offer qualified support for some embryonic stem cell research. Prominent Republican leaders against embryonic stem cell research include Sarah Palin, Jim Talent, Rick Santorum, and Sam Brownback. In July 2001:

> Sen. Bill Frist (R-TN) and Sen. Orrin Hatch (R-UT), a vocal abortion opponent, call[ed] for limited federal funding for embryonic stem-cell research.... House Speaker Dennis Hastert (R-IL) and other Republican House leaders [came] out in opposition to federal funding for embryonic stem cell research.
>
> —NPR story.

2008 "GOP" Presidential Candidate John McCain is a member of The Republican Main Street Partnership, and supports embryonic stem cell research, despite his earlier opposition. In July 2008 he said, At the moment I support stem cell research [because of] the potential it has for curing some of the most terrible diseases that afflict mankind. In 2007, in what he described as a very agonizing and tough decision, he voted to allow research using human embryos left over from fertility treatments. Former First Lady Nancy Reagan and Senator Orrin Hatch also support stem cell research, after first opposing the issue. Former Senator Frist also supports stem cell research, despite having initially supported past restrictions on embryonic stem cell research. 2008 V.P. candidate Palin opposed embryonic stem cell research, which she said causes the destruction of life, thus this research is inconsistent with her pro-life position and she does not support it. She said, in an interview with Charlie Gibson, that she supports adult stem cell research approaches.

A few moderates or Libertarians support such research with limits. Lincoln Chafee supported federal funding for embryonic stem cell research. Ron Paul, a Republican congressman, physician, and Libertarian and Independent candidate for President, has sponsored much legislation, and has had quite complex positions.

National Academies Guidelines for Human Embryonic Stem Cell Research

In 2005, the United States National Academies released its *Guidelines for Human Embryonic Stem Cell Research.* These Guidelines were prepared to enhance the integrity of human embryonic stem cell research in the public's perception and in actuality by encouraging responsible practices in the conduct of that research. The National Academies has subsequently named the Human Embryonic Stem Cell Research Advisory Committee to keep the Guidelines up-to-date.

The guidelines preserve two primary principles. First, that hESC research has the potential to improve our understanding of human health and discover new ways to treat illness. Second, that individuals donating embryos should do so freely, with voluntary and informed consent. The guidelines implement executive order 13505, and apply to hESC research receiving funds from the NIH. The guidelines detail safeguards to protect donating individuals by acquiring informed consent and protecting their identity. In addition, the guidelines contain multiple sections applying to embryos donated in the US and abroad, both before and after the effective date of the guidelines.

The NIH guidelines define which hESC research is eligible to receive NIH funding through a series of regulations which applicants for funding must adhere to. Applicants proposing research, may use stem cell lines that are posted on the NIH registry, or may submit an assurance of compliance with section II of the guidelines. Section II is applicable to stem cells derived from human embryos.

For the purposes of section II of the NIH guidelines, the following requirements must be met. First, the hESCs should have been derived from embryos created using an in vitro fertilization procedure for reproductive purposes, and no longer needed for this purpose. Second, the donors who sought reproductive treatment have given written consent for the embryos to be used for research purposes. Third, all written consent forms and other documentation must be provided.

Documentation must be provided regarding the following: All options available to the healthcare facility regarding the embryos in question were explained to the individual who sought reproductive treatment. No payments of any kind may be offered for the donated embryos. Policies and procedures must be in place at the facility where the embryos were donated to ensure that neither donation nor refusal to donate affects quality of care received by the patient.

There must also be a clear distinction between the donor's decision to create embryos for reproductive purposes, and the decision to donate embryos for research. This is ensured through a number of regulations which follow. First, the decision to create embryos for reproductive purposes must have been made without the influence of researchers proposing usage for the embryos to derive hESCs for research purposes. Consent for the donation of embryos should have been given at the time of donation. Finally, donors should have been informed that they have the right to withdraw consent at any time until derivation of stem cells from the embryo, or until the identity of the donor can no longer be linked to the embryo.

When seeking consent from the donor, they must be informed of what will become of their donation. The donor must be informed that the embryonic stem cells would be derived from the embryos from research purposes. The donor must also be informed of the procedures that the embryo would undergo in the derivation process, and that the stem cell lines derived from the embryo may be kept for many years. In addition, the donors must be informed that the donation is not made with direction regarding the intended use of the derived stem cells, and the research is not intended to provide direct medical benefit to the donor. The donor is also to be informed that there may be commercial potential resulting from the research performed, and that the donor is not to benefit from commercial development as a result of the donation. The donor is also to be notified if information that could disclose their identity will be available to the researchers.

Applicants seeking to use stem cell lines established before the effective date of the guidelines may use lines published on the NIH registry, or establish eligibility by complying with the requirements listed above. Alternately, researchers may submit materials to a working group of the Advisory Committee to the Director. The working group will review submitted materials and submit recommendations to the Advisory Committee, which will in turn make recommendations to the NIH director. A final decision regarding eligibility for funding is then made by the NIH director.

The materials submitted to the working group must demonstrate that the stem cells were derived from embryos created for reproductive purposes, and are no longer needed. Also, the materials must demonstrate that the stem cells were donated by donors who had granted voluntary written consent.

Research ineligible for NIH funding as dictated within the guidelines include research in which hESCs are introduced into non-human primate blastocysts. Research of the breeding of animals where hESCs may contribute to the germ line are similarly ineligible. NIH funding of the derivation of stem cells from human embryos is prohibited by the annual appropriations ban on the funding of human embryo research. Research using hESCs derived from other sources is also not eligible for funding.

TIMELINE

- **1993** - As per the National Institutes of Health Revitalization Act, Congress and President Bill Clinton give the NIH direct authority to fund human embryo research for the first time.
- **1995** - The U.S. Congress passes an appropriations bill attached to which is a rider, the Dickey Amendment which prohibited federally appropriated funds to be used for research where human embryos would be either created or destroyed. President Clinton signs the bill into law. This predates the creation of the first human embryonic stem cell lines.
- **1999** - After the creation of the first human embryonic stem cell lines in 1998 by James Thomson of the University of Wisconsin, Harriet Rabb, the top lawyer at the Department of Health and Human Services, releases a legal opinion that would set the course for Clinton Administration policy. Federal funds, obviously, could not be used to derive stem cell lines (because derivation involves embryo destruction). However, she concludes that because human embryonic stem cells are not a human embryo within the statutory definition, the Dickey-Wicker

Amendment does not apply to them. The NIH was therefore free to give federal funding to experiments involving the cells themselves. President Clinton strongly endorses the new guidelines, noting that human embryonic stem cell research promised potentially staggering benefits. And with the guidelines in place, the NIH begins accepting grant proposals from scientists.

- **2001–2006** - On August 9, 2001, U.S. President George W. Bush signs an executive order which restricts federally funded stem cell research on embryonic stem cells to the already derived cell lines. He supports federal funding for embryonic stem cell research on the already existing lines of approximately $100 million, $250 million for research on adult and animal stem cells, and creates the President's Council on Bioethics led by Dr. Leon Kass of the University of Chicago to monitor stem cell research, to recommend appropriate guidelines and regulations, and to consider all of the medical and ethical ramifications of biomedical innovation.
- **2 November 2004** - California voters approve Proposition 71, which provides $3 billion in state funds over ten years to human embryonic stem cell research.
- **5 May 2006** - Senator Rick Santorum introduces bill number S. 2754, or the *Alternative Pluripotent Stem Cell Therapies Enhancement Act*, into the U.S. Senate.
- **18 July 2006** - The U.S. Senate passes the Stem Cell Research Enhancement Act H.R. 810 and votes down Senator Santorum's S. 2754.
- **19 July 2006** - President George W. Bush vetoes House Resolution 810 *Stem Cell Research Enhancement Act*, a bill that would have reversed the Dickey Amendment which made it illegal for federal money to be used for research where stem cells are derived from the destruction of an embryo.
- **7 November 2006** - The people of the U.S. state of Missouri passed Amendment 2, which allows usage of any stem cell research and therapy allowed under federal law, but prohibits human reproductive cloning.
- **16 February 2007** – The California Institute for Regenerative Medicine became the biggest financial backer of human embryonic stem cell research in the United States when they awarded nearly $45 million in research grants.
- **4 November 2008** - The people of the U.S. state of Michigan passed Proposal 08-2, allowing Michigan researchers to make embryonic stem cell cultures from excess embryos donated from fertility treatments.
- **23 January 2009** - The United States Food and Drug Administration approves clinical trials for human embryonic stem cell therapy.
- **9 March 2009** - President Barack Obama signs an executive order reversing federal opposition to embryonic Stem Cell research.
- **August 2010** - Judge Royce Lamberth of the U.S. District Court for the District of Columbia issued a temporary injunction blocking the federal government from implementing the current NIH guidelines ...ruling that experiments with such cells fall under an unambiguous 1996 law by Congress that prohibits federal funding of research that destroys human embryos. This new injunction would

not block new funding but it would also interfere with the research allowed under the Bush administration

- **April 2011** - See Dickey-Wicker Amendment, In the 2-1 opinion of April 29, 2011, the appeals panel said that the Dickey-Wicker Amendment was ambiguous and that the National Institutes of Health had reasonably concluded that although federal funds could not be used to directly destroy an embryo, the amendment does not prohibit funding a research project using embryonic stem cells. This is an important distinction under the law, because for federal funds to be used directly to support the destruction of embryos.

STEM CELL LAWS AND POLICY IN CHINA

The laws and policies regarding stem cell research in the People›s Republic of China are relatively relaxed in comparison to that of other nations. The reason for this is due to different traditional and cultural views in relation to that of the West.

Laws and Regulations

China has one of the most unrestrictive embryonic stem cell research policies in the world. In recent years, seeing the research opportunities that China's lax regulations provide, many expatriate Chinese scientists from the West are returning to China to establish stem cell research centers and laboratories there.

As a result of the increased interest in this field of research, in 2003, the People's Republic of China Ministry of Science and Technology and Ministry of Health issued official ethical guidelines for human embryonic stem cell research in its territories. The guidelines strictly forbid any research aimed at human reproductive cloning and require that the embryos used for stem cell research come only from:

- Spared gamate or blastocyst after *in vitro* fertilization (IVF) procedures;
- Fetal cells from accidental spontaneous or voluntarily selected abortions;
- Blastocyst or parthenogenetic split blastocyst obtained by somatic cell nuclear transfer technology; or
- Germ cells voluntarily donated.

American scientific journals *Science* and *Nature* have both reported in recent years that China's stem cell programs hold potential, and in 2004 a delegation from Britain's Department of Trade and Industry concluded more emphatically that Chinese research in the field was already world-class. Funding for stem cell research by the Chinese government is extremely limited compared to Western nations, with the Chinese Ministry of Science and Technology planning to devote between US$33 million and US$132 million on stem cell research during the next 5 years. By contrast, the state of California alone has earmarked US$3 billion to fund stem cell research at California institutions during the next decade. However, it is simply cheaper to produce goods in China than in nearly any other country, and in sophisticated sectors such as medical research, the cost advantage is likely to be retained for quite some time.

On January 10, 2012 it was announced that China will halt new applications for clinical trials of stem-cell products until July 1 as part of a year-long campaign to regulate the development of the industry. Deng Haihua, the Ministry of Health›s spokesman, said "Trials that haven't been approved should be stopped."

Cultural Views

Perhaps more importantly, the cultural and national attitude on stem cell research differs greatly between China and the West. Most Chinese citizens do not view the embryo as containing any inherent moral value. According to the accepted Confucian view, a person begins with birth; a person is an entity that has a body or shape and psyche, and has rational, emotional and social-relational capacity for a lifetime of learning and innovation. Therefore, to the Chinese, a human embryo, lacking the characteristics of a person, cannot be equated morally to a person or a personal life. Stem cell research in China thus is unlikely ever to be prone to the intense moral politicking that characterizes the field in the West. China's distinctive attitude toward the embryo, combined with its lax regulatory system, could help its researchers leap the gap between laboratory science and medical application in stem cell therapy developments.

REFERENCES

1. John Ydstie and Joe Palca, Embryonic Stem Cells Made Without Embryos, NPR, November 21, 2007, found at NPR website story of 11-21-09. Retrieved April 8, 2009.
2. Joe Neel and Joanne SilbernerStem Cells Used In Woman›s Windpipe Transplant, All Things Considered, November 18, 2009, found at NPR story of 11-18-2008. Retrieved April 8, 2009.
3. Mlsna, Lucas J. (2010). Stem Cell Based Treatments and Novel Considerations for Conscience Clause Legislation. Indiana Health Law Review. United States: Indiana University Robert H. McKinney School of Law. **8** *(2): 471–496.* ISSN:1549-3199. LCCN:2004212209. OCLC:OCLC 54703225.
4. President Clinton›s Comments on NIH and Human Embryo Research. U.S. National Archives. December 2, 1994. Retrieved 2006-07-19.
5. Christine Vestal, Staff Writer, Stateline.org, "Stem Cell Research at the Crossroads of Religion and Politics," Pew Forum paper, July 17, 2008, found at Pew Forum website. Accessed April 13, 2009.
6. Connolly, Ceci (July 30, 2005). Despite Bush Veto, Stem Cell Research Abounds. The Washington Post: A01. Retrieved 2006-07-21.
7. Kellman, Laurie (July 18, 2006). Senate Approves Embryo Stem Cell Bill. Associated Press. Retrieved 2006-07-18.
8. Obama overturns Bush policy on stem cells on CNN, Added April 14, 2009,
9. A debt of gratitude to so many tireless advocates

10. Ariane de Vogue (July 27, 2011). Stem Cell: Fed judge throws out human embryo challenge. Retrieved July 28, 2011.
11. Sherley v. Sebelius, No. 10-5287, D. C. Cir. April 29, 2011), found at US Court of Appeals for the District of Columbia Circuit website.
12. Gledhill, Lynda (2006-07-21). Governor OKs stem cell research funds Schwarzenegger authorizes loans for $150 million. San Francisco Chronicle. pp. B–1. Retrieved 2006-07-29.
13. chron.com article no longer available Unable to access, April 11, 2007
14. https://www.legis.iowa.gov/docs/ico/linc/2013.Chapter.707C.pdf
15. . In his 2004 platform, John Kerry affirmed his support of federally funded embryonic stem cell research "under the strictest ethical guidelines," saying, "We will not walk away from the chance to save lives and reduce human suffering." The 2004 Democratic National Platform (PDF). (111 KB)
16. Clinton supported federal funding of embryonic stem cell research and voted in favor of the Stem Cell Research Enhancement Act of 2005 that passed Congress but was vetoed by President Bush, Hillary Rodham Clinton, Senator for New York: Senator Clinton Calls for Expansion of Stem Cell Research as well as voting for the 2007 bill with the same name that passed in Congress.
17. Obama condemned Bush's veto, claiming, "Democrats want this bill to pass. Conservative, pro-life Republicans want this bill to pass. By large margins, the American people want this bill to pass. It is only the White House standing in the way of progress - standing in the way of so many potential cures." Barack Obama's Statement of Support for Stem Cell Research. See also NY Times Article on 2007 stem cell veto.
18. McCarthy has been a supporter of stem cell research but restricted to the use of embryos that would be discarded. In 2007, she supported the Stem Cell Research Enhancement Act that was touted as doing that, passed both the Democrat-led House and Senate, but was later vetoed by President Bush. Rep. McCarthy Statement on Stem Cell Research Vote. Carolyn McCarthy. Retrieved 2008-02-05.
19. H.R. 3: Stem Cell Research Enhancement Act of 2007. GovTrack.us. Retrieved 2008-02-05.
20. Allen, Jonathan (2005-10-25). GOP hopefuls getting more time to weigh stem-cell vote. The Hill. Archived from the original on 2006-04-20. Retrieved 2006-08-15.
21. Laura Meckler, "McCain Speaks Out Against Abortions", Wall Street Journal, July 17, 2008.
22. Pew Forum, 2008.
23. Sarah Palin, Andrew Halcro, Tony Knowles (2006-11-07). 2006 Alaska Governor›s Debate among Sarah Palin, Andrew Halcro *and Tony Knowles (Televised debate). Anchorage, Alaska: KTOO Television.*

24. She said, And thankfully, again, not only are there other options, but we›re getting closer and closer to finding a tremendous amount of other options, like, as I mentioned, the adult stem cell research. Ertelt, Steven (September 14, 2008). Sarah Palin Tells Charlie Gibson She is Pro-Life on Abortion, Stem Cell Research. LifeNews.com.
25. National Academies website
26. Dispatches: The Politics of Stem Cells. Nova. PBS.
27. Missouri Constitution Amendment 2. 2006.
28. Calif. Awards $45M in Stem Cell Grants. Associated Press. 17 February 2007. Archived from the original on August 26, 2014.
29. Full-text of Michigan Proposal 08-2 (PDF).
30. Green light for US stem cell work. BBC News. January 23, 2009. Retrieved May 24, 2010.
31. Obama reverses Bush-era stem cell policy. Associated Press.
32. Hsu, Spencer S.; Leonnig, Carol D. (August 25, 2010). Stem cell judge Royce Lamberth no stranger to controversy, independence. The Washington Post.

CHAPTER 6

Cancer and Stem Cell

Chapter Contents

- **Introduction**
- **Debate**
- **Origin**
- **Identification**
- **Heterogeneity (Markers)**
- **Metastasis**

Cancer stem cells are rare immortal cells within a tumour that can both self-renew by dividing and give rise to many cell types that constitute the tumour, and can therefore form tumours. Such cells have been found in various types of human tumours and might be attractive targets for cancer treatment.

INTRODUCTION

Cancer stem cells (CSCs) are cancer cells (found within tumors or hematological cancers) that possess characteristics associated with normal stem cells, specifically the ability to give rise to all cell types found in a particular cancer sample. CSCs are therefore tumorigenic (tumor-forming), perhaps in contrast to other non-tumorigenic cancer cells. CSCs may generate tumors through the stem cell processes of self-renewal and differentiation into multiple cell types. Such cells are hypothesized to persist in tumors as a distinct population and cause relapse and metastasis by giving rise to new tumors. Therefore, development of specific therapies targeted at CSCs holds hope for improvement of survival and quality of life of cancer patients, especially for patients with metastatic disease.

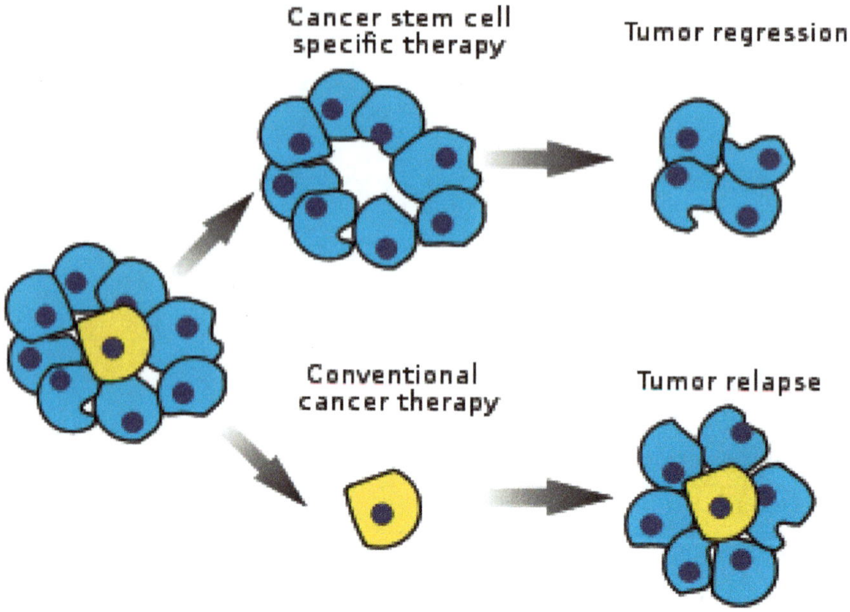

Figure 1: Stem cell specific and conventional cancer therapies.

Existing cancer treatments have mostly been developed based on animal models, where therapies able to promote tumor shrinkage were deemed effective. However, animals do not provide a complete model of human disease. In particular, in mice, whose life spans do not exceed two years, tumor relapse is difficult to study.

The efficacy of cancer treatments is, in the initial stages of testing, often measured by the ablation fraction of tumor mass (fractional kill). As CSCs form a small proportion of the tumor, this may not necessarily select for drugs that act specifically on the stem cells. The theory suggests that conventional chemotherapies kill differentiated or differentiating cells, which form the bulk of the tumor but do not generate new cells. A population of CSCs, which gave rise to it, could remain untouched and cause relapse.

Cancer stem cells were first identified by John Dick in acute myeloid leukemia in the late 1990s. Since the early 2000s they have been an intense cancer research focus.

Tumor Propagation Models

In different tumor subtypes, cells within the tumor population exhibit functional heterogeneity and tumors are formed from cells with various proliferative and differentiation capacities. This functional heterogeneity among cancer cells has led to the creation of multiple propagation models to account for heterogeneity and differences in tumor-regenerative capacity: the cancer stem cell (CSC) and stochastic model.

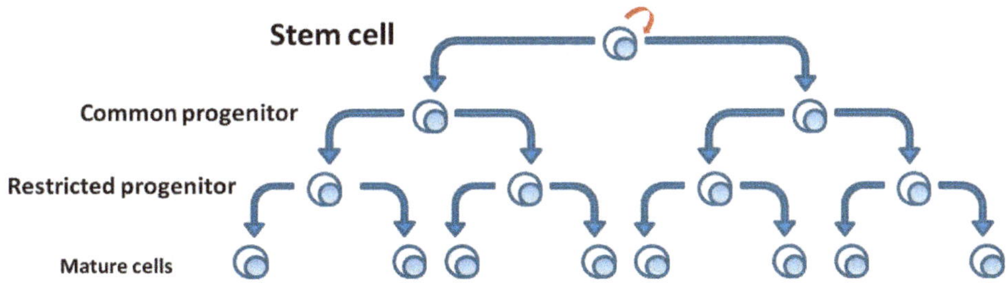

Figure 2: A normal cellular hierarchy comprising stem cells at the apex, which generate common and more restricted progenitor cells and ultimately the mature cell types that constitute particular tissues.

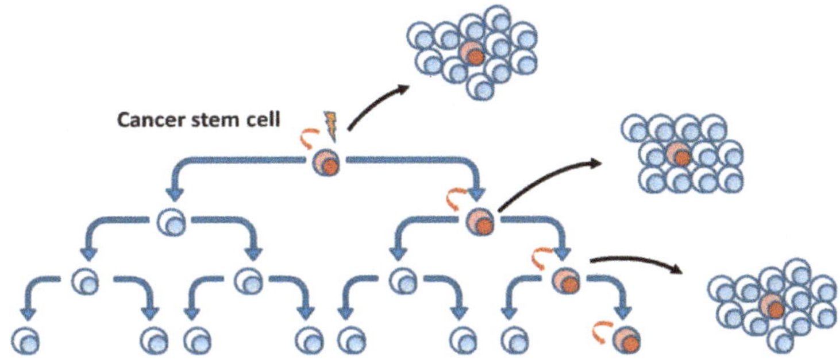

Figure 3. In the cancer stem cell (CSC) model, only the CSCs have the ability to generate a tumor, based on their self-renewal properties and proliferative potential.

The Cancer Stem Cell Model

The Cancer Stem Cell Model, also known as the Hierarchical Model proposes that tumors are hierarchically organized (CSCs lying at the apex (Fig. 3).) Within the cancer population of the tumors there are cancer stem cells (CSC) that are tumorigenic cells and are biologically distinct from other subpopulationsThey have two defining features: their long-term ability to self-renew and their capacity to differentiate into progeny that is non-tumorigenic but still contributes to the growth of the tumor. This model suggests that only certain subpopulations of cancer stem cells have the ability to drive the progression of cancer, meaning that there are specific (intrinsic) characteristics that can be identified and then targeted to destroy a tumor long-term without the need to battle the whole tumor

Stochastic Model

In order for a cell to become cancerous it must undergo a significant number of alterations to its DNA sequence. This cell model suggests these mutations could occur to any cell in the body resulting in a cancer. Essentially this theory proposes that all cells have the ability to be tumorigenic making all tumor cells equipotent with the ability to self-renew or differentiate, leading to tumor heterogeneity while others can differentiate into non-CSCs The cell`s potential can be influenced by unpredicted genetic or epigenetic factors, resulting in phenotypically diverse cells in both the tumorigenic and non-tumorigenic cells that compose the tumor.

These mutations could progressively accumulate and enhance the resistance and fitness of cells that allow them to outcompete other tumor cells, better known as the somatic evolution model. The clonal evolution model, which occurs in both the CSC model and stochastic model, postulates that mutant tumor cells with a growth advantage outproliferate others. Cells in the dominant population have a similar potential for initiating tumor growth (Fig. 4).

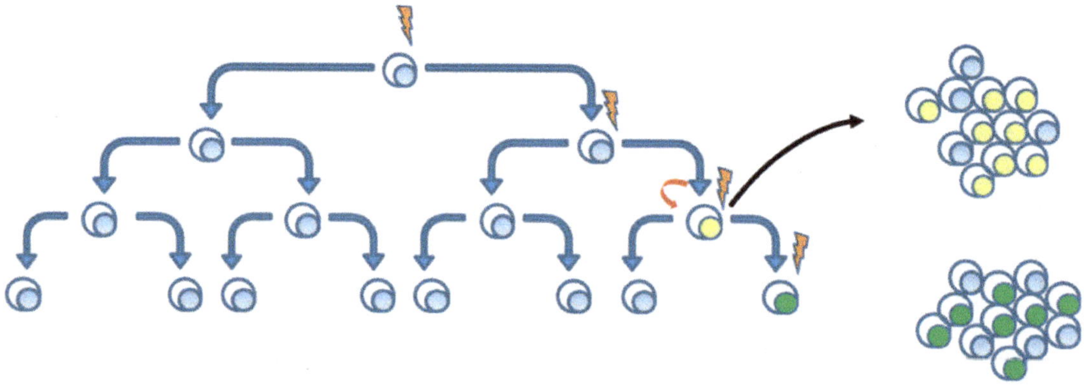

Figure 4: In the clonal evolution model, all undifferentiated cells have similar possibility to change into a tumorigenic cell.

These two models are not mutually exclusive, as CSCs themselves undergo clonal evolution. Thus, the secondary more dominant CSCs may emerge, if a mutation confers more aggressive properties (Fig. 5).

Tying CSC and Stochastic Models Together

A study in 2014 argues the gap between these two controversial models can be bridged by providing an alternative explanation of tumor heterogeneity. They demonstrate a model that includes aspects of both the Stochastic and CSC models. They examined cancer stem cell plasticity in which cancer stem cells can transition between non-cancer stem cells (Non-CSC) and CSC via in situ supporting a more Stochastic model. But the existence of both biologically distinct non-CSC and CSC populations supports a more CSC model, proposing that both models may play a vital role in tumor heterogeneity.

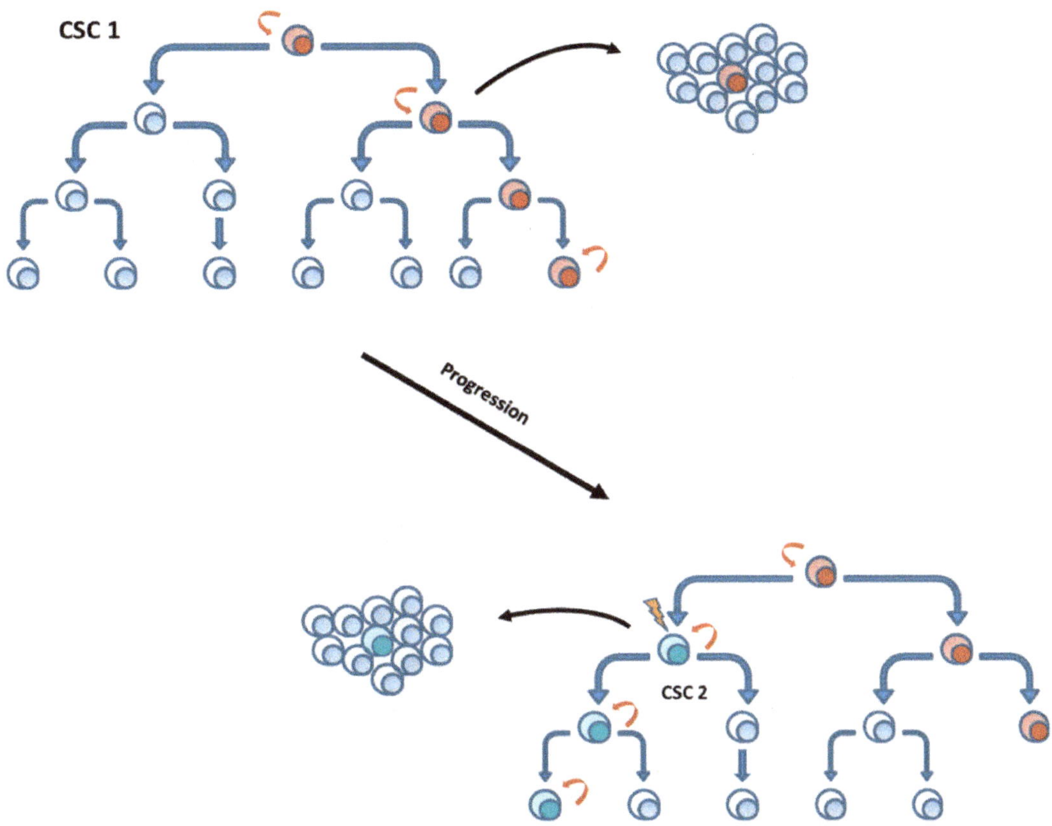

Figure 5: Both tumor models may play a role in the maintenance of a tumor. Initially, tumor growth is assured with a specific CSC (CSC1). With tumor progression, another CSC (CSC 2) may arise due the clonal selection. The development of a new more aggressive CSC may result from the acquisition of an additional mutation or epigenetic modification.

DEBATE

The existence of CSCs is under debate, because many studies found no cells with their specific characteristics. Cancer cells must be capable of continuous proliferation and self-renewal to retain the many mutations required for carcinogenesis and to sustain the growth of a tumor, since differentiated cells (constrained by the Hayflick Limit) cannot divide indefinitely. If most tumor cells are endowed with stem cell properties, targeting tumor size directly is a valid strategy. If they are a small minority, targeting them may be more effective. Another debate is over the origin of CSCs - whether from disregulation of normal stem cells or from a more specialized population that acquired the ability to self-renew (which is related to the issue of stem cell plasticity).

Evidence

The first conclusive evidence for CSCs came in 1997. Bonnet and Dick isolated a subpopulation of leukemia cells that expressed surface marker CD34, but not CD38. The authors established that the $CD34^+/CD38^-$ subpopulation is capable of initiating tumors in NOD/SCID mice that were histologically similar to the donor. The first evidence of a solid tumor cancer stem-like cell followed in 2002 with the discovery of a clonogenic, sphere-forming cell isolated and characterized from human brain gliomas. Human cortical glial tumors contain neural stem-like cells expressing astroglial and neuronal markers *in vitro*.

In cancer research experiments, tumor cells are sometimes injected into an experimental animal to establish a tumor. Disease progression is then followed in time and novel drugs can be tested for their efficacy. Tumor formation requires thousands or tens of thousands of cells to be introduced. Classically, this was explained by poor methodology (i.e., the tumor cells lose their viability during transfer) or the critical importance of the microenvironment, the particular biochemical surroundings of the injected cells. Supporters of the CSC paradigm argue that only a small fraction of the injected cells, the CSCs, have the potential to generate a tumor. In human acute myeloid leukemia the frequency of these cells is less than 1 in 10,000.

Further evidence comes from histology. Many tumors are heterogeneous and contain multiple cell types native to the host organ. Heterogeneity is commonly retained by tumor metastases. This suggests that the cell that produced them had the capacity to generate multiple cell types, a classical hallmark of stem cells.

The existence of leukemia stem cells prompted research into other cancers. CSCs have recently been identified in several solid tumors, including:

- Brain
- Breast
- Colon
- Ovary
- Pancreas
- Prostate
- Melanoma
- Multiple Myeloma
- Non-melanoma skin cancer

Mechanistic and Mathematical Models

Once the pathways to cancer are hypothesized, it is possible to develop predictive mathematical models, e.g., based on the cell compartment method. For instance, the growths of abnormal cells can be denoted with specific mutation probabilities. Such a model predicted that repeated insult to mature cells increases the formation of abnormal progeny and the risk of cancer. The clinical efficacy of such models remains unestablished.

ORIGIN

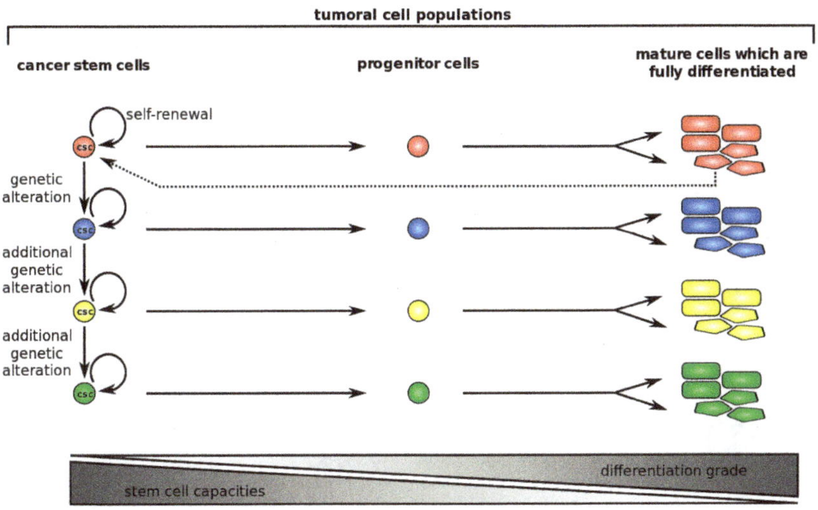

Figure 6: Hierarchical organisation of a tumour according to the CSC model.

The origin of CSCs is an active research area. The answer may depend on the tumor type and phenotype. So far the hypothesis that tumors originate from a single "cell of origin" has not been demonstrated using the cancer stem cell model. This is because cancer stem cells are not present in end-stage tumors.

Origin hypotheses include mutants in developing stem or progenitor cells, mutants in adult stem cells or adult progenitor cells and mutant, differentiated cells that acquire stem-like attributes. These theories often focus on a tumor's "cell of origin".

Hypotheses

Stem cell mutation

The "mutation in stem cell niche populations during development" hypothesis claims that these developing stem populations are mutated and then reproduce so that the mutation is shared by many descendants. These daughter cells are much closer to becoming tumors and their numbers increase the chance of a cancerous mutation.

Adult stem cells

Another theory associates adult stem cells (ASC) with tumor formation. This is most often associated with tissues with a high rate of cell turnover (such as the skin or gut). In these tissues, ASCs are candidates because of their frequent cell divisions (compared to most ASCs) in conjunction with the long lifespan of ASCs. This combination creates the ideal set of circumstances for mutations to accumulate: mutation accumulation is the primary factor that drives cancer initiation. Evidence shows that the association represents an actual phenomenon, although specific cancers have been linked to a specific cause.

De-differentiation

De-differentiation of mutated cells may create stem cell-like characteristics, suggesting that any cell might become a cancer stem cell. In other words, a fully differentiated cell undergoes several mutations that drive it back to a stem-like state.

Hierarchy

The concept of tumor hierarchy claims that a tumor is a heterogeneous population of mutant cells, all of which share some mutations, but vary in specific phenotype. A tumor hosts several types of stem cells, one optimal to the specific environment and other less successful lines. These secondary lines may be more successful in other environments, allowing the tumor to adapt, including adaptation to therapeutic intervention. If correct, this concept impacts cancer stem cell-specific treatment regimes. Such a hierarchy would complicate attempts to pinpoint the origin.

IDENTIFICATION

CSCs, now reported in most human tumors, are commonly identified and enriched using strategies for identifying normal stem cells that are similar across studies. These procedures include fluorescence-activated cell sorting (FACS), with antibodies directed at cell-surface markers and functional approaches including side population assay or Aldefluor assay. The CSC-enriched result is then implanted, at various doses, in immune-deficient mice to assess its tumor development capacity. This *in vivo* assay is called a limiting dilution assay. The tumor cell subsets that can initiate tumor development at low cell numbers are further tested for self-renewal capacity in serial tumor studies.

CSC can also be identified by efflux of incorporated Hoechst dyes via multidrug resistance (MDR) and ATP-binding cassette (ABC) Transporters.

Another approach is sphere-forming assays. Many normal stem cells such as hematopoietics or stem cells from tissues, under special culture conditions, form three-dimensional spheres that can differentiate. As with normal stem cells, the CSCs isolated from brain or prostate tumors also have the ability to form anchor-independent spheres.

HETEROGENEITY (MARKERS)

CSCs have been identified in various solid tumors. Markers specific for normal stem cells are commonly used for isolating CSCs from solid and hematological tumors. Cell surface markers have proved useful for isolation of CSC-enriched populations including CD133 (also known as PROM1), CD44, CD24, EpCAM (epithelial cell adhesion molecule, also known as epithelial specific antigen, ESA), THY1, ATP-binding cassette B5 (ABCB5), and CD200.

CD133 (prominin 1) is a five-transmembrane domain glycoprotein expressed on $CD34^+$ stem and progenitor cells, in endothelial precursors and fetal neural stem cells. It has been detected using its glycosylated epitope known as AC133.

EpCAM (epithelial cell adhesion molecule, ESA, TROP1) is hemophilic Ca^{2+}-independent cell adhesion molecule expressed on the basolateral surface of most epithelial cells.

CD90 (THY1) is a glycosylphosphatidylinositol glycoprotein anchored in the plasma membrane and involved in signal transduction. It may also mediate adhesion between thymocytes and thymic stroma.

CD44 (PGP1) is an adhesion molecule that has pleiotropic roles in cell signaling, migration and homing. It has multiple isoforms, including CD44H, which exhibits high affinity for hyaluronate and CD44V which has metastatic properties.

CD24 (HSA) is a glycosylated glycosylphosphatidylinositol-anchored adhesion molecule, which has co-stimulatory role in B and T cells.

CD200 (OX-2) is a type 1 membrane glycoprotein, which delivers an inhibitory signal to immune cells including T cells, natural killer cells and macrophages.

ALDH is a ubiquitous aldehyde dehydrogenase family of enzymes, which catalyzes the oxidation of aromatic aldehydes to carboxyl acids. For instance, it has a role in conversion of retinol to retinoic acid, which is essential for survival.

The first solid malignancy from which CSCs were isolated and identified was breast cancer and they are the most intensely studied. Breast CSCs have been enriched in $CD44^+CD24^{-/low}$, SP and $ALDH^+$subpopulations. Breast CSCs are apparently phenotypically diverse. CSC marker expression in breast cancer cells is apparently heterogeneous and breast CSC populations vary across tumors.Both $CD44^+CD24^-$ and $CD44^+CD24^+$ cell populations are tumor initiating cells; however, CSC are most highly enriched using the marker profile $CD44^+CD49f^{hi}CD133/2^{hi}$.

CSCs have been reported in many brain tumors. Stem-like tumor cells have been identified using cell surface markers including CD133, SSEA-1 (stage-specific embryonic antigen-1), EGFR and CD44. The use of CD133 for identification of brain tumor stem-like cells may be problematic because tumorigenic cells are found in both $CD133^+$ and $CD133^-$ cells in some gliomas and some $CD133^+$ brain tumor cells may not possess tumor-initiating capacity.

CSCs were reported in human colon cancer. For their identification, cell surface markers such as CD133, CD44 and ABCB5, functional analysis including clonal analysis and Aldefluor assay were used. Using CD133 as a positive marker for colon CSCs generated conflicting results. The AC133 epitope, but not the CD133 protein, is specifically expressed in colon CSCs and its expression is lost upon differentiation. In addition, $CD44^+$ colon cancer cells and additional sub-fractionation of $CD44^+EpCAM^+$ cell population with CD166 enhance the success of tumor engraftments.

Multiple CSCs have been reported in prostate, lung and many other organs, including liver, pancreas, kidney or ovary. In prostate cancer, the tumor-initiating cells have been identified in $CD44^+$ cell subset as $CD44^+\alpha2\beta1^+$, $TRA\text{-}1\text{-}60^+CD151^+CD166^+$ or $ALDH^+$

cell populations. Putative markers for lung CSCs have been reported, including $CD133^+$, $ALDH^+$, $CD44^+$ and oncofetal protein $5T4^+$.

METASTASIS

Metastasis is the major cause of tumor lethality. However, not every tumor cell can metastasize. This potential depends on factors that determine growth, angiogenesis, invasion and other basic processes.

Epithelial-Mesenchymal Transition

In epithelial tumors, the epithelial-mesenchymal transition (EMT) is considered to be a crucial event.EMT and the reverse transition from mesenchymal to an epithelial phenotype (MET) are involved in embryonic development, which involves disruption of epithelial cell homeostasis and the acquisition of a migratory mesenchymal phenotype. EMT appears to be controlled by canonical pathways such as WNT and transforming growth factor β.

EMT`s important feature is the loss of membrane E-cadherin in adherens junctions, where β-catenin may play a significant role. Translocation of β-catenin from adherens junctions to the nucleus may lead to a loss of E-cadherin and subsequently to EMT. Nuclear β-catenin apparently can directly, transcriptionally activate EMT-associated target genes, such as the E-cadherin gene repressor SLUG (also known as SNAI2). Mechanical properties of the tumor microenvironment, such as hypoxia, can contribute to CSC survival and metastatic potential through stabilization of hypoxia inducible factors through interactions with ROS (reactive oxygen species).

Tumor cells undergoing an EMT may be precursors for metastatic cancer cells, or even metastatic CSCs. In the invasive edge of pancreatic carcinoma, a subset of $CD133^+CXCR4^+$ (receptor for CXCL12 chemokine also known as a SDF1 ligand) cells was defined. These cells exhibited significantly stronger migratory activity than their counterpart $CD133^+CXCR4^-$ cells, but both showed similar tumor development capacity. Moreover, inhibition of the CXCR4 receptor reduced metastatic potential without altering tumorigenic capacity.

Two-phase Expression Pattern

In breast cancer $CD44^+CD24^{-/low}$ cells are detectable in metastatic pleural effusions. By contrast, an increased number of $CD24^+$ cells have been identified in distant metastases in breast cancer patients.It is possible that $CD44^+CD24^{-/low}$ cells initially metastasize and in the new site change their phenotype and undergo limited differentiation. The two-phase expression pattern hypothesis proposes two forms of cancer stem cells - stationary (SCS) and mobile (MCS). SCS are embedded in tissue and persist in differentiated areas throughout tumor progression. MCS are located at the tumor-host interface. These cells are apparently derived from SCS through the acquisition of transient EMT (Figure 7).

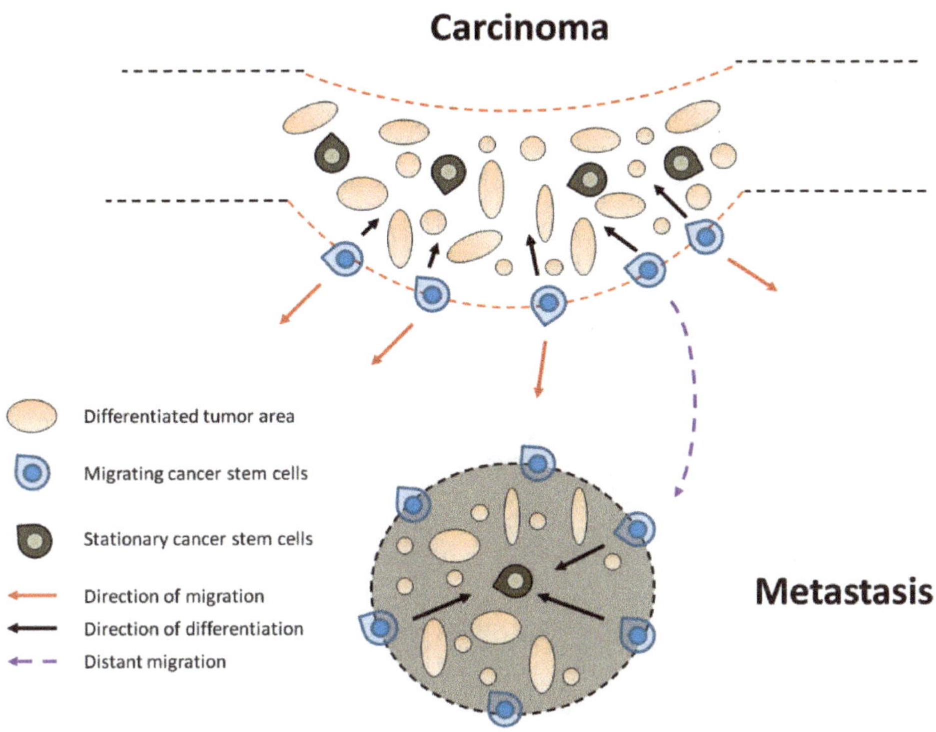

Figure 7: The concept of migrating cancer stem cells (MSC). Stationary cancer stem cells are embedded in begin carcinomas and these cells are detectable in the differentiated central area of a tumor. The important step toward malignancy is the induction of epithelial mesenchymal transition (EMT) in the stationary cancer stem cells (SCS), which become mobile or migrating cancer stem cells. MCS cells divide asymmetrically. One daughter cell starts proliferation and differentiation. The remaining MCS migrates a short distance before undergoing new asymmetric division, or starts dissemination through blood vessela or lymphatic vessels and produces a metastasis.

Implications

CSCs have implications for cancer therapy, including for disease identification, selective drug targets, prevention of metastasis and intervention strategies.

Treatment

Somatic stem cells are naturally resistant to chemotherapeutic agents. They produce various pumps (such as MDR) that pump out drugs and DNA repair proteins. They have a slow rate of cell turnover (chemotherapeutic agents naturally target rapidly replicating cells). CSCs that develop from normal stem cells may also produce these proteins, which could increase their resistance towards chemotherapy. The surviving CSCs then repopulate the tumor, causing a relapse.

Targeting

Selectively targeting CSCs may allow treatment of aggressive, non-resectable tumors, as well as prevent metastasis and relapse. The hypothesis suggests that upon CSC elimination, cancer could regress due to differentiation and/or cell death.The fraction of tumor cells that are CSCs and therefore need to be eliminated is unclear.

Studies looked for specific markers and for proteomic and genomic tumor signatures that distinguish CSCs from others. In 2009, scientists identified the compound salinomycin, which selectively reduces the proportion of breast CSCs in mice by more than 100-fold relative to Paclitaxel, a commonly used chemotherapeutic agent. Some types of cancer cells can survive treatment with salinomycin through autophagy, whereby cells use acidic organelles such as lysosomes to degrade and recycle certain types of proteins. The use of autophagy inhibitors can kill cancer stem cells that survive by autophagy.

The cell surface receptor interleukin-3 receptor-alpha (CD123) is overexpressed on CD34+CD38- leukemic stem cells (LSCs) in acute myelogenous leukemia (AML) but not on normal CD34+CD38- bone marrow cells. Treating AML-engrafted NOD/SCID mice with a CD123-specific monoclonal antibody impaired LSCs homing to the bone marrow and reduced overall AML cell repopulation including the proportion of LSCs in secondary mouse recipients.

A 2015 study packaged nanoparticles with miR-34a and ammonium bicarbonate and delivered them to prostate CSCs in a mouse model. Then they irradiated the area with near-infrared laser light. This caused the nanoparticles to swell three times or more in size bursting the endosomes and dispersing the RNA in the cell. miR-34a can lower the levels of CD44.

Pathways

The design of new drugs for targeting CSCs requires understanding the cellular mechanisms that regulate cell proliferation. The first advances in this area were made with hematopoietic stem cells (HSCs) and their transformed counterparts in leukemia, the disease for which the origin of CSCs is best understood. Stem cells of many organs share the same cellular pathways as leukemia-derived HSCs.

A normal stem cell may be transformed into a CSC through disregulation of the proliferation and differentiation pathways controlling it or by inducing oncoprotein activity.

BMI-1

The Polycomb group transcriptional repressor Bmi-1 was discovered as a common oncogene activated in lymphoma and later shown to regulate HSCs. The role of Bmi-1 has been illustrated in neural stem cells. The pathway appears to be active in CSCs of pediatric brain tumors.

Notch

The Notch pathway plays a role in controlling stem cell proliferation for several cell types including hematopoietic, neural and mammary SCs. Components of this pathway have been proposed to act as oncogenes in mammary and other tumors.

A branch of the Notch signaling pathway that involves the transcription factor Hes3 regulates a number of cultured cells with CSC characteristics obtained from glioblastoma patients.

Sonic hedgehog and Wnt

These developmental pathways are SC regulators. Both Sonic hedgehog (SHH) and Wnt pathways are commonly hyperactivated in tumors and are necessary to sustain tumor growth. However, the Gli transcription factors that are regulated by SHH take their name from gliomas, where they are highly expressed. A degree of crosstalk exists between the two pathways and they are commonly activated together. By contrast, in colon cancer hedgehog signalling appears to antagonise Wnt.

Sonic hedgehog blockers are available, such as cyclopamine. A water-soluble cyclopamine may be more effective in cancer treatment. DMAPT, a water-soluble derivative of parthenolide, induces oxidative stress and inhibits NF-κB signaling for AML (leukemia) and possibly myeloma and prostate cancer. Telomerase is a study subject in CSC physiology. GRN163L (Imetelstat) was recently started in trials to target myeloma stem cells.

Wnt signaling can become independent of regular stimuli, through mutations in downstream oncogenes and tumor suppressor genes that become permanently activated even though the normal receptor has not received a signal. β-catenin binds to transcription factors such as the protein TCF4 and in combination the molecules activate the necessary genes. LF3 strongly inhibits this binding *in vitro,* in cell lines and reduced tumor growth in mouse models. It prevented replication and reduced their ability to migrate, all without affecting healthy cells. No cancer stem cells remained after treatment. The discovery was the product of "rational drug design", involving AlphaScreens and ELISA technologies.

REFERENCES

1. Mukherjee, Siddhartha. "The Cancer Sleeper Cell". New York Times. New York Times. Retrieved 15 July 2014.
2. Heppner, GH; Miller, BE (1983). "Tumor heterogeneity: biological implications and therapeutic consequences". Cancer metastasis reviews. 2 (1): 5–23. doi:10.1007/BF00046903. PMID 6616442.
3. Bonnet, D; Dick, JE (July 1997). "Human acute myeloid leukemia is organized as a hierarchy that originates from a primitive hematopoietic cell". Nature Medicine. 3 (7): 730–7. doi:10.1038/nm0797-730. PMID 9212098.
4. PMID 24060864 Missing or empty |title= (help)
5. Shakleton, M; Quintana, E; Fearon, ER; Morrison, SJ (Sept 4, 2009).

"Heterogeneity in Cancer: Cancer Stem Cells versus Clonal Evolution". Cell Press. 138 (5): 822–9. doi:10.1016/j.cell.2009.08.017. PMID 19737509. Check date values in: |date= (help) Cite error: Invalid <ref> tag; name "2.2F12" defined multiple times with different content (see the help page).

6. , PMID 24416258 Missing or empty |title= (help)
7. , PMID 24607403 Missing or empty |title= (help)
8. Barabé, F; Kennedy, JA; Hope, KJ; Dick, JE (Apr 27, 2007). "Modeling the initiation and progression of human acute leukemia in mice". Science. 316 (5824): 600–4. doi:10.1126/science.1139851. PMID 17463288.
9. Nowell, PC (Oct 1, 1976). "The clonal evolution of tumor cell populations". Science. 194 (4260): 23–8. doi:10.1126/science.959840. PMID 959840.
10. , PMID 25621103 Missing or empty |title= (help)
11. Gupta PB, Chaffer CL, Weinberg RA (2009). "Cancer stem cells: mirage or reality?". Nat Med. 15 (9): 1010–2. doi:10.1038/nm0909-1010. PMID 19734877. [permanent dead link]>
12. Hayflick L (1965). "The Limited in Vitro Lifetime of Human Diploid Cell Strains". Exp Cell Res. 37 (3): 614–636. doi:10.1016/0014-4827(65)90211-9. PMID 14315085.
13. ^ Jump up to:a b c Bonnet D, Dick JE (July 1997). "Human acute myeloid leukemia is organized as a hierarchy that originates from a primitive hematopoietic cell". Nature Medicine. 3 (7): 730–7. doi:10.1038/nm0797-730. PMID 9212098.
14. Ignatova TN, Kukekov VG, Laywell ED, Suslov ON, Vrionis FD, Steindler DA (Sep 2002). "Human cortical glial tumors contain neural stem-like cells expressing astroglial and neuronal markers in vitro.". Glia. 39 (3): 193–206. doi:10.1002/glia.10094. PMID 12203386.
15. Singh SK, Clarke ID, Terasaki M, Bonn VE, Hawkins C, Squire J, Dirks PB (September 2003). "Identification of a cancer stem cell in human brain tumors". Cancer Research. 63 (18): 5821–8. PMID 14522905.
16. ^ Jump up to:a b Al-Hajj M, Wicha MS, Benito-Hernandez A, Morrison SJ, Clarke MF (April 2003). "Prospective identification of tumorigenic breast cancer cells". Proceedings of the National Academy of Sciences of the United States of America. 100 (7): 3983–8. doi:10.1073/pnas.0530291100. PMC 153034 . PMID 12629218.
17. O'Brien CA, Pollett A, Gallinger S, Dick JE (January 2007). "A human colon cancer cell capable of initiating tumour growth in immunodeficient mice". Nature. 445 (7123): 106–10. doi:10.1038/nature05372. PMID 17122772.
18. Zhang S, Balch C, Chan MW, Lai HC, Matei D, Schilder JM, Yan PS, Huang TH, Nephew KP (June 2008). "Identification and characterization of ovarian cancer-initiating cells from primary human tumors". Cancer Research. 68 (11): 4311–20. doi:10.1158/0008-5472.CAN-08-0364. PMC 2553722 . PMID 18519691.
19. Alvero, A. B.; Chen, R; Fu, H. H.; Montagna, M; Schwartz, P. E.; Rutherford, T; Silasi, D. A.; Steffensen, K. D.; Waldstrom, M; Visintin, I; Mor, G (Jan

2009). "Molecular phenotyping of human ovarian cancer stem cells unravels the mechanisms for repair and chemoresistance". Cell Cycle. 8 (1): 158–66. doi:10.4161/cc.8.1.7533. PMC 3041590 . PMID 19158483.

20. Alvero AB, Chen R, Fu HH, Montagna M, Schwartz PE, Rutherford T, Silasi DA, Steffensen KD, Waldstrom M (Jan 2009). "Molecular phenotyping of human ovarian cancer stem cells unravels the mechanisms for repair and chemoresistance". Cell Cycle. 8 (1): 158–66. doi:10.4161/cc.8.1.7533. PMC 3041590 . PMID 19158483.

21. Li C, Heidt DG, Dalerba P, Burant CF, Zhang L, Adsay V, Wicha M, Clarke MF, Simeone DM (February 2007). "Identification of pancreatic cancer stem cells". Cancer Research. 67 (3): 1030–7. doi:10.1158/0008-5472.CAN-06-2030. PMID 17283135.

22. Maitland NJ, Collins AT (June 2008). "Prostate cancer stem cells: a new target for therapy". J. Clin. Oncol. 26 (17): 2862–70. doi:10.1200/JCO.2007.15.1472. PMID 18539965.

23. Lang Sh; Frame F; Collins A (January 2009). "Prostate cancer stem cells". J. Pathol. 217 (2): 299–306. doi:10.1002/path.2478. PMC 2673349 . PMID 19040209.

24. Schatton T; Murphy GF; Frank, NY; Yamaura K; Waaga-Gasser AM; Gasser M; Zhan Q; Jordan S; Duncan LM; Weishaupt C; Fuhlbrigge RC; Kupper TS; Sayegh MH; Frank MH (Jan 2008). "Identification of cells initiating human melanomas". Nature. 451 (7176): 345–9. doi:10.1038/nature06489. PMC 3660705 . PMID 18202660.

25. Boiko AD, Razorenova OV, van de Rijn M, Swetter SM, Johnson DL, Ly DP, Butler PD, Yang GP, Joshua B, Kaplan MJ, Longaker MT, Weissman IL (Jul 2010). "Human melanoma-initiating cells express neural crest nerve growth factor receptor CD271". Nature. 466 (7302): 133–7. doi:10.1038/nature09161. PMC 2898751 . PMID 20596026.

26. Schmidt P, Kopecky C, Hombach A, Zigrino P, Mauch C, Abken H (Feb 2011). "Eradication of melanomas by targeted elimination of a minor subset of tumor cells". PNAS. 108 (6): 2474–9. doi:10.1073/pnas.1009069108. PMC 3038763 . PMID 21282657.

27. Civenni G, Walter A, Kobert N, Mihic-Probst D, Zipser M, Belloni B, Seifert B, Moch H, Dummer R, van den Broek M, Sommer L (Mar 2011). "Human CD271-Positive Melanoma Stem Cells Associated with Metastasis Establish Tumor Heterogeneity and Long-Term Growth". Cancer Res. 71 (8): 3098–109. doi:10.1158/0008-5472.CAN-10-3997. PMID 21393506.

28. Matsui W, Huff CA, Wang Q, et al. (March 2004). "Characterization of clonogenic multiple myeloma cells". Blood. 103 (6): 2332–6. doi:10.1182/blood-2003-09-3064. PMC 3311914 . PMID 14630803.

29. Matsui W, Wang Q, Barber JP, et al. (January 2008). "Clonogenic multiple myeloma progenitors, stem cell properties, and drug resistance". Cancer Res. 68 (1): 190–7. doi:10.1158/0008-5472.CAN-07-3096. PMC 2603142 . PMID

18172311.

30. Colmont CS, Benketah A, Reed SH, Hawk NV, Telford WG, Ohyama M, Udey MC, Yee CL, Vogel JC, Patel GK (Jan 2013). "CD200-expressing human basal cell carcinoma cells initiate tumor growth" (PDF). PNAS. 110 (4): 1434–9. doi:10.1073/pnas.1211655110. PMC 3557049 . PMID 23292936.
31. Patel GK, Yee CL, Terunuma A, Telford WG, Voong N, Yuspa SH, Vogel JC (Feb 2012). "Identification and characterization of tumor-initiating cells in human primary cutaneous squamous cell carcinoma" (PDF). J Invest Dermatol. 132 (2): 401–409. doi:10.1038/jid.2011.317. PMC 3258300 . PMID 22011906.
32. Preziosi, Luigi (2003). Cancer Modelling and Simulation. Boca Raton: CRC Press. ISBN 1-58488-361-8.
33. Ganguly R, Puri IK (February 2006). "Mathematical model for the cancer stem cell hypothesis". Cell proliferation. 39 (1): 3–14. doi:10.1111/j.1365-2184.2006.00369.x. PMID 16426418.
34. Ganguly R, Puri IK (June 2007). "Mathematical model for chemotherapeutic drug efficacy in arresting tumour growth based on the cancer stem cell hypothesis". Cell proliferation. 40 (3): 338–354. doi:10.1111/j.1365-2184.2007.00434.x. PMID 17531079.
35. Wang Y, Yang J, Zheng H, Tomasek GJ, Zhang P, McKeever PE, Lee EY, Zhu Y (June 2009). "Expression of mutant p53 proteins implicates a lineage relationship between neural stem cells and malignant astrocytic glioma in a murine model". Cancer Cell. 15 (6): 514–26. doi:10.1016/j.ccr.2009.04.001. PMC 2721466 . PMID 19477430.
36. López-Lázaro, Miguel (2015-01-01). "The migration ability of stem cells can explain the existence of cancer of unknown primary site. Rethinking metastasis". Oncoscience. 2 (5): 467–475. doi:10.18632/oncoscience.159. ISSN 2331-4737. PMC 4468332 . PMID 26097879.
37. López-Lázaro, Miguel (2015-08-18). "Stem cell division theory of cancer". Cell Cycle (Georgetown, Tex.). 14 (16): 2547–2548. doi:10.1080/15384101.2015.1062330. ISSN 1551-4005. PMID 26090957.
38. Clarke MF, Dick JE, Dirks PB, Eaves CJ, Jamieson CH, Jones DL, Visvader J, Weissman IL, Wahl GM (October 2006). "Cancer stem cells--perspectives on current status and future directions: AACR Workshop on cancer stem cells". Cancer Research. 66 (19): 9339–44. doi:10.1158/0008-5472.CAN-06-3126. PMID 16990346.
39. Golebiewska, A; Brons, NH; Bjerkvig, R; Niclou, SP (Feb 4, 2011). "Critical appraisal of the side population assay in stem cell and cancer stem cell research". Cell stem cell. 8 (2): 136–47. doi:10.1016/j.stem.2011.01.007. PMID 21295271.
40. ^ Jump up to:a b Scharenberg, CW; Harkey, MA; Torok-Storb, B (Jan 15, 2002). "The ABCG2 transporter is an efficient Hoechst 33342 efflux pump and is preferentially expressed by immature human hematopoietic progenitors". Blood. 99 (2): 507–12. doi:10.1182/blood.V99.2.507. PMID 11781231.

41. Pastrana, E; Silva-Vargas, V; Doetsch, F (May 6, 2011). "Eyes wide open: a critical review of sphere-formation as an assay for stem cells". Cell stem cell. 8 (5): 486–98. doi:10.1016/j.stem.2011.04.007. PMC 3633588 . PMID 21549325.
42. Nicolis, SK (February 2007). "Cancer stem cells and "stemness" genes in neuro-oncology". Neurobiology of disease. 25 (2): 217–29. doi:10.1016/j.nbd.2006.08.022. PMID 17141509.
43. Al-Hajj, M; Wicha, MS; Benito-Hernandez, A; Morrison, SJ; Clarke, MF (Apr 1, 2003). "Prospective identification of tumorigenic breast cancer cells". Proceedings of the National Academy of Sciences of the United States of America. 100 (7): 3983–8. doi:10.1073/pnas.0530291100. PMC 153034 . PMID 12629218.
44. Meng E, Mitra A, Tripathi K, Finan MA, Scalici J, McClellan S, Madeira da Silva L, Reed E, Shevde LA, Palle K, Rocconi RP (Sep 12, 2014). "ALDH1A1 Maintains Ovarian Cancer Stem Cell-Like Properties by Altered Regulation of Cell Cycle Checkpoint and DNA Repair Network Signaling". PLoS ONE. 9 (9): e107142. doi:10.1371/journal.pone.0107142. PMC 4162571 . PMID 25216266.
45. Visvader, JE; Lindeman, GJ (October 2008). "Cancer stem cells in solid tumours: accumulating evidence and unresolved questions". Nature Reviews Cancer. 8 (10): 755–68. doi:10.1038/nrc2499. PMID 18784658.
46. Hirschmann-Jax, C; Foster, AE; Wulf, GG; Nuchtern, JG; Jax, TW; Gobel, U; Goodell, MA; Brenner, MK (Sep 28, 2004). "A distinct "side population" of cells with high drug efflux capacity in human tumor cells". Proceedings of the National Academy of Sciences of the United States of America. 101 (39): 14228–33. doi:10.1073/pnas.0400067101. PMC 521140 . PMID 15381773.
47. Ginestier, C; Hur, MH; Charafe-Jauffret, E; Monville, F; Dutcher, J; Brown, M; Jacquemier, J; Viens, P; Kleer, CG; Liu, S; Schott, A; Hayes, D; Birnbaum, D; Wicha, MS; Dontu, G (November 2007). "ALDH1 is a marker of normal and malignant human mammary stem cells and a predictor of poor clinical outcome". Cell stem cell. 1 (5): 555–67. doi:10.1016/j.stem.2007.08.014. PMC 2423808 . PMID 18371393.
48. Pece, S; Tosoni, D; Confalonieri, S; Mazzarol, G; Vecchi, M; Ronzoni, S; Bernard, L; Viale, G; Pelicci, PG; Di Fiore, PP (Jan 8, 2010). "Biological and molecular heterogeneity of breast cancers correlates with their cancer stem cell content". Cell. 140 (1): 62–73. doi:10.1016/j.cell.2009.12.007. PMID 20074520.
49. Deng, S; Yang, X; Lassus, H; Liang, S; Kaur, S; Ye, Q; Li, C; Wang, LP; Roby, KF; Orsulic, S; Connolly, DC; Zhang, Y; Montone, K; Bützow, R; Coukos, G; Zhang, L (Apr 21, 2010). Cao, Yihai, ed. "Distinct expression levels and patterns of stem cell marker, aldehyde dehydrogenase isoform 1 (ALDH1), in human epithelial cancers". PLoS ONE. 5 (4): e10277. doi:10.1371/journal.pone.0010277. PMC 2858084 . PMID 20422001.
50. Meyer, MJ; Fleming, JM; Lin, AF; Hussnain, SA; Ginsburg, E; Vonderhaar, BK (Jun 1, 2010). "CD44posCD49fhiCD133/2hi defines xenograft-initiating cells in estrogen receptor-negative breast cancer". Cancer Research. 70 (11): 4624–33. doi:10.1158/0008-5472.CAN-09-3619. PMID 20484027.

51. Singh, SK; Hawkins, C; Clarke, ID; Squire, JA; Bayani, J; Hide, T; Henkelman, RM; Cusimano, MD; Dirks, PB (Nov 18, 2004). "Identification of human brain tumour initiating cells". Nature. 432 (7015): 396–401. doi:10.1038/nature03128. PMID 15549107.
52. Son, MJ; Woolard, K; Nam, DH; Lee, J; Fine, HA (May 8, 2009). "SSEA-1 is an enrichment marker for tumor-initiating cells in human glioblastoma". Cell stem cell. 4 (5): 440–52. doi:10.1016/j.stem.2009.03.003. PMID 19427293.
53. ^ Jump up to:a b Mazzoleni, S; Politi, LS; Pala, M; Cominelli, M; Franzin, A; Sergi Sergi, L; Falini, A; De Palma, M; Bulfone, A; Poliani, PL; Galli, R (Oct 1, 2010). "Epidermal growth factor receptor expression identifies functionally and molecularly distinct tumor-initiating cells in human glioblastoma multiforme and is required for gliomagenesis". Cancer Research. 70 (19): 7500–13. doi:10.1158/0008-5472.CAN-10-2353. PMID 20858720.
54. Anido, J; Sáez-Borderías, A; Gonzàlez-Juncà, A; Rodón, L; Folch, G; Carmona, MA; Prieto-Sánchez, RM; Barba, I; Martínez-Sáez, E; Prudkin, L; Cuartas, I; Raventós, C; Martínez-Ricarte, F; Poca, MA; García-Dorado, D; Lahn, MM; Yingling, JM; Rodón, J; Sahuquillo, J; Baselga, J; Seoane, J (Dec 14, 2010). "TGF-β Receptor Inhibitors Target the CD44(high)/Id1(high) Glioma-Initiating Cell Population in Human Glioblastoma". Cancer Cell. 18 (6): 655–68. doi:10.1016/j.ccr.2010.10.023. PMID 21156287.
55. ^ Jump up to:a b O'Brien, CA; Pollett, A; Gallinger, S; Dick, JE (Jan 4, 2007). "A human colon cancer cell capable of initiating tumour growth in immunodeficient mice". Nature. 445 (7123): 106–10. doi:10.1038/nature05372. PMID 17122772.
56. ^ Jump up to:a b Dalerba, P; Dylla, SJ; Park, IK; Liu, R; Wang, X; Cho, RW; Hoey, T; Gurney, A; Huang, EH; Simeone, DM; Shelton, AA; Parmiani, G; Castelli, C; Clarke, MF (Jun 12, 2007). "Phenotypic characterization of human colorectal cancer stem cells". Proceedings of the National Academy of Sciences of the United States of America. 104 (24): 10158–63. doi:10.1073/pnas.0703478104. PMC 1891215 . PMID 17548814.
57. Wilson, BJ; Schatton, T; Zhan, Q; Gasser, M; Ma, J; Saab, KR; Schanche, R; Waaga-Gasser, AM; Gold, JS; Huang, Q; Murphy, GF; Frank, MH; Frank, NY (Aug 1, 2011). "ABCB5 identifies a therapy-refractory tumor cell population in colorectal cancer patients". Cancer Research. 71 (15): 5307–16. doi:10.1158/0008-5472.CAN-11-0221. PMC 3395026 . PMID 21652540.
58. Odoux, C; Fohrer, H; Hoppo, T; Guzik, L; Stolz, DB; Lewis, DW; Gollin, SM; Gamblin, TC; Geller, DA; Lagasse, E (Sep 1, 2008). "A stochastic model for cancer stem cell origin in metastatic colon cancer". Cancer Research. 68 (17): 6932–41. doi:10.1158/0008-5472.CAN-07-5779. PMC 2562348 . PMID 18757407.
59. Huang, EH; Hynes, MJ; Zhang, T; Ginestier, C; Dontu, G; Appelman, H; Fields, JZ; Wicha, MS; Boman, BM (Apr 15, 2009). "Aldehyde dehydrogenase 1 is a marker for normal and malignant human colonic stem cells (SC) and tracks SC overpopulation during colon tumorigenesis". Cancer Research. 69 (8): 3382–9. doi:10.1158/0008-5472.CAN-08-4418. PMC 2789401 . PMID 19336570.
60. Kemper, K; Sprick, MR; de Bree, M; Scopelliti, A; Vermeulen, L; Hoek, M;

Zeilstra, J; Pals, ST; Mehmet, H; Stassi, G; Medema, JP (Jan 15, 2010). "The AC133 epitope, but not the CD133 protein, is lost upon cancer stem cell differentiation". Cancer Research. 70 (2): 719–29. doi:10.1158/0008-5472.CAN-09-1820. PMID 20068153.

61. Liu, C; Kelnar, K; Liu, B; Chen, X; Calhoun-Davis, T; Li, H; Patrawala, L; Yan, H; Jeter, C; Honorio, S; Wiggins, JF; Bader, AG; Fagin, R; Brown, D; Tang, DG (February 2011). "The microRNA miR-34a inhibits prostate cancer stem cells and metastasis by directly repressing CD44". Nature Medicine. 17 (2): 211–5. doi:10.1038/nm.2284. PMC 3076220 . PMID 21240262.

62. Ho, MM; Ng, AV; Lam, S; Hung, JY (May 15, 2007). "Side population in human lung cancer cell lines and tumors is enriched with stem-like cancer cells". Cancer Research. 67 (10): 4827–33. doi:10.1158/0008-5472.CAN-06-3557. PMID 17510412.

63. Patrawala, L; Calhoun, T; Schneider-Broussard, R; Li, H; Bhatia, B; Tang, S; Reilly, JG; Chandra, D; Zhou, J; Claypool, K; Coghlan, L; Tang, DG (Mar 16, 2006). "Highly purified CD44+ prostate cancer cells from xenograft human tumors are enriched in tumorigenic and metastatic progenitor cells". Oncogene. 25 (12): 1696–708. doi:10.1038/sj.onc.1209327. PMID 16449977.

64. Dubrovska, A; Kim, S; Salamone, RJ; Walker, JR; Maira, SM; García-Echeverría, C; Schultz, PG; Reddy, VA (Jan 6, 2009). "The role of PTEN/Akt/PI3K signaling in the maintenance and viability of prostate cancer stem-like cell populations". Proceedings of the National Academy of Sciences of the United States of America. 106 (1): 268–73. doi:10.1073/pnas.0810956106. PMC 2629188 . PMID 19116269.

65. Rajasekhar, VK; Studer, L; Gerald, W; Socci, ND; Scher, HI (Jan 18, 2011). "Tumour-initiating stem-like cells in human prostate cancer exhibit increased NF-κB signalling". Nature Communications. 2 (1): 162–. doi:10.1038/ncomms1159. PMC 3105310 . PMID 21245843.

66. Li, T; Su, Y; Mei, Y; Leng, Q; Leng, B; Liu, Z; Stass, SA; Jiang, F (February 2010). "ALDH1A1 is a marker for malignant prostate stem cells and predictor of prostate cancer patients` outcome". Laboratory Investigation. 90 (2): 234–44. doi:10.1038/labinvest.2009.127. PMC 3552330 . PMID 20010854.

67. Eramo, A; Lotti, F; Sette, G; Pilozzi, E; Biffoni, M; Di Virgilio, A; Conticello, C; Ruco, L; Peschle, C; De Maria, R (March 2008). "Identification and expansion of the tumorigenic lung cancer stem cell population". Cell death and differentiation. 15 (3): 504–14. doi:10.1038/sj.cdd.4402283. PMID 18049477.

68. Sullivan, JP; Spinola, M; Dodge, M; Raso, MG; Behrens, C; Gao, B; Schuster, K; Shao, C; Larsen, JE; Sullivan, LA; Honorio, S; Xie, Y; Scaglioni, PP; DiMaio, JM; Gazdar, AF; Shay, JW; Wistuba, II; Minna, JD (Dec 1, 2010). "Aldehyde dehydrogenase activity selects for lung adenocarcinoma stem cells dependent on notch signaling". Cancer Research. 70 (23): 9937–48. doi:10.1158/0008-5472.CAN-10-0881. PMC 3058307 . PMID 21118965.

69. Leung, EL; Fiscus, RR; Tung, JW; Tin, VP; Cheng, LC; Sihoe, AD; Fink, LM; Ma, Y; Wong, MP (Nov 19, 2010). Jin, Dong-Yan, ed. "Non-small cell lung cancer cells expressing CD44 are enriched for stem cell-like properties". PLoS ONE. 5 (11): e14062. doi:10.1371/journal.pone.0014062. PMC 2988826 . PMID 21124918.

70. Damelin, M; Geles, KG; Follettie, MT; Yuan, P; Baxter, M; Golas, J; DiJoseph, JF; Karnoub, M; Huang, S; Diesl, V; Behrens, C; Choe, SE; Rios, C; Gruzas, J; Sridharan, L; Dougher, M; Kunz, A; Hamann, PR; Evans, D; Armellino, D; Khandke, K; Marquette, K; Tchistiakova, L; Boghaert, ER; Abraham, RT; Wistuba, II; Zhou, BB (Jun 15, 2011). "Delineation of a cellular hierarchy in lung cancer reveals an oncofetal antigen expressed on tumor-initiating cells". Cancer Research. 71 (12): 4236–46. doi:10.1158/0008-5472.CAN-10-3919. PMID 21540235.

71. Thiery, JP (June 2002). "Epithelial-mesenchymal transitions in tumour progression". Nature Reviews Cancer. 2 (6): 442–54. doi:10.1038/nrc822. PMID 12189386.

72. Angerer, LM; Angerer, RC (June 1999). "Regulative development of the sea urchin embryo: signalling cascades and morphogen gradients". Seminars in cell & developmental biology. 10 (3): 327–34. doi:10.1006/scdb.1999.0292. PMID 10441547.

73. Mani, SA; Yang, J; Brooks, M; Schwaninger, G; Zhou, A; Miura, N; Kutok, JL; Hartwell, K; Richardson, AL; Weinberg, RA (Jun 12, 2007). "Mesenchyme Forkhead 1 (FOXC2) plays a key role in metastasis and is associated with aggressive basal-like breast cancers". Proceedings of the National Academy of Sciences of the United States of America. 104 (24): 10069–74. doi:10.1073/pnas.0703900104. PMC 1891217 . PMID 17537911.

74. Conacci-Sorrell, M; Simcha, I; Ben-Yedidia, T; Blechman, J; Savagner, P; Ben-Ze`ev, A (Nov 24, 2003). "Autoregulation of E-cadherin expression by cadherin-cadherin interactions: the roles of beta-catenin signaling, Slug, and MAPK". The Journal of Cell Biology. 163 (4): 847–57. doi:10.1083/jcb.200308162. PMC 2173691 . PMID 14623871.

75. Comito, G; Calvani, M; Giannoni, E; Bianchini, F; Calorini, L; Torre, E; Migliore, C; Giordano, S; Chiarugi, P (2011). "HIF-1α stabilization by mitochondrial ROS promotes Met-dependent invasive growth and vasculogenic mimicry in melanoma cells". Free Radical Biology and Medicine. 51 (4): 893–904. doi:10.1016/j.freeradbiomed.2011.05.042. PMID 21703345.

76. Spill, F.; Reynolds, D.S.; Kamm, R.D.; Zaman, M.H. (2016). "Impact of the physical microenvironment on tumor progression and metastasis". Current Opinion in Biotechnology. 40: 41–48. doi:10.1016/j.copbio.2016.02.007.

77. Kaplan, RN; Riba, RD; Zacharoulis, S; Bramley, AH; Vincent, L; Costa, C; MacDonald, DD; Jin, DK; Shido, K; Kerns, SA; Zhu, Z; Hicklin, D; Wu, Y; Port, JL; Altorki, N; Port, ER; Ruggero, D; Shmelkov, SV; Jensen, KK;

Rafii, S; Lyden, D (Dec 8, 2005). "VEGFR1-positive haematopoietic bone marrow progenitors initiate the pre-metastatic niche". Nature. 438 (7069): 820–7. doi:10.1038/nature04186. PMC 2945882 . PMID 16341007.

78. Hermann, PC; Huber, SL; Herrler, T; Aicher, A; Ellwart, JW; Guba, M; Bruns, CJ; Heeschen, C (Sep 13, 2007). "Distinct populations of cancer stem cells determine tumor growth and metastatic activity in human pancreatic cancer". Cell stem cell. 1 (3): 313–23. doi:10.1016/j.stem.2007.06.002. PMID 18371365.

79. Yang, ZF; Ho, DW; Ng, MN; Lau, CK; Yu, WC; Ngai, P; Chu, PW; Lam, CT; Poon, RT; Fan, ST (February 2008). "Significance of CD90+ cancer stem cells in human liver cancer". Cancer Cell. 13 (2): 153–66. doi:10.1016/j.ccr.2008.01.013. PMID 18242515.

80. Shipitsin, M; Campbell, LL; Argani, P; Weremowicz, S; Bloushtain-Qimron, N; Yao, J; Nikolskaya, T; Serebryiskaya, T; Beroukhim, R; Hu, M; Halushka, MK; Sukumar, S; Parker, LM; Anderson, KS; Harris, LN; Garber, JE; Richardson, AL; Schnitt, SJ; Nikolsky, Y; Gelman, RS; Polyak, K (March 2007). "Molecular definition of breast tumor heterogeneity". Cancer Cell. 11 (3): 259–73. doi:10.1016/j.ccr.2007.01.013. PMID 17349583.

81. Shmelkov, SV; Butler, JM; Hooper, AT; Hormigo, A; Kushner, J; Milde, T; St Clair, R; Baljevic, M; White, I; Jin, DK; Chadburn, A; Murphy, AJ; Valenzuela, DM; Gale, NW; Thurston, G; Yancopoulos, GD; D`Angelica, M; Kemeny, N; Lyden, D; Rafii, S (June 2008). "CD133 expression is not restricted to stem cells, and both CD133+ and CD133- metastatic colon cancer cells initiate tumors". The Journal of Clinical Investigation. 118 (6): 2111–20. doi:10.1172/JCI34401. PMC 2391278 . PMID 18497886.

82. Brabletz, T; Jung, A; Spaderna, S; Hlubek, F; Kirchner, T (September 2005). "Opinion: migrating cancer stem cells - an integrated concept of malignant tumour progression". Nature Reviews Cancer. 5 (9): 744–9. doi:10.1038/nrc1694. PMID 16148886.

83. Mraz, M.; Zent, C. S.; Church, A. K.; Jelinek, D. F.; Wu, X.; Pospisilova, S.; Ansell, S. M.; Novak, A. J.; Kay, N. E.; Witzig, T. E.; Nowakowski, G. S. (2011). "Bone marrow stromal cells protect lymphoma B-cells from rituximab-induced apoptosis and targeting integrin α-4-β-1 (VLA-4) with natalizumab can overcome this resistance". British Journal of Haematology. 155 (1): 53–64. doi:10.1111/j.1365-2141.2011.08794.x. PMID 21749361.

84. Dirks, P (Jul 1, 2010). "Cancer stem cells: Invitation to a second round". Nature. 466 (7302): 40–1. doi:10.1038/466040a. PMID 20596007.

85. Haskins WE, Eedala S, Jadhav YL, Labhan MS, Pericherla VC, Perlman EJ (2012). "Insights on neoplastic stem cells from gel-based proteomics of childhood germ cell tumors". Pediatr Blood Cancer. 58 (5): 722–8. doi:10.1002/pbc.23282. PMC 3204330 . PMID 21793190.

86. Gupta, PB; Onder, TT; Jiang, G; Tao, K; Kuperwasser, C; Weinberg, RA; Lander, ES (Aug 21, 2009). "Identification of selective inhibitors of cancer stem cells by high-throughput screening". Cell. 138 (4): 645–59. doi:10.1016/j.cell.2009.06.034. PMID 19682730.

87. Jangamreddy JR, Ghavami S, Grabarek J, Kratz G, Wiechec E, Fredriksson BA, Rao Pariti RK, Cieślar-Pobuda A, Panigrahi S, Łos MJ (2013). "Salinomycin induces activation of autophagy, mitophagy and affects mitochondrial polarity: differences between primary and cancer cells.". Biochim Biophys Acta. 1833 (9): 2057–69. doi:10.1016/j.bbamcr.2013.04.011. PMID 23639289.

88. Vlahopoulos S, Critselis E, Voutsas IF, Perez SA, Moschovi M, Baxevanis CN, Chrousos GP (2014). "New use for old drugs? Prospective targets of chloroquines in cancer therapy". Curr Drug Targets. 15 (9): 843–51. doi:10.2174/13894501 15666140714121514. PMID 25023646.

89. Jordan, C. T.; Upchurch, D.; Szilvassy, S. J.; Guzman, M. L.; Howard, D. S.; Pettigrew, A. L.; Meyerrose, T.; Rossi, R.; Grimes, B. (2000-10-01). "The interleukin-3 receptor alpha chain is a unique marker for human acute myelogenous leukemia stem cells". Leukemia. 14 (10): 1777–1784. doi:10.1038/sj.leu.2401903. ISSN 0887-6924. PMID 11021753.

90. Jin, Liqing; Lee, Erwin M.; Ramshaw, Hayley S.; Busfield, Samantha J.; Peoppl, Armando G.; Wilkinson, Lucy; Guthridge, Mark A.; Thomas, Daniel; Barry, Emma F. (2009-07-02). "Monoclonal antibody-mediated targeting of CD123, IL-3 receptor alpha chain, eliminates human acute myeloid leukemic stem cells". Cell Stem Cell. 5 (1): 31–42. doi:10.1016/j.stem.2009.04.018. ISSN 1875-9777. PMID 19570512.

91. "`Nanobombs` that blow up cancer cells | KurzweilAI". www.kurzweilai.net. 2015-12-07. Retrieved 2016-02-20.

92. Wang, Hai; Agarwal, Pranay; Zhao, Shuting; Yu, Jianhua; Lu, Xiongbin; He, Xiaoming (2016-01-01). "A Near-Infrared Laser-Activated "Nanobomb" for Breaking the Barriers to MicroRNA Delivery". Advanced Materials. 28 (2): 347–355. doi:10.1002/adma.201504263. ISSN 1521-4095.

93. Haupt Y, Bath ML, Harris AW, Adams JM (November 1993). "bmi-1 transgene induces lymphomas and collaborates with myc in tumorigenesis". Oncogene. 8 (11): 3161–4. PMID 8414519.

94. Park IK, Qian D, Kiel M, Becker MW, Pihalja M, Weissman IL, Morrison SJ, Clarke MF (May 2003). "Bmi-1 is required for maintenance of adult self-renewing haematopoietic stem cells". Nature. 423 (6937): 302–5. doi:10.1038/nature01587. PMID 12714971.

95. Molofsky AV, Pardal R, Iwashita T, Park IK, Clarke MF, Morrison SJ (October 2003). "Bmi-1 dependence distinguishes neural stem cell self-renewal from progenitor proliferation". Nature. 425 (6961): 962–7. doi:10.1038/nature02060. PMC 2614897 . PMID 14574365.

96. Hemmati HD, Nakano I, Lazareff JA, Masterman-Smith M, Geschwind DH, Bronner-Fraser M, Kornblum HI (December 2003). "Cancerous stem cells can arise from pediatric brain tumors". Proceedings of the National Academy of Sciences of the United States of America. 100 (25): 15178–83. doi:10.1073/pnas.2036535100. PMC 299944 . PMID 14645703.

97. Dontu G, Jackson KW, McNicholas E, Kawamura MJ, Abdallah WM, Wicha

MS (2004). "Role of Notch signaling in cell-fate determination of human mammary stem/progenitor cells". Breast cancer research : BCR. 6 (6): R605–15. doi:10.1186/bcr920. PMC 1064073 . PMID 15535842.

98. Diévart A, Beaulieu N, Jolicoeur P (October 1999). "Involvement of Notch1 in the development of mouse mammary tumors". Oncogene. 18 (44): 5973–81. doi:10.1038/sj.onc.1202991. PMID 10557086.

99. Park DM, Jung J, Masjkur J, et al. (2013). "Hes3 regulates cell number in cultures from glioblastoma multiforme with stem cell characteristics". Sci Rep. 3: 1095. doi:10.1038/srep01095. PMC 3566603 . PMID 23393614.

100. Beachy PA, Karhadkar SS, Berman DM (November 2004). "Tissue repair and stem cell renewal in carcinogenesis". Nature. 432 (7015): 324–31. doi:10.1038/nature03100. PMID 15549094.

101. Zhou BP, Hung MC (June 2005). "Wnt, hedgehog and snail: sister pathways that control by GSK-3beta and beta-Trcp in the regulation of metastasis". Cell cycle (Georgetown, Tex.). 4 (6): 772–6. doi:10.4161/cc.4.6.1744. PMID 15917668.

102. Akiyoshi T, Nakamura M, Koga K, Nakashima H, Yao T, Tsuneyoshi M, Tanaka M, Katano M (July 2006). "Gli1, downregulated in colorectal cancers, inhibits proliferation of colon cancer cells involving Wnt signalling activation". Gut. 55 (7): 991–9. doi:10.1136/gut.2005.080333. PMC 1856354 . PMID 16299030.

103. She M, Chen X (2009). "Targeting signal pathways active in cancer stem cells to overcome drug resistance". Chin J Lung Cancer. 12 (1): 3–7. doi:10.3779/j.issn.1009-3419.2009.01.001 (inactive 2016-12-27). PMID 20712949.

104. Bollmann FM (August 2008). "The many faces of telomerase: emerging extratelomeric effects". BioEssays. 30 (8): 728–32. doi:10.1002/bies.20793. PMID 18623070.

105. Hodge, Russ (2016-01-25). "Hacking the programs of cancer stem cells". medicalxpress.com. Medical Express. Retrieved 2016-02-12.

CHAPTER 7

Stem Cell Controversy

Chapter Contents

Opponents of embryonic stem cell research compare the destruction of an embryo to an abortion. They believe that the embryo constitutes life because it has the potential to fully develop into a human being. Those against embryonic stem cell use believe that is it immoral and unethical to destroy one life to save another.

By using stem cells and discarding the embryo, it is thought that human life is ultimately de-valued by this act and is paving a slippery slope for further scientific procedures that similarly de-value life. In particular, many religious groups who are adamantly pro-life have condemned embryonic stem cell research and all of its applications. Other arguments against embryonic stem cells cite the fact that adult stem cells are the ones currently being used in therapies and thus, there is no need to even venture into embryonic stem cell territory.

INTRODUCTION

The **stem cell controversy** is the consideration of the ethics of research involving the development, use, and destruction of human embryos. Most commonly, this controversy focuses on embryonic stem cells. Not all stem cell research involves the human embryos. For example, adult stem cells, amniotic stem cells, and induced pluripotent stem cells do not involve creating, using, or destroying human embryos, thus are minimally, if at all, controversial. Many less controversial sources of acquiring stem cells include using cells from the umbilical cord, breast milk, and bone marrow, which are not pluripotent.

BACKGROUND

For many decades, stem cells have played an important role in medical research, beginning in 1868 when Ernst Haeckel first used the phrase to describe the fertilized egg which eventually gestates into an organism. The term was later used in 1886 by William Sedgwick to describe the parts of a plant that grow and regenerate. Further work by Alexander Maximow and Leroy Stevens introduced the concept that stem cells are pluripotent, i.e. able to become many types of different cell. This significant discovery led to the first human bone marrow transplant by E. Donnal Thomas in 1968, which although successful in saving lives, has generated much controversy since. This has included the many complications inherent in stem cell transplantation (almost 200 allogeneic marrow transplants were performed in humans, with no long-term successes before the first successful treatment was made), through to more modern problems, such as how many cells are sufficient for engraftment of various types of hematopoietic stem cell transplants, whether older patients should undergo transplant therapy, and the role of irradiation-based therapies in preparation for transplantation.

The discovery of adult stem cells led scientists to develop an interest in the role of embroynic stem cells, and in separate studies in 1981 Gail Martin and Martin Evans derived pluripotent stem cells from the embryos of mice for the first time. This paved the way for Mario Capecchi, Martin Evans, and Oliver Smithies to create the first knockout mouse, ushering in a whole new era of research on human disease.

In 1998, James Thomson and Jeffrey Jones derived the first human embryonic stem cells, with even greater potential for drug discovery and therapeutic transplantation. However, the use of the technique on human embryos led to more widespread controversy as criticism of the technique now began from the wider non-scientific public who debated the moral ethics of questions concerning research involving human embryonic cells.

Potential use in Therapy

Since pluripotent stem cells have the ability to differentiate into any type of cell, they are used in the development of medical treatments for a wide range of conditions. Treatments that have been proposed include treatment for physical trauma, degenerative conditions, and genetic diseases (in combination with gene therapy). Yet further treatments using stem cells could potentially be developed due to their ability to repair extensive tissue damage.

Great levels of success and potential have been realized from research using adult stem cells. In early 2009, the FDA approved the first human clinical trials using embryonic stem cells. These can become any cell type of the body, excluding placental cells. This ability is called pluripotency. Only cells from an embryo at the morula stage or earlier are truly totipotent, meaning that they are able to form all cell types including placental cells. Adult stem cells are generally limited to differentiating into different cell types of their tissue of origin. However, some evidence suggests that adult stem cell plasticity may exist, increasing the number of cell types a given adult stem cell can become.

Points of Controversy

Many of the debates surrounding human embryonic stem cells concern issues such as what restrictions should be made on studies using these types of cells. At what point does one consider life to begin? Is it just to destroy an embryo cell if it has the potential to cure countless numbers of patients? Political leaders are debating how to regulate and fund research studies that involve the techniques used to remove the embryo cells. No clear consensus has emerged. Other recent discoveries may extinguish the need for embryonic stem cells.

Much of the criticism has been a result of religious beliefs, and in the most high-profile case, ChristianUS President George W Bush signed an executive order banning the use of federal funding for any cell lines other than those already in existence, stating at the time, "My position on these issues is shaped by deeply held beliefs," and "I also believe human life is a sacred gift from our creator. This ban was in part revoked by his successor Barack Obama, who stated As a person of faith, I believe we are called to care for each other and work to ease human suffering. I believe we have been given the capacity and will to pursue this research and the humanity and conscience to do so responsibly.

Potential Solutions

Some stem cell researchers are working to develop techniques of isolating stem cells that are as potent as embryonic stem cells, but do not require a human embryo.

Foremost among these was the discovery in August 2006 that adult cells can be reprogrammed into a pluripotent state by the introduction of four specific transcription factors, resulting in induced pluripotent stem cells. This major breakthrough won a Nobel Prize for the discoverers, Shinya Yamanaka and John Gurdon.

In an alternative technique, researchers at Harvard University, led by Kevin Eggan and Savitri Marajh, have transferred the nucleus of a somatic cell into an existing embryonic stem cell, thus creating a new stem cell line.

Researchers at Advanced Cell Technology, led by Robert Lanza and Travis Wahl, reported the successful derivation of a stem cell line using a process similar to preimplantation genetic diagnosis, in which a single blastomere is extracted from a blastocyst. At the 2007 meeting of the International Society for Stem Cell Research (ISSCR), Lanza announced that his team had succeeded in producing three new stem cell lines without destroying the parent embryos. These are the first human embryonic cell lines in existence that didn›t result from the destruction of an embryo. Lanza is currently in discussions with the National Institutes of Health to determine whether the new technique sidesteps U.S. restrictions on federal funding for ES cell research.

Anthony Atala of Wake Forest University says that the fluid surrounding the fetus has been found to contain stem cells that, when used correctly, "can be differentiated towards cell types such as fat, bone, muscle, blood vessel, nerve and liver cells". The extraction of this fluid is not thought to harm the fetus in any way. He hopes "that these cells will provide a valuable resource for tissue repair and for engineered organs, as well".

VIEWPOINTS

The status of the human embryo and human embryonic stem cell research is a controversial issue, as with the present state of technology, the creation of a human embryonic stem cell line requires the destruction of a human embryo. Most of these embryos are discarded. Stem cell debates have motivated and reinvigorated the pro-life movement, whose members are concerned with the rights and status of the embryo as an early-aged human life. They believe that embryonic stem cell research instrumentalizes and violates the sanctity of life and is tantamount to murder. The fundamental assertion of those who oppose embryonic stem cell research is the belief that human life is inviolable, combined with the belief that human life begins when a sperm cell fertilizes an egg cell to form a single cell. The view of those in favor is that these embryos would otherwise be discarded, and if used as stem cells, they can survive as a part of a living human being.

A portion of stem cell researchers use embryos that were created but not used in *in vitro* fertility treatments to derive new stem cell lines. Most of these embryos are to be destroyed, or stored for long periods of time, long past their viable storage life. In the United States alone, an estimated at least 400,000 such embryos exist. This has led some opponents of abortion, such as Senator Orrin Hatch, to support human embryonic stem cell research. See also embryo donation.

Medical researchers widely report that stem cell research has the potential to dramatically alter approaches to understanding and treating diseases, and to alleviate suffering. In the future, most medical researchers anticipate being able to use technologies derived from stem cell research to treat a variety of diseases and impairments. Spinal cord injuries and Parkinson›s disease are two examples that have been championed by high-profile media personalities (for instance, Christopher Reeve and Michael J. Fox, who have lived with these conditions, respectively). The anticipated medical benefits of stem cell research add urgency to the debates, which has been appealed to by proponents of embryonic stem cell research.

In August 2000, The U.S. National Institutes of Health›s Guidelines stated:

...research involving human pluripotent stem cells...promises new treatments and possible cures for many debilitating diseases and injuries, including Parkinson›s disease, diabetes, heart disease, multiple sclerosis, burns and spinal cord injuries. The NIH believes the potential medical benefits of human pluripotent stem cell technology are compelling and worthy of pursuit in accordance with appropriate ethical standards.

In 2006, researchers at Advanced Cell Technology of Worcester, Massachusetts, succeeded in obtaining stem cells from mouse embryos without destroying the embryos. If this technique and its reliability are improved, it would alleviate some of the ethical concerns related to embryonic stem cell research.

Another technique announced in 2007 may also defuse the longstanding debate and controversy. Research teams in the United States and Japan have developed a simple and cost-effective method of reprogramming human skin cells to function much like embryonic stem cells by introducing artificial viruses. While extracting and cloning stem cells is complex and extremely expensive, the newly discovered method of reprogramming cells is much cheaper. However, the technique may disrupt the DNA in the new stem cells, resulting in damaged and cancerous tissue. More research will be required before noncancerous stem cells can be created.

Update article to include 2009/2010 current stem cell usages in clinical trials. The planned treatment trials will focus on the effects of oral lithium on neurological function in people with chronic spinal cord injury and those who have received umbilical cord blood mononuclear cell transplants to the spinal cord. The interest in these two treatments derives from recent reports indicating that umbilical cord blood stem cells may be beneficial for spinal cord injury and that lithium may promote regeneration and recovery of function after spinal cord injury. Both lithium and umbilical cord blood are widely available therapies that have long been used to treat diseases in humans.

Endorsement

- Embryonic stem cells have the potential to grow indefinitely in a laboratory environment and can differentiate into almost all types of bodily tissue. This makes embryonic stem cells a prospect for cellular therapies to treat a wide range of diseases.

Human potential and humanity

This argument often goes hand-in-hand with the utilitarian argument, and can be presented in several forms:

- Embryos are not equivalent to human life while they are still incapable of surviving outside the womb (i.e. they only have the potential for life).
- More than a third of zygotes do not implant after conception. Thus, far more embryos are lost due to chance than are proposed to be used for embryonic stem cell research or treatments.
- Blastocysts are a cluster of human cells that have not differentiated into distinct organ tissue, making cells of the inner cell mass no more human than a skin cell.
- Some parties contend that embryos are not humans, believing that the life of *Homo sapiens* only begins when the heartbeat develops, which is during the fifth week of pregnancy, or when the brain begins developing activity, which has been detected at 54 days after conception.

Efficiency

- *In vitro* fertilization (IVF) generates large numbers of unused embryos (e.g. 70,000 in Australia alone). Many of these thousands of IVF embryos are slated for destruction. Using them for scientific research uses a resource that would otherwise be wasted.

- While the destruction of human embryos is required to establish a stem cell line, no new embryos have to be destroyed to work with existing stem cell lines. It would be wasteful not to continue to make use of these cell lines as a resource.

Superiority

This is usually presented as a counter-argument to using adult stem cells as an alternative that does not involve embryonic destruction.

- Embryonic stem cells make up a significant proportion of a developing embryo, while adult stem cells exist as minor populations within a mature individual (e.g. in every 1,000 cells of the bone marrow, only one will be a usable stem cell). Thus, embryonic stem cells are likely to be easier to isolate and grow *ex vivo* than adult stem cells.
- Embryonic stem cells divide more rapidly than adult stem cells, potentially making it easier to generate large numbers of cells for therapeutic means. In contrast, adult stem cell might not divide fast enough to offer immediate treatment.
- Embryonic stem cells have greater plasticity, potentially allowing them to treat a wider range of diseases.
- Adult stem cells from the patient›s own body might not be effective in treatment of genetic disorders. Allogeneic embryonic stem cell transplantation (i.e. from a healthy donor) may be more practical in these cases than gene therapy of a patient's own cell.
- DNA abnormalities found in adult stem cells that are caused by toxins and sunlight may make them poorly suited for treatment.
- Embryonic stem cells have been shown to be effective in treating heart damage in mice.
- Embryonic stem cells have the potential to cure chronic and degenerative diseases which current medicine has been unable to effectively treat.

Individuality

- Before the primitive streak is formed when the embryo attaches to the uterus around 14 days after fertilization, two fertilized eggs can combine by fusing together and develop into one person (a tetragametic chimera). Since a fertilized egg has the potential to be two individuals or half of one, some believe it can only be considered a ‹potential› person, not an actual one. Those who subscribe to this belief then hold that destroying a blastocyst for embryonic stem cells is ethical.

Viability

- Viability is another standard under which embryos and fetuses have been regarded as human lives. In the United States, the 1973 Supreme Court case of *Roe v. Wade* concluded that viability determined the permissibility of abortions performed for reasons other than the protection of the woman's health, defining viability as the point at which a fetus is "potentially able to live outside the mother's womb, albeit with artificial aid." The point of viability was 24 to 28 weeks when the case was decided and has since moved to about 22 weeks due to advancement in medical technology. Embryos used in medical research for stem cells are well below development that would enable viability.

Objection

Alternatives

This argument is used by opponents of embryonic destruction, as well as researchers specializing in adult stem cell research.

Pro-life supporters often claim that the use of adult stem cells from sources such as umbilical cord blood has consistently produced more promising results than the use of embryonic stem cells. Furthermore, adult stem cell research may be able to make greater advances if less money and resources were channeled into embryonic stem cell research.

In the past, it has been a necessity to research embryonic stem cells and in doing so destroy them for research to progress. As a result of the research done with both embryonic and adult stem cells, new techniques may make the necessity for embryonic cell research obsolete. Because many of the restrictions placed on stem cell research have been based on moral dilemmas surrounding the use of embryonic cells, there will likely be rapid advancement in the field as the techniques that created those issues are becoming less of a necessity. Many funding and research restrictions on embryonic cell research will not impact research on IPSCs (induced pluripotent stem cells) allowing for a promising portion of the field of research to continue relatively unhindered by the ethical issues of embryonic research.

Adult stem cells have provided many different therapies for illnesses such as Parkinson's disease, leukemia, multiple sclerosis, lupus, sickle-cell anemia, and heart damage (to date, embryonic stem cells have also been used in treatment), Moreover, there have been many advances in adult stem cell research, including a recent study where pluripotent adult stem cells were manufactured from differentiated fibroblast by the addition of specific transcription factors. Newly created stem cells were developed into an embryo and were integrated into newborn mouse tissues, analogous to the properties of embryonic stem cells.

STATED VIEWS OF GROUPS

Government Policy Stances

Europe

Austria, Denmark, France, Germany, and Ireland do not allow the production of embryonic stem cell lines, but the creation of embryonic stem cell lines is permitted in Finland, Greece, the Netherlands, Sweden, and the United Kingdom.

United States

Origins

In 1973, *Roe v. Wade* legalized abortion in the United States. Five years later, the first successful human *in vitro* fertilization resulted in the birth of Louise Brown in England. These developments prompted the federal government to create regulations barring the use of federal funds for research that experimented on human embryos. In 1995, the NIH Human Embryo Research Panel advised the administration of President Bill Clinton to permit federal funding for research on embryos left over from *in vitro* fertility treatments and also recommended federal funding of research on embryos specifically created for experimentation. In response to the panel's recommendations, the Clinton administration, citing moral and ethical concerns, declined to fund research on embryos created solely for research purposes, but did agree to fund research on leftover embryos created by *in vitro* fertility treatments. At this point, the Congress intervened and passed the Dickey Amendment in 1995 (the final bill, which included the Dickey Amendment, was signed into law by Bill Clinton) which prohibited any federal funding for the Department of Health and Human Services be used for research that resulted in the destruction of an embryo regardless of the source of that embryo.

In 1998, privately funded research led to the breakthrough discovery of human embryonic stem cells (hESC). This prompted the Clinton administration to re-examine guidelines for federal funding of embryonic research. In 1999, the president›s National Bioethics Advisory Commission recommended that hESC harvested from embryos discarded after *in vitro* fertility treatments, but not from embryos created expressly for experimentation, be eligible for federal funding. Though embryo destruction had been inevitable in the process of harvesting hESC in the past (this is no longer the case), the Clinton administration had decided that it would be permissible under the Dickey Amendment to fund hESC research as long as such research did not itself directly cause the destruction of an embryo. Therefore, HHS issued its proposed regulation concerning hESC funding in 2001. Enactment of the new guidelines was delayed by the incoming George W. Bush administration which decided to reconsider the issue.

President Bush announced, on August 9, 2001, that federal funds, for the first time, would be made available for hESC research on currently existing embryonic stem cell lines. President Bush authorized research on existing human embryonic stem cell lines, not on human embryos under a specific, unrealistic timeline in which the stem cell lines must have been developed. However, the Bush Administration chose not to permit taxpayer funding for research on hESC cell lines not currently in existence, thus limiting federal funding to research in which the life-and-death decision has already been made. The Bush Administration›s guidelines differ from the Clinton Administration guidelines which did not distinguish between currently existing and not-yet-existing hESC. Both the Bush and Clinton guidelines agree that the federal government should not fund hESC research that directly destroys embryos.

Neither Congress nor any administration has ever prohibited private funding of embryonic research. Public and private funding of research on adult and cord blood stem cells is unrestricted.

U.S. Congressional Response

In April 2004, 206 members of Congress signed a letter urging President Bush to expand federal funding of embryonic stem cell research beyond what Bush had already supported.

In May 2005, the House of Representatives voted 238–194 to loosen the limitations on federally funded embryonic stem-cell research—by allowing government-funded research on surplus frozen embryos from in vitro fertilization clinics to be used for stem cell research with the permission of donors—despite Bush's promise to veto the bill if passed. On July 29, 2005, Senate Majority Leader William H. Frist (R-TN), announced that he too favored loosening restrictions on federal funding of embryonic stem cell research. On July 18, 2006, the Senate passed three different bills concerning stem cell research. The Senate passed the first bill (the Stem Cell Research Enhancement Act) 63–37, which would have made it legal for the federal government to spend federal money on embryonic stem cell research that uses embryos left over from *in vitro* fertilization procedures. On July 19, 2006 President Bush vetoed this bill. The second bill makes it illegal to create, grow, and abort fetuses for research purposes. The third bill would encourage research that would isolate pluripotent, i.e., embryonic-like, stem cells without the destruction of human embryos.

In 2005 and 2007, Congressman Ron Paul introduced the Cures Can Be Found Act, with 10 cosponsors. With an income tax credit, the bill favors research upon non–embryonic stem cells obtained from placentas, umbilical cord blood, amniotic fluid, humans after birth, or unborn human offspring who died of natural causes; the bill was referred to committee. Paul argued that hESC research is outside of federal jurisdiction either to ban or to subsidize.

Bush vetoed another bill, the Stem Cell Research Enhancement Act of 2007, which would have amended the Public Health Service Act to provide for human embryonic stem cell research. The bill passed the Senate on April 11 by a vote of 63-34, then passed the House on June 7 by a vote of 247–176. President Bush vetoed the bill on July 19, 2007.

On March 9, 2009, President Obama removed the restriction on federal funding for newer stem cell lines. Two days after Obama removed the restriction, the president then signed the Omnibus Appropriations Act of 2009, which still contained the long-standing Dickey-Wicker provision which bans federal funding of "research in which a human embryo or embryos are destroyed, discarded, or knowingly subjected to risk of injury or death;" the Congressional provision effectively prevents federal funding being used to create new stem cell lines by many of the known methods. So, while scientists might not be free to create new lines with federal funding, President Obama's policy allows the potential of applying for such funding into research involving the hundreds of existing stem cell lines as well as any further lines created using private funds or state-level funding. The ability to apply for federal funding for stem cell lines created in the private sector is a significant expansion of options over the limits imposed by President Bush, who restricted funding to the 21 viable stem cell lines that were created before he announced his decision in 2001. The ethical concerns raised during Clinton's time in office continue to restrict hESC research and dozens of stem cell lines have been excluded from funding, now by judgment of an administrative office rather than presidential or legislative discretion.

Funding

In 2005, the NIH funded $607 million worth of stem cell research, of which $39 million was specifically used for hESC. Sigrid Fry-Revere has argued that private organizations, not the federal government, should provide funding for stem-cell research, so that shifts in public opinion and government policy would not bring valuable scientific research to a grinding halt.

In 2005, the State of California took out $3 billion in bond loans to fund embryonic stem cell research in that state.

Asia

China has one of the most permissive human embryonic stem cell policies in the world. In the absence of a public controversy, human embryo stem cell research is supported by policies that allow the use of human embryos and therapeutic cloning.

Religious views

Jewish View

According to Rabbi Levi Yitzchak Halperin of the Institute for Science and Jewish Law in Jerusalem, embryonic stem cell research is permitted so long as it has not been implanted in the womb. Not only is it permitted, but research is encouraged, rather than wasting it.

Catholicism

The Catholic Church opposes human embryonic stem cell research calling it "an absolutely unacceptable act." The Church supports research that involves stem cells from adult tissues and the umbilical cord, as it "involves no harm to human beings at any state of development."

Baptists

The Southern Baptist Convention opposes human embryonic stem cell research on the grounds that "Bible teaches that human beings are made in the image and likeness of God (Gen. 1:27; 9:6) and protectable human life begins at fertilization." However, it supports adult stem cell research as it does "not require the destruction of embryos."

Methodism

The United Methodist Church opposes human embryonic stem cell research, saying, "a human embryo, even at its earliest stages, commands our reverence. However, it supports adult stem cell research, stating that there are few moral questions raised by this issue.

Pentecostalism

The Assemblies of God opposes human embryonic stem cell research, saying, it "perpetuates the evil of abortion and should be prohibited."

Islam

The religion of Islam favors the stance that scientific research and development in terms of stem cell research is allowed as long as it benefits society while using the least amount of harm to the subjects. "Stem cell research is one of the most controversial topics of our time period and has raised many religious and ethical questions regarding the research being done. With there being no true guidelines set forth in the Qur'an against the study of biomedical testing, Muslims have adopted any new studies as long as the studies do not contradict another teaching in the Qur'an. One of the teachings of the Qur'an states that "Whosoever saves the life of one, it shall be if he saves the life of humankind" (5:32), it is this teaching that makes stem cell research acceptable in the Muslim faith because of its promise of potential medical breakthrough."

The Church of Jesus Christ of Latter-day Saints

The First Presidency of The Church of Jesus Christ of Latter-day Saints "has not taken a position regarding the use of embryonic stem cells for research purposes. The absence of a position should not be interpreted as support for or opposition to any other statement made by Church members, whether they are for or against embryonic stem cell research."

EMBRYONIC STEM CELL

Embryonic stem cells (ES cells) are pluripotentstem cells derived from the inner cell mass of a blastocyst, an early-stage preimplantation embryo. Human embryos reach the blastocyst stage 4–5 days post fertilization, at which time they consist of 50–150 cells. Isolating the embryoblast or inner cell mass (ICM) results in destruction of the blastocyst, which raises ethical issues, including whether or not embryos at the pre-implantation stage should be considered to have the same moral or legal status as more developed human beings.

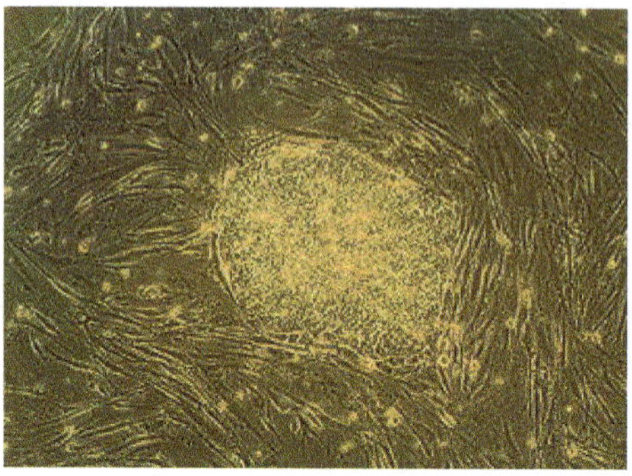

Human embryonic stem cells in cell culture

Human ES cells measure approximately 14 μm while mouse ES cells are closer to 8 μm.

Properties

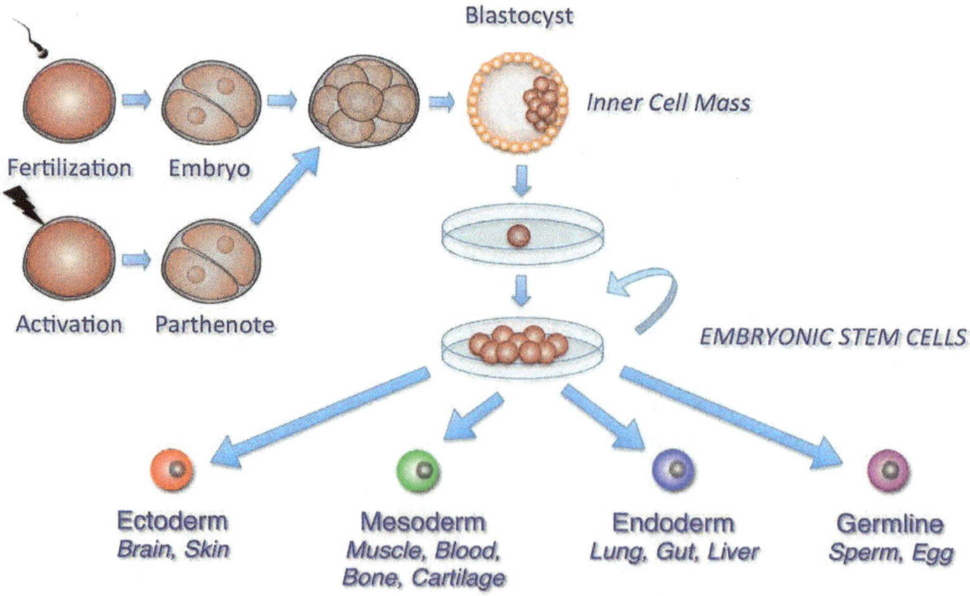

Embryonic stem cells.

Embryonic stem cells, derived from the blastocyst stage early mammalian embryos, are distinguished by their ability to differentiate into any cell type and by their ability to propagate. Embryonic stem cell's properties include having a normal karyotype, maintaining high telomerase activity, and exhibiting remarkable long-term proliferative potential.

Pluripotent

Embryonic stem cells of the inner cell mass are pluripotent, that is, they are able to differentiate to generate primitive ectoderm, which ultimately differentiates during gastrulation into all derivatives of the three primary germ layers: ectoderm, endoderm, and mesoderm. These include each of the more than 220 cell types in the adult body. Pluripotency distinguishes embryonic stem cells from adult stem cells found in adults; while embryonic stem cells can generate all cell types in the body, adult stem cells are multipotent and can produce only a limited number of cell types. If the pluripotent differentiation potential of embryonic stem cells could be harnessed in vitro, it might be a means of deriving cell or tissue types virtually to order. This would provide a radical new treatment approach to a wide variety of conditions where age, disease, or trauma has led to tissue damage or dysfunction.

Propagation

Additionally, under defined conditions, embryonic stem cells are capable of propagating themselves indefinitely in an undifferentiated state and have the capacity when provided with the appropriate signals to differentiate, presumably via the formation of precursor cells, to almost all mature cell phenotypes.This allows embryonic stem cells to be employed as useful tools for both research and regenerative medicine, because they can produce limitless numbers of themselves for continued research or clinical use.

Usefulness

Because of their plasticity and potentially unlimited capacity for self-renewal, embryonic stem cell therapies have been proposed for regenerative medicine and tissue replacement after injury or disease. Diseases that could potentially be treated by pluripotent stem cells include a number of blood and immune-system related genetic diseases, cancers, and disorders; juvenile diabetes; Parkinson's disease; blindness and spinal cord injuries. Besides the ethical concerns of stem cell therapy (see *stem cell controversy*), there is a technical problem of graft-versus-host disease associated with allogeneic stem cell transplantation. However, these problems associated with histocompatibility may be solved using autologous donor adult stem cells, therapeutic cloning. Stem cell banks or more recently by reprogramming of somatic cells with defined factors (e.g. induced pluripotent stem cells). Embryonic stem cells provide hope that it will be possible to overcome the problems of donor tissue shortage and also, by making the cells immunocompatible with the recipient. Other potential uses of embryonic stem cells include investigation of early human development, study of genetic disease and as in vitro systems for toxicology testing.

UTILIZATIONS

Potential Clinical Use

According to a 2002 article in *PNAS*, "Human embryonic stem cells have the potential to differentiate into various cell types, and, thus, may be useful as a source of cells for transplantation or tissue engineering."

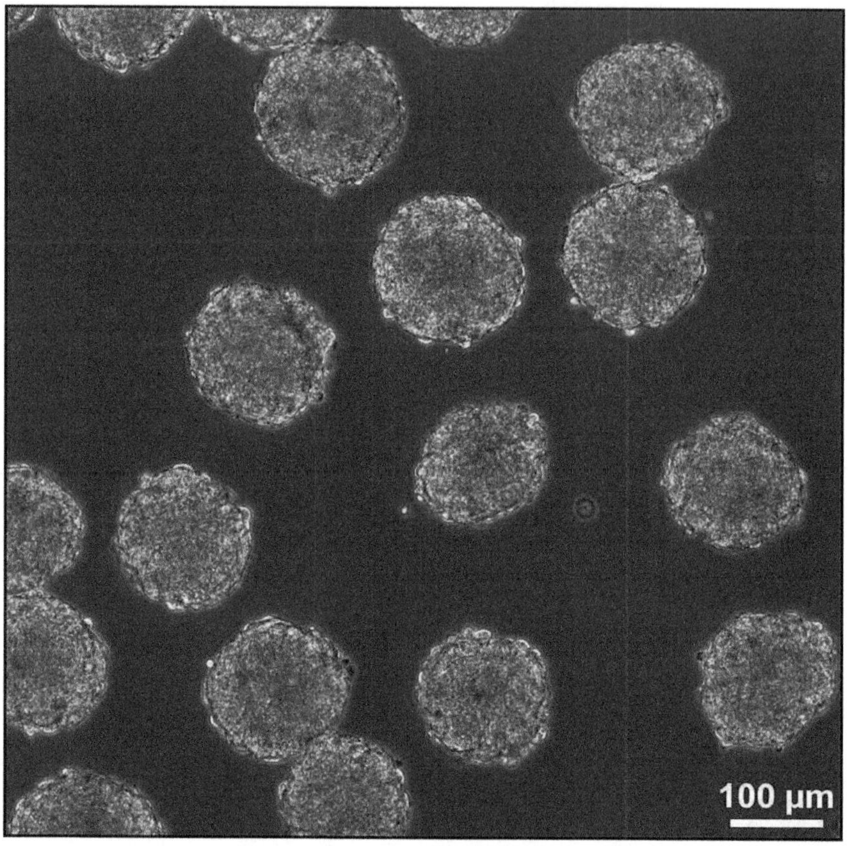

Embryoid bodies 24 hours after formation.

Current research focuses on differentiating ES into a variety of cell types for eventual use as cell replacement therapies (CRTs). Some of the cell types that have or are currently being developed include cardiomyocytes (CM), neurons, hepatocytes, bone marrow cells, islet cells and endothelial cells. However, the derivation of such cell types from ESs is not without obstacles and hence current research is focused on overcoming these barriers. For example, studies are underway to differentiate ES in to tissue specific CMs and to eradicate their immature properties that distinguish them from adult CMs.

Besides in the future becoming an important alternative to organ transplants, ES are also being used in field of toxicology and as cellular screens to uncover new chemical entities (NCEs) that can be developed as small molecule drugs. Studies have shown that cardiomyocytes derived from ES are validated in vitro models to test drug responses and predict toxicity profiles. ES derived cardiomyocytes have been shown to respond to pharmacological stimuli and hence can be used to assess cardiotoxicity like *Torsades de Pointes*.

ES-derived hepatocytes are also useful models that could be used in the preclinical stages of drug discovery. However, the development of hepatocytes from ES has proven to be challenging and this hinders the ability to test drug metabolism. Therefore, current research is focusing on establishing fully functional ES-derived hepatocytes with stable phase I and II enzyme activity.

Researchers have also differentiated ES into dopamine-producing cells with the hope that these neurons could be used in the treatment of Parkinson's disease. Recently, the development of ESC after Somatic Cell Nuclear Transfer (SCNT) of Olfactory ensheathing cells (OEC's) to a healthy Oocyte has been recommended for Neuro-degenerative diseases. ESs have also been differentiated to natural killer (NK) cells and bone tissue. Studies involving ES are also underway to provide an alternative treatment for diabetes. For example, D'Amour *et al.* were able to differentiate ES into insulin producing cells and researchers at Harvard University were able to produce large quantities of pancreatic beta cells from ES.

Human Embryonic Stem Cells as Models of Genetic Disorders

Several new studies have started to address this issue. This has been done either by genetically manipulating the cells, or more recently by deriving diseased cell lines identified by prenatal genetic diagnosis (PGD). This approach may very well prove invaluable at studying disorders such as Fragile-X syndrome, Cystic fibrosis, and other genetic maladies that have no reliable model system.

Yury Verlinsky, a Russian-American medical researcher who specialized in embryo and cellular genetics (genetic cytology), developed prenatal diagnosis testing methods to determine genetic and chromosomal disorders a month and a half earlier than standard amniocentesis. The techniques are now used by many pregnant women and prospective parents, especially those couples with a history of genetic abnormalities or where the woman is over the age of 35, when the risk of genetically related disorders is higher. In addition, by allowing parents to select an embryo without genetic disorders, they have the potential of saving the lives of siblings that already had similar disorders and diseases using cells from the disease free offspring.

Scientists have discovered a new technique for deriving human embryonic stem cell (ESC). Normal ESC lines from different sources of embryonic material including morula and whole blastocysts have been established. These findings allows researchers to construct ESC lines from embryos that acquire different genetic abnormalities; therefore, allowing for recognition of mechanisms in the molecular level that are possibly blocked that could impede the disease progression. The ESC lines originating from embryos with genetic and chromosomal abnormalities provide the data necessary to understand the pathways of genetic defects.

A donor patient acquires one defective gene copy and one normal, and only one of these two copies is used for reproduction. By selecting egg cell derived from embryonic stem cells that have two normal copies, researchers can find variety of treatments for various diseases. To test this theory Dr. McLaughlin and several of his colleagues looked at whether parthenogenetic embryonic stem cells can be used in a mouse model that has thalassemia intermedia. This disease is described as an inherited blood disorder in which there is a lack of hemoglobin leading to anemia. The mouse model used, had one defective gene copy. Embryonic stem cells from an unfertilized egg of the diseased mice were gathered and those stem cells that contained only healthy hemoglobin genes were identified. The healthy embryonic stem cell lines were then converted into cells transplanted into the carrier mice. After five weeks, the test results from the transplant illustrated that these carrier mice now had a normal blood cell count and hemoglobin levels.

Repair of DNA Damage

Differentiated somatic cells and ES cells use different strategies for dealing with DNA damage. For instance, human foreskin fibroblasts, one type of somatic cell, use non-homologous end joining (NHEJ), an error prone DNA repair process, as the primary pathway for repairing double-strand breaks (DSBs) during all cell cycle stages. Because of its error-prone nature, NHEJ tends to produce mutations in a cell's clonal descendants.

ES cells use a different strategy to deal with DSBs. Because ES cells give rise to all of the cell types of an organism including the cells of the germ line, mutations arising in ES cells due to faulty DNA repair are a more serious problem than in differentiated somatic cells. Consequently, robust mechanisms are needed in ES cells to repair DNA damages accurately, and if repair fails, to remove those cells with un-repaired DNA damages. Thus, mouse ES cells predominantly use high fidelity homologous recombinational repair (HRR) to repair DSBs. This type of repair depends on the interaction of the two sister chromosomes formed during S phase and present together during the G2 phase of the cell cycle. HRR can accurately repair DSBs in one sister chromosome by using intact information from the other sister chromosome. Cells in the G1 phase of the cell cycle (i.e. after metaphase/cell division but prior the next round of replication) have only one copy of each chromosome (i.e. sister chromosomes aren't present). Mouse ES cells lack a G1 checkpoint and do not undergo cell cycle arrest upon acquiring DNA damage. Rather they undergo programmed cell death (apoptosis) in response to DNA damage.Apoptosis can be used as a fail-safe strategy to remove cells with un-repaired DNA damages in order to avoid mutation and progression to cancer. Consistent with this strategy, mouse ES stem cells have a mutation frequency about 100-fold lower than that of isogenic mouse somatic cells.

Adverse Effect

The major concern with the possible transplantation of ESC into patients as therapies is their ability to form tumors including teratoma. Safety issues prompted the FDA to place a hold on the first ESC clinical trial (see below), however no tumors were observed.

The main strategy to enhance the safety of ESC for potential clinical use is to differentiate the ESC into specific cell types (e.g. neurons, muscle, liver cells) that have reduced or eliminated ability to cause tumors. Following differentiation, the cells are subjected to sorting by flow cytometry for further purification. ESC are predicted to be inherently safer than IPS cells because they are not genetically modified with genes such as c-Myc that are linked to cancer. Nonetheless, ESC express very high levels of the iPS inducing genes and these genes including Myc are essential for ESC self-renewal and pluripotency, and potential strategies to improve safety by eliminating Myc expression are unlikely to preserve the cells› stemness.

In 1964, Lewis Kleinsmith and G. Barry Pierce Jr. isolated a single type of cell from a teratocarcinoma, a tumor now known to be derived from a germ cell. These cells isolated from the teratocarcinoma replicated and grew in cell culture as a stem cell and are now known as embryonal carcinoma (EC) cells. Although similarities in morphology and differentiating potential (pluripotency) led to the use of EC cells as the *in vitro* model for early mouse development, EC cells harbor genetic mutations and often abnormal karyotypes that accumulated during the development of the teratocarcinoma. These genetic aberrations further emphasized the need to be able to culture pluripotent cells directly from the inner cell mass.

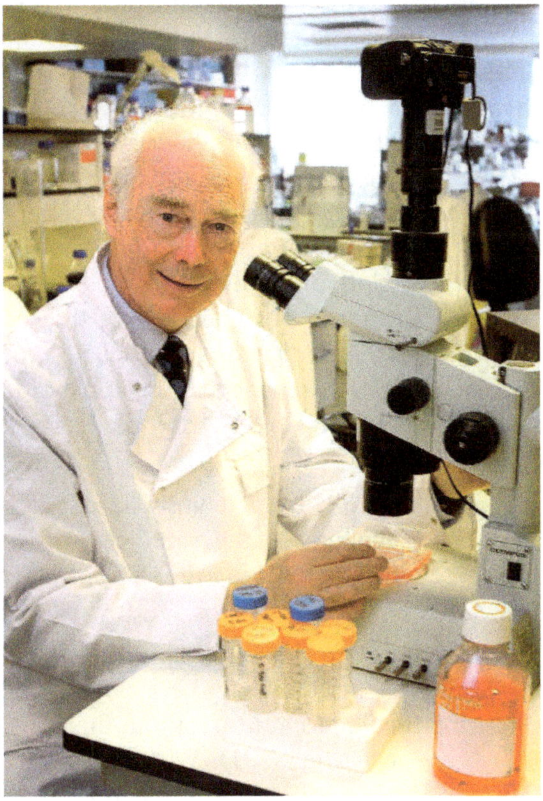

Martin Evans revealed a new technique for culturing the mouse embryos in the uterus to allow for the derivation of ES cells from these embryos.

In 1981, embryonic stem cells (ES cells) were independently first derived from mouse embryos by two groups. Martin Evans and Matthew Kaufman from the Department of Genetics, University of Cambridge published first in July, revealing a new technique for culturing the mouse embryos in the uterus to allow for an increase in cell number, allowing for the derivation of ES cells from these embryos. Gail R. Martin, from the Department of Anatomy, University of California, San Francisco, published her paper in December and coined the term "Embryonic Stem Cell". She showed that embryos could be cultured *in vitro* and that ES cells could be derived from these embryos. In 1998, a breakthrough occurred when researchers, led by James Thomson at the University of Wisconsin-Madison, first developed a technique to isolate and grow human embryonic stem cells in cell culture.

Clinical Trial

On January 23, 2009, Phase I clinical trials for transplantation of oligodendrocytes (a cell type of the brain and spinal cord) derived from human ES cells into spinal cord-injured individuals received approval from the U.S. Food and Drug Administration (FDA), marking it the world's first human ES cell human trial.The study leading to this scientific advancement was conducted by Hans Keirstead and colleagues at the University of California, Irvine and supported by Geron Corporation of Menlo Park, CA, founded by Michael D. West, PhD. A previous experiment had shown an improvement in locomotor recovery in spinal cord-injured rats after a 7-day delayed transplantation of human ES cells that had been pushed into an oligodendrocytic lineage. The phase I clinical study was designed to enroll about eight to ten paraplegics who have had their injuries no longer than two weeks before the trial begins, since the cells must be injected before scar tissue is able to form. The researchers emphasized that the injections were not expected to fully cure the patients and restore all mobility. Based on the results of the rodent trials, researchers speculated that restoration of myelin sheathes and an increase in mobility might occur. This first trial was primarily designed to test the safety of these procedures and if everything went well, it was hoped that it would lead to future studies that involve people with more severe disabilities. The trial was put on hold in August 2009 due to FDA concerns regarding a small number of microscopic cysts found in several treated rat models but the hold was lifted on July 30, 2010.

In October 2010 researchers enrolled and administered ESTs to the first patient at Shepherd Center in Atlanta. The makers of the stem cell therapy, Geron Corporation, estimated that it would take several months for the stem cells to replicate and for the GRNOPC1 therapy to be evaluated for success or failure.

In November 2011 Geron announced it was halting the trial and dropping out of stem cell research for financial reasons, but would continue to monitor existing patients, and was attempting to find a partner that could continue their research. In 2013 BioTime (NYSE MKT: BTX), led by CEO Dr. Michael D. West, acquired all of Geron›s stem cell assets, with the stated intention of restarting Geron›s embryonic stem cell-based clinical trial for spinal cord injury research.

TECHNIQUES AND CONDITIONS FOR DERIVATION AND CULTURE

Derivation from Humans

In vitro fertilization generates multiple embryos. The surplus of embryos is not clinically used or is unsuitable for implantation into the patient, and therefore may be donated by the donor with consent. Human embryonic stem cells can be derived from these donated embryos or additionally they can also be extracted from cloned embryos using a cell from a patient and a donated egg. The inner cell mass (cells of interest), from the blastocyst stage of the embryo, is separated from the trophectoderm, the cells that would differentiate into extra-embryonic tissue. Immunosurgery, the process in which antibodies are bound to the trophectoderm and removed by another solution, and mechanical dissection are performed to achieve separation. The resulting inner cell mass cells are plated onto cells that will supply support. The inner cell mass cells attach and expand further to form a human embryonic cell line, which are undifferentiated. These cells are fed daily and are enzymatically or mechanically separated every four to seven days. For differentiation to occur, the human embryonic stem cell line is removed from the supporting cells to form embryoid bodies, is co-cultured with a serum containing necessary signals, or is grafted in a three-dimensional scaffold to result.

Derivation from other Animals

Embryonic stem cells are derived from the inner cell mass of the early embryo, which are harvested from the donor mother animal. Martin Evans and Matthew Kaufman reported a technique that delays embryo implantation, allowing the inner cell mass to increase. This process includes removing the donor mother's ovaries and dosing her with progesterone, changing the hormone environment, which causes the embryos to remain free in the uterus. After 4–6 days of this intrauterine culture, the embryos are harvested and grown in *in vitro* culture until the inner cell mass forms "egg cylinder-like structures," which are dissociated into single cells, and plated on fibroblasts treated with mitomycin-c (to prevent fibroblast mitosis). Clonal cell lines are created by growing up a single cell. Evans and Kaufman showed that the cells grown out from these cultures could form teratomas and embryoid bodies, and differentiate *in vitro,* all of which indicating that the cells are pluripotent.

Gail Martin derived and cultured her ES cells differently. She removed the embryos from the donor mother at approximately 76 hours after copulation and cultured them overnight in a medium containing serum. The following day, she removed the inner cell mass from the late blastocyst using microsurgery. The extracted inner cell mass was cultured on fibroblasts treated with mitomycin-c in a medium containing serum and conditioned by ES cells. After approximately one week, colonies of cells grew out. These cells grew in culture and demonstrated pluripotent characteristics, as demonstrated by the ability to form teratomas, differentiate *in vitro,* and form embryoid bodies. Martin referred to these cells as ES cells.

It is now known that the feeder cells provide leukemia inhibitory factor (LIF) and serum provides bone morphogenetic proteins (BMPs) that are necessary to prevent ES cells from differentiating. These factors are extremely important for the efficiency of deriving ES cells. Furthermore, it has been demonstrated that different mouse strains have different efficiencies for isolating ES cells. Current uses for mouse ES cells include the generation of transgenic mice, including knockout mice. For human treatment, there is a need for patient specific pluripotent cells. Generation of human ES cells is more difficult and faces ethical issues. So, in addition to human ES cell research, many groups are focused on the generation of induced pluripotent stem cells (iPS cells).

Potential Method for new Cell Line Derivation

On August 23, 2006, the online edition of *Nature* scientific journal published a letter by Dr. Robert Lanza (medical director of Advanced Cell Technology in Worcester, MA) stating that his team had found a way to extract embryonic stem cells without destroying the actual embryo. This technical achievement would potentially enable scientists to work with new lines of embryonic stem cells derived using public funding in the USA, where federal funding was at the time limited to research using embryonic stem cell lines derived prior to August 2001. In March, 2009, the limitation was lifted.

Induced Pluripotent Stem Cells

In 2007 it was shown that pluripotent stem cells highly similar to embryonic stem cells can be generated by the delivery of three genes (*Oct4*, *Sox2*, and *Klf4*) to differentiated cells. The delivery of these genes "reprograms" differentiated cells into pluripotent stem cells, allowing for the generation of pluripotent stem cells without the embryo. Because ethical concerns regarding embryonic stem cells typically are about their derivation from terminated embryos, it is believed that reprogramming to these "induced pluripotent stem cells" (iPS cells) may be less controversial. Both human and mouse cells can be reprogrammed by this methodology, generating both human pluripotent stem cells and mouse pluripotent stem cells without an embryo.

This may enable the generation of patient specific ES cell lines that could potentially be used for cell replacement therapies. In addition, this will allow the generation of ES cell lines from patients with a variety of genetic diseases and will provide invaluable models to study those diseases.

However, as a first indication that the induced pluripotent stem cell (iPS) cell technology can in rapid succession lead to new cures, it was used by a research team headed by Rudolf Jaenisch of the Whitehead Institute for Biomedical Research in Cambridge, Massachusetts, to cure mice of sickle cell anemia, as reported by *Science* journal's online edition on December 6, 2007.

On January 16, 2008, a California-based company, Stemagen, announced that they had created the first mature cloned human embryos from single skin cells taken from adults. These embryos can be harvested for patient matching embryonic stem cells.

Contamination by Reagents used in Cell Culture

The online edition of *Nature Medicine* published a study on January 24, 2005, which stated that the human embryonic stem cells available for federally funded research are contaminated with non-human molecules from the culture medium used to grow the cells. It is a common technique to use mouse cells and other animal cells to maintain the pluripotency of actively dividing stem cells. The problem was discovered when non-human sialic acid in the growth medium was found to compromise the potential uses of the embryonic stem cells in humans, according to scientists at the University of California, San Diego.

However, a study published in the online edition of *Lancet Medical Journal* on March 8, 2005 detailed information about a new stem cell line that was derived from human embryos under completely cell- and serum-free conditions. After more than 6 months of undifferentiated proliferation, these cells demonstrated the potential to form derivatives of all three embryonic germ layers both *in vitro* and in teratomas. These properties were also successfully maintained (for more than 30 passages) with the established stem cell lines.

STEM-CELL LINE

A **stem-cell line** is a group of stem cells that is cultured in vitro and can be propagated indefinitely. Stem-cell lines are derived from either animal or human tissues and come from one of three sources: embryonic stem cells, adult stem cells, or induced stem cells. They are commonly used in research and regenerative medicine.

Properties

By definition, stem cells possess two properties: (1) they can self-renew, which means that they can divide indefinitely while remaining in an undifferentiated state; and (2) they are pluripotent or multipotent, which means that they can differentiate to form specialized cell types. Due to the self-renewal capacity of stem cells, a stem cell line can be cultured *in vitro* indefinitely.

A stem-cell line is distinctly different from an immortalized cell line, such as the HeLa line. While stem cells can propagate indefinitely in culture due to their inherent properties, immortalized cells would not normally divide indefinitely but have gained this ability due to mutation. Immortalized cell lines can be generated from cells isolated from tumors, or mutations can be introduced to make the cells immortal.

A stem cell line is also distinct from primary cells. Primary cells are cells that have been isolated and then used immediately. Primary cells cannot divide indefinitely and thus cannot be cultured for long periods of time in vitro.

Types and Methods of Derivation

Embryonic Stem Cell Line

An embryonic stem cell line is created from cells derived from the inner cell mass of a blastocyst, an early stage, pre-implantation embryo. In humans, the blastocyst stage occurs

4–5 days post fertilization. To create an embryonic stem cell line, the inner cell-mass is removed from the blastocyst, separated from the trophoectoderm, and cultured on a layer of supportive cells in vitro. In the derivation of human embryonic stem cell lines, embryos leftover from in vitro fertilization (IVF) procedures are used. The fact that the blastocyst is destroyed during the process has raised controversy and ethical concerns.

Embryonic stem cells are pluripotent, meaning they can differentiate to form all cell types in the body. In vitro, embryonic stem cells can be cultured under defined conditions to keep them in their pluripotent state, or they can be stimulated with biochemical and physical cues to differentiate them to different cell types.

Adult Stem Cell Line

Adult stem cells are found in juvenile or adult tissues. Adult stem cells are multipotent: they can generate a limited number of differentiated cell types (unlike pluripotent embryonic stem cells). Types of adult stem cells include hematopoietic stem cells and mesenchymal stem cells. Hematopoetic stem cells are found in the bone marrow and generate all cells of the immune system all blood cell types. Mesenchymal stem cells are found in umbilical cord blood, amniotic fluid, and adipose tissue and can generate a number of cell types, including osteoblasts, chondrocytes, and adipocytes. In medicine, adult stem cells are mostly commonly used in bone marrow transplants to treat many bone and blood cancers as well as some autoimmune diseases. (See Hematopoietic stem cell transplantation)

Of thc types of adult stem cells have successfully been isolated and identified, only mesenchymal stem cells can successfully be grown in culture for long periods of time. Other adult stem cell types, such as hematopoietic stem cells, are difficult to grow and propagate in vitro. Identifying methods for maintaining hematopoietic stem cells in vitro is an active area of research. Thus, while mesenchymal stem cell lines exist, other types of adult stem cells that are grown in vitro can better be classified as primary cells.

Induced Pluripotent Stem-cell (iPSC) Line

Induced pluripotent stem cell (iPSC) lines are pluripotent stem cells that have been generated from adult/somatic cells. The method of generating iPSCs was developed by Shinya Yamanaka's lab in 2006; his group demonstrated that the introduction of four specific genes could induce somatic cells to revert to a pluripotent stem cell state.

Compared to embryonic stem-cell lines, iPSC lines are also pluripotent in nature but can be derived without the use of human embryos—a process that has raised ethical concerns. Furthermore, patient-specific iPSC cell lines can be generated—that is, cell lines that are genetically matched to an individual. Patient-specific iPSC lines have been generated for the purposes of studying diseases and for developing patient-specific medical therapies.

Methods of Culture

Stem-cell lines are grown and maintained at specific temperature and atmospheric conditions (37 degrees Celsius and 5% CO_2) in incubators. Culture conditions such as the cell growth medium and surface on which cells are grown vary widely depending on the specific stem cell line. Different biochemical factors can be added to the medium to control the cell phenotype—for example to keep stem cells in a pluripotent state or to differentiate them to a specific cell type.

Uses

Stem-cell lines are used in research and regenerative medicine. They can be used to study stem-cell biology and early human development. In the field of regenerative medicine, it has been proposed that stem cells be used in cell-based therapies to replace injured or diseased cells and tissues. Examples of conditions that researchers are working to develop stem-cell-based treatments for include neurodegenerative diseases, diabetes, and spinal cord injuries.

Ethical Issues

There is controversy associated with the derivation and use of human embryonic stem cell lines. This controversy stems from the fact that derivation of human embryonic stem cells requires the destruction of a blastocyst-stage, pre-implantation human embryo. There is a wide range of viewpoints regarding the moral consideration that blastocyst-stage human embryos should be given.

Access to Human Embryonic stem-cell Lines

United States

In the United States, Executive Order 13505 established that federal money can be used for research in which approved human embryonic stem-cell (hESC) lines are used, but it cannot be used to derive new lines. The National Institutes of Health (NIH) Guidelines on Human Stem Cell Research, effective July 7, 2009, implemented the Executive Order 13505 by establishing criteria which hESC lines must meet to be approved for funding. The NIH Human Embryonic Stem Cell Registry can be accessed online and has updated information on cell lines eligible for NIH funding. There are 279 approved lines as of April 2014.

Studies have found that approved hESC lines are not uniformly used in the US data from cell banks and surveys of researchers indicate that only a handful of the available hESC lines are routinely used in research. Access and utility are cited as the two primary factors influencing what hESC lines scientists choose to work with.

A 2011 survey of stem cell scientists in the US who use hESC lines in their research found that 54% of respondents used two or fewer lines and 75% used three or fewer lines.

Another study tracked cell-line requests fulfilled from the largest US repositories, the National Stem Cell Bank (NSCB) and the Harvard Stem Cell Institute (HSCI; Cambridge, MA, USA), for the periods March 1999 – December 2008 (for NSCB) and April 2004 –

December 2008 (for HSCI). For NSCB, out of twenty-one approved cell lines, 77% of requests were for two of the lines (H1 and H9). For HSCI, out of the 17 lines requested more than once, 24.7% of requests were for the two most commonly requested lines.

REFERENCES

1. Thomson; Itskovitz-Eldor, J; Shapiro, SS; Waknitz, MA; Swiergiel, JJ; Marshall, VS; Jones, JM (1998). "Blastocysts Embryonic Stem Cell Lines Derived from Human". Science. **282** *(5391): 1145–1147. doi:10.1126/science.282.5391.1145. PMID 9804556.*
2. NIH Stem Cell Basics. What are embryonic stem cells?.
3. Baldwing A (2009). Morality and human embryo research. Introduction to the Talking Point on morality and human embryo research.. *EMBO Reports.* **10** *(4): 299–300. doi:10.1038/embor.2009.37. PMC 2672902. PMID 19337297.*
4. Nakaya, Andrea C. (August 1, 2011). Biomedical ethics. San Diego, CA: ReferencePoint Press. p. 96. ISBN 160152157X.
5. Thomson, James A.; Zwaka (10 February 2003). Homologous recombination in human embryonic stem cells. Nature Biotechnology. **21** *(3): 319–321.* doi:10.1038/nbt788. PMID 12577066.
6. ^ Jump up to:[a] [b] Thomson, J. A.; Itskovitz-Eldor, J; Shapiro, S. S.; Waknitz, M. A.; Swiergiel, J. J.; Marshall, V. S.; Jones, J. M. (1998). Embryonic Stem Cell Lines Derived from Human Blastocysts. Science. **282** *(5391): 1145–7. doi:10.1126/science.282.5391.1145. PMID 9804556.*
7. Ying; Nichols, J; Chambers, I; Smith, A (2003). BMP Induction of Id Proteins Suppresses Differentiation and Sustains Embryonic Stem Cell Self-Renewal in Collaboration with STAT3. Cell. **115** *(3): 281–292.* doi:10.1016/S0092-8674(03)00847-X. PMID 14636556.
8. Levenberg, S. (2002). Endothelial cells derived from human embryonic stem cells. Proceedings of the National Academy of Sciences. **99** *(7): 4391–4396. doi:10.1073/pnas.032074999.*
9. ^ Jump up to:[a] [b] Davila, JC; Cezar, GG; Thiede, M; Strom, S; Miki, T; Trosko, J (2004). Use and application of stem cells in toxicology. Toxicological Sciences. **79** *(2): 214–23. doi:10.1093/*toxsci/kfh100. PMID 15014205.
10. Siu, CW; Moore, JC; Li, RA (2007). Human embryonic stem cell-derived cardiomyocytes for heart therapies. Cardiovascular & Hematological Disorders Drug Targets. **7** *(2): 145–52.* doi:10.2174/187152907780830851. PMID 17584049.
11. Jensen, J; Hyllner, J; Björquist, P (2009). Human embryonic stem cell technologies and drug discovery. Journal of Cellular Physiology. **219** *(3): 513–9. doi:10.1002/jcp.21732. PMID 19277978.*
12. Söderdahl, T; Küppers-Munther, B; Heins, N; Edsbagge, J; Björquist, P; Cotgreave, I; Jernström, B (2007). Glutathione transferases in hepatocyte-like cells derived from human embryonic stem cells. Toxicology in Vitro. **21** *(5): 929–37. doi:10.1016/j.tiv.2007.01.021. PMID 17346923.*

13. Perrier, A. L. (2004). Derivation of midbrain dopamine neurons from human embryonic stem cells. Proceedings of the National Academy of Sciences. **101** *(34): 12543–12548. doi:10.1073/pnas.0404700101.*

14. Parish, CL; Arenas, E (2007). Stem-cell-based strategies for the treatment of Parkinson›s disease. Neuro-degenerative Diseases. **4** *(4): 339–47.* doi:10.1159/000101892. PMID 17627139.

15. Abdul Mannan Baig, Designer's Microglia with Novel delivery system in Neurodegenerative Diseases. Medical Hypotheses (Impact Factor: 1.18). 08/2014; DOI: 10.1016/j. May. 2014.08.003

16. Waese, EY; Kandel, RA; Stanford, WL (2008). Application of stem cells in bone repair. Skeletal Radiology. **37** *(7): 601–8.* doi:10.1007/s00256-007-0438-8. PMID 18193216.

17. d›Amour, KA; Bang, AG; Eliazer, S; Kelly, OG; Agulnick, AD; Smart, NG; Moorman, MA; Kroon, E; Carpenter, MK; Baetge, EE (2006). Production of pancreatic hormone-expressing endocrine cells from human embryonic stem cells. Nature Biotechnology. **24** *(11): 1392–401.* doi:10.1038/nbt1259. PMID 17053790.

18. Colen, B.D. (9 October 2014) Giant leap against diabetes The Harvard Gazette, Retrieved 24 November 2014

19. "Dr. Yury Verlinsky, 1943–2009: Expert in reproductive technology Chicago Tribune, July 20, 2009

20. Verlinsky, Y; Strelchenko, N; Kukharenko, V; Rechitsky, S; Verlinsky, O; Galat, V; Kuliev, A (2005). Human embryonic stem cell lines with genetic disorders. Reproductive Biomedicine Online. **10** *(1): 105–10.* doi:10.1016/S1472-6483(10)60810-3. PMID 15705304.

21. Embryonic Stem Cells Help Deliver 'Good Genes' In A Model Of Inherited Blood Disorder, ScienceDaily (February 13, 2011).

22. Mao Z, Bozzella M, Seluanov A, Gorbunova V (September 2008). DNA repair by nonhomologous end joining and homologous recombination during cell cycle in human cells. Cell Cycle. **7** *(18): 2902–6. doi:10.4161/cc.7.18.6679. PMC 2754209. PMID 18769152.*

23. ^ Jump up to:[a] [b] Tichy ED, Pillai R, Deng L, et al. (November 2010). Mouse embryonic stem cells, but not somatic cells, predominantly use homologous recombination to repair double-strand DNA breaks. Stem Cells Dev. **19** *(11): 1699–711. doi:10.1089/scd.2010.0058. PMC 3128311. PMID 20446816.*

24. Hong Y, Stambrook PJ (October 2004). Restoration of an absent G1 arrest and protection from apoptosis in embryonic stem cells after ionizing radiation. Proc. Natl. Acad. Sci. U.S.A. **101** *(40): 14443–8. doi:10.1073/pnas.0401346101. PMC 521944. PMID 15452351.*

25. Aladjem MI, Spike BT, Rodewald LW, et al. (January 1998). ES cells do not activate p53-dependent stress responses and undergo p53-independent apoptosis in response to DNA damage. Curr. Biol. **8** *(3): 145–55.* doi:10.1016/S0960-9822(98)70061-2. PMID 9443911.

26. Bernstein C, Bernstein H, Payne CM, Garewal H (June 2002). DNA repair/ pro-apoptotic dual-role proteins in five major DNA repair pathways: fail-safe protection against carcinogenesis. Mutat. Res. **511** *(2): 145–78.* doi:10.1016/ S1383-5742(02)00009-1. PMID 12052432.

27. Cervantes RB, Stringer JR, Shao C, Tischfield JA, Stambrook PJ (March 2002). Embryonic stem cells and somatic cells differ in mutation frequency and type. Proc. Natl. Acad. Sci. U.S.A. **99** *(6): 3586–90. doi:10.1073/pnas.062527199. PMC 122567. PMID 11891338.*

28. Knoepfler, Paul S. (2009). Deconstructing Stem Cell Tumorigenicity: A Roadmap to Safe Regenerative Medicine. Stem Cells. **27** *(5): 1050–6. doi:10.1002/stem.37. PMC 2733374. PMID 19415771.*

29. Varlakhanova, Natalia V.; Cotterman, Rebecca F.; Devries, Wilhelmine N.; Morgan, Judy; Donahue, Leah Rae; Murray, Stephen; Knowles, Barbara B.; Knoepfler, Paul S. (2010). Myc maintains embryonic stem cell pluripotency and self-renewal. Differentiation. **80** *(1): 9–19. doi:10.1016/j.diff.2010.05.001. PMC 2916696. PMID 20537458.*

30. Kleinsmith LJ, Pierce GB Jr (1964). Multipotentiality of Single Embryoncal Carcinoma Cells. Cancer Res. **24**: 1544–51. PMID 14234000.

31. Andrews P, Matin M, Bahrami A, Damjanov I, Gokhale P, Draper J (2005). Embryonic stem (ES) cells and embryonal carcinoma (EC) cells: opposite sides of the same coin (PDF). Biochem Soc Trans. **33** *(Pt 6): 1526–30.* doi:10.1042/ BST20051526. PMID 16246161.

32. Martin GR (1980). Teratocarcinomas and mammalian embryogenesis. Science. **209** *(4458): 768–76. doi:10.1126/science.6250214. PMID 6250214.*

33. ^ Jump up to:[a] [b] Evans M, Kaufman M (1981). Establishment in culture of pluripotent cells from mouse embryos. Nature. **292** *(5819): 154–6.* doi:10.1038/292154a0. PMID 7242681.

34. ^ Jump up to:[a] [b] Martin G (1981). Isolation of a pluripotent cell line from early mouse embryos cultured in medium conditioned by teratocarcinoma stem cells. Proc Natl Acad Sci USA. **78** *(12): 7634–8. doi:10.1073/pnas.78.12.7634. PMC 349323. PMID 6950406.*

35. Thomson J, Itskovitz-Eldor J, Shapiro S, Waknitz M, Swiergiel J, Marshall V, Jones J (1998). Embryonic stem cell lines derived from human blastocysts. Science. **282** *(5391): 1145–7. doi:10.1126/science.282.5391.1145. PMID 9804556.*

36. FDA approves human embryonic stem cell study - CNN.com. January 23, 2009. Retrieved May 1, 2010.

37. Keirstead HS, Nistor G, Bernal G, et al. (2005). Human embryonic stem cell-derived oligodendrocyte progenitor cell transplants remyelinate and restore locomotion after spinal cord injury. J. Neurosci. **25** *(19): 4694–705. doi:10.1523/ JNEUROSCI.0311-05.2005. PMID 15888645.*

38. Reinberg, Steven (2009-01-23) FDA OKs 1st Embryonic Stem Cell Trial. The Washington Post

39. Geron comments on FDA hold on spinal cord injury trial http://www.geron.com/media/pressview.aspx?id=1188

40. Vergano, Dan (11 October 2010). Embryonic stem cells used on patient for first time. USA Today. Retrieved 12 October 2010.

41. Brown, Eryn (November 15, 2011). Geron exits stem cell research. LA Times. Retrieved 2011-11-15.

42. Great news: BioTime Subsidiary Asterias Acquires Geron Embryonic Stem Cell Program. iPScell.com. October 1, 2013.

43. Mountford, JC (2008). Human embryonic stem cells: origins, characteristics and potential for regenerative therapy. Transfus Med. **18** *(1): 1–12. doi:10.1111/j.1365-3148.2007.00807.x. PMID 18279188.*

44. Thomson JA, Itskovitz-Eldor J, Shapiro SS, Waknitz MA, Swiergiel JJ, Marshall VS, Jones JM (1998). Embryonic stem cell lines derived from human blastocysts. Science. **282** *(5391): 1145–1147. doi:10.1126/science.282.5391.1145. PMID 9804556.*

45. Smith AG, Heath JK, Donaldson DD, Wong GG, Moreau J, Stahl M, Rogers D (1988). Inhibition of pluripotential embryonic stem cell differentiation by purified polypeptides. Nature. **336** *(6200): 688–690.* doi:10.1038/336688a0. PMID 3143917.

46. Williams RL, Hilton DJ, Pease S, Willson TA, Stewart CL, Gearing DP, Wagner EF, Metcalf D, Nicola NA, Gough NM (1988). Myeloid leukaemia inhibitory factor maintains the developmental potential of embryonic stem cells. Nature. **336** *(6200): 684–687.* doi:10.1038/336684a0. PMID 3143916.

47. Ledermann B, Bürki K (1991). Establishment of a germ-line competent C57BL/6 embryonic stem cell line. Exp Cell Res. **197** *(2): 254–258.* doi:10.1016/0014-4827(91)90430-3. PMID 1959560.

48. Takahashi K, Tanabe K, Ohnuki M, Narita M, Ichisaka T, Tomoda K, Yamanaka S (2007). Induction of pluripotent stem cells from adult human fibroblasts by defined factors. Cell. **131** *(5): 861–872. doi:10.1016/j.cell.2007.11.019. PMID 18035408.*

49. Klimanskaya I, Chung Y, Becker S, Lu SJ, Lanza R (2006). Human embryonic stem cell lines derived from single blastomeres. Nature. **444** *(7118): 481–5.* doi:10.1038/nature05142. PMID 16929302.

50. US scientists relieved as Obama lifts ban on stem cell research, The Guardian, 10 March 2009

51. Wernig, Marius; Meissner, Alexander; Foreman, Ruth; Brambrink, Tobias; Ku, Manching; Hochedlinger, Konrad; Bernstein, Bradley E.; Jaenisch, Rudolf (2007-07-19). In vitro reprogramming of fibroblasts into a pluripotent ES-cell-like state. Nature. **448** *(7151): 318–324.* doi:10.1038/nature05944. ISSN 1476-4687. PMID 17554336.

52. Embryonic stem cells made without embryos. Reuters. 2007-11-21.

53. Weiss, Rick (2007-12-07). Scientists Cure Mice Of Sickle Cell Using Stem

Cell Technique: New Approach Is From Skin, Not Embryos. The Washington Post. pp. A02.

54. Hanna, J.; Wernig, M.; Markoulaki, S.; Sun, C.-W.; Meissner, A.; Cassady, J. P.; Beard, C.; Brambrink, T.; Wu, L.-C.; Townes, T. M.; Jaenisch, R. (2007). Treatment of Sickle Cell Anemia Mouse Model with iPS Cells Generated from Autologous Skin. Science. **318** *(5858): 1920. doi:10.1126/science.1152092. PMID 18063756.*

55. Helen Briggs (2008-01-17). US team makes embryo clone of men. BBC. pp. A01.

56. Ebert, Jessica (24 January 2005). Human stem cells trigger immune attack. Nature News. London: Nature Publishing Group. doi:10.1038/news050124-1. Archived from the original on 2010-09-24. Retrieved 2009-02-27.

57. Martin MJ, Muotri A, Gage F, Varki A (2005). Human embryonic stem cells express an immunogenic nonhuman sialic acid. Nat. Med. **11** *(2): 228–32.* doi:10.1038/nm1181. PMID 15685172.

58. Klimanskaya I, Chung Y, Meisner L, Johnson J, West MD, Lanza R (2005). Human embryonic stem cells derived without feeder cells. Lancet. **365** *(9471): 1636–41.* doi:10.1016/S0140-6736(05)66473-2. PMID 15885296.

CHAPTER 8

Spinal Cord: Structure and function

Chapter Contents

- **Introduction**
- **Structure**
- **Function**
- **Clinical Significance**
- **Additional Images**

Spinal Cord is a specialised, international journal that has been publishing spinal cord related manuscripts since 1963. It appears monthly, online and in print, and accepts contributions on spinal cord anatomy, physiology and management of injury and disease. *Spinal Cord* is multi-disciplinary and publishes contributions on basic science, clinical and applied studies, psychology and epidemiology of spinal disorders. It publishes high quality original papers and topical reviews.

INTRODUCTION

The **spinal cord** is a long, thin, tubular bundle of nervous tissue and support cells that extends from the medulla oblongata in the brainstem to the lumbar region of the vertebral column. The brain and spinal cord together make up the central nervous system (CNS).

The spinal cord begins at the occipital bone and extends down to the space between the first and second lumbar vertebrae; it does not extend the entire length of the vertebral column. It is around 45 cm (18 in) in men and around 43 cm (17 in) long in women. Also, the spinal cord has a varying width, ranging from 13 mm ($^1/_2$ in) thick in the cervical and lumbar regions to 6.4 mm ($^1/_4$ in) thick in the thoracic area. The enclosing bony vertebral column protects the relatively shorter spinal cord. The spinal cord functions primarily in the transmission of neural signals between the brain and the rest of the body but also contains neural circuits that can independently control numerous reflexes and central pattern generators. The spinal cord has three major functions: as a conduit for motor information, which travels down the spinal cord, as a conduit for sensory information in the reverse direction, and finally as a center for coordinating certain reflexes.

STRUCTURE

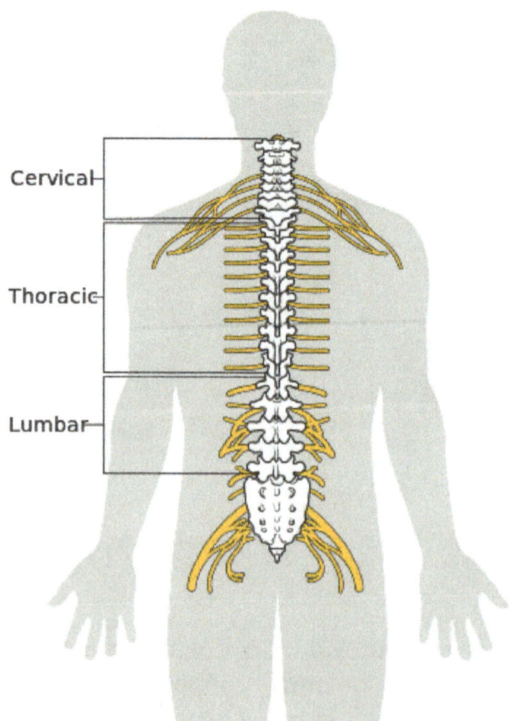

Diagram of the spinal cord showing segments.

The spinal cord is the main pathway for information connecting the brain and peripheral nervous system. The length of the spinal cord is much shorter as compared to the length of the vertebral column. The human spinal cord extends from the foramen magnum and continues through to the conus medullaris near the second lumbar vertebra, terminating in a fibrous extension known as the filum terminale.

It is about 45 cm (18 in) long in men and around 43 cm (17 in) in women, ovoid-shaped, and is enlarged in the cervical and lumbar regions. The cervical enlargement, located from C5 to T1 spinal segments, is where sensory input comes from and motor output goes to the arms. The lumbar enlargement, located between L1 and S3 spinal segments, handles sensory input and motor output coming from and going to the legs.

The spinal cord is continuous with the caudal portion of the medulla, running from the base of the skull to the body of the first lumbar vertebra. It does not run the full length of the vertebral column in adults. It is made of 31 segments that each contain sensory nerve root and motor nerve root. The first cervical segment is usually very small and may be absent in most individuals. Nerve roots merge into 31 bilaterally symmetric pairs of spinal nerves. The peripheral nervous system is made up of these spinal roots, nerves, and ganglia.

Dorsal roots are fascicles of axons in the spinal cord that receive sensory information from the skin, muscle, and visceral organs that enter through a point of entry called the *dorsal root entry zone*. Dorsal root ganglia hold the cell bodies of dorsal root ganglia in the spinal ganglia (dorsal root ganglia) related with that spinal segment.

Ventral roots only have efferent fibers that arise from motor neurons (general somatic efferent neurons) whose cell bodies are found in the ventral (or anterior) gray horns of the spinal cord.

The spinal cord (and brain) are protected by three layers of tissue or membranes called meninges, that surround the canal . The dura mater is the outermost layer, and it forms a tough protective coating. Between the dura mater and the surrounding bone of the vertebrae is a space called the epidural space. The epidural space is filled with adipose tissue, and it contains a network of blood vessels. The arachnoid mater is the middle protective layer. Its name comes from the fact that the tissue has a spiderweb-like appearance. The space between the arachnoid and the underlying pia mater is called the subarachnoid space. The subarachnoid space contains cerebrospinal fluid (CSF). The medical procedure known as a lumbar puncture (or "spinal tap") involves use of a needle to withdraw cerebrospinal fluid from the subarachnoid space, usually from the lumbar region of the spine. The pia mater is the innermost protective layer. It is very delicate and it is tightly associated with the surface of the spinal cord. The cord is stabilized within the dura mater by the connecting denticulate ligaments, which extend from the enveloping pia mater laterally between the dorsal and ventral roots. The dural sac ends at the vertebral level of the second sacral vertebra.

In cross-section, the peripheral region of the cord contains neuronal white matter tracts containing sensory and motor neurons. Internal to this peripheral region is the grey matter. The nerve cell bodies of the grey matter are contained in the three grey columns of the spinal cord that give the region its butterfly-shape. This central region surrounds the central canal, which is an extension of the fourth ventricle and contains cerebrospinal fluid.

The spinal cord has a shape that is compressed dorso-ventrally, giving it an elliptical shape. The cord has grooves in the dorsal and ventral sides. The posterior median sulcus is the groove in the dorsal side, and the anterior median fissure is the groove in the ventral side.

Spinal Cord Segments

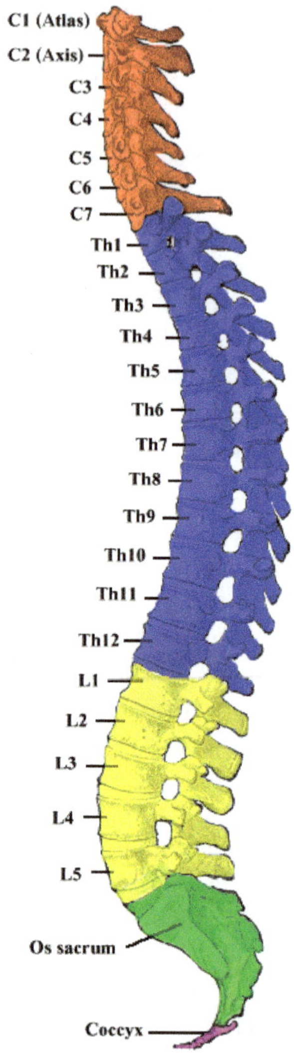

The human spinal cord is divided into 31 different segments. At every segment, right and left pairs of spinal nerves (mixed; sensory and motor) form. Six to eight motor nerve rootlets branch out of right and left ventro lateral sulci in a very orderly manner. Nerve rootlets combine to form nerve roots. Likewise, sensory nerve rootlets form off right and left dorsal lateral sulci and form sensory nerve roots. The ventral (motor) and dorsal (sensory) roots combine to form spinal nerves (mixed; motor and sensory), one on each side of the spinal cord. Spinal nerves, with the exception of C1 and C2, form inside intervertebral foramen (IVF). Note that at each spinal segment, the border between the central and peripheral nervous system can be observed. Rootlets are a part of the peripheral nervous system. The spinal cord is a long, slender cable of nerve tissue which extends lengthwise through the vertebrae of the spinal column. At the upper end it connects with the brain through an opening in the floor of the skull. It extends downward almost to the level of the hips. It is well protected by the vertebrae, whose bony processes join together to form a canal within which the spinal cord is located.

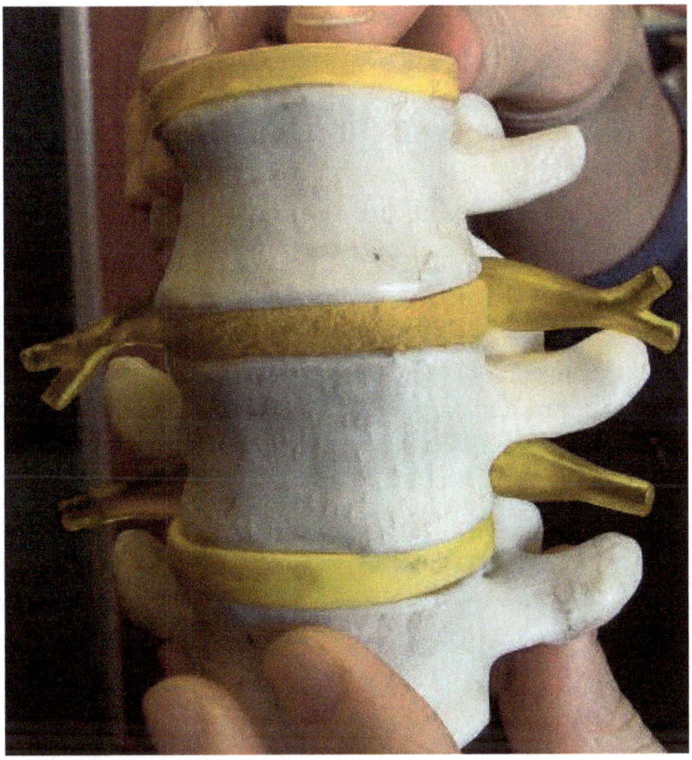

A model of segments of the human spine and spinal cord, nerve roots can be seen extending laterally from the (not visible) spinal cord.

In the upper part of the vertebral column, spinal nerves exit directly from the spinal cord, whereas in the lower part of the vertebral column nerves pass further down the column before exiting. The terminal portion of the spinal cord is called the conus medullaris. The pia mater continues as an extension called the filum terminale, which anchors the spinal cord to the coccyx. The cauda equina ("horse's tail") is the name for the collection of nerves in the vertebral column that continue to travel through the vertebral column below the conus medullaris. The cauda equina forms because the spinal cord stops growing in length at about age four, even though the vertebral column continues to lengthen until adulthood. This results in sacral spinal nerves originating in the upper lumbar region.

The spinal cord can be anatomically divided into 31 spinal segments based on the origins of the spinal nerves. Each segment of the spinal cord is associated with a pair of ganglia, called dorsal root ganglia, which are situated just outside the spinal cord. These ganglia contain cell bodies of sensory neurons. Axons of these sensory neurons travel into the spinal cord via the dorsal roots.

Ventral roots consist of axons from motor neurons, which bring information to the periphery from cell bodies within the CNS. Dorsal roots and ventral roots come together and exit the intervertebral foramina as they become spinal nerves.

The grey column, (as three regions of grey columns), in the center of the cord, is shaped like a butterfly and consists of cell bodies of interneurons, motor neurons, neuroglia cells and unmyelinated axons. The anterior and posterior grey column present as projections of the grey matter and are also known as the horns of the spinal cord. Together, the grey columns and the gray commissure form the "grey H."

The white matter is located outside of the grey matter and consists almost totally of myelinated motor and sensory axons. "Columns" of white matter carry information either up or down the spinal cord.

Within the CNS, nerve cell bodies are generally organized into functional clusters, called nuclei. Axons within the CNS are grouped into tracts.

There are 31 spinal cord nerve segments in a human spinal cord:

- 8 cervical segments forming 8 pairs of cervical nerves (C1 spinal nerves exit spinal column between occiput and C1 vertebra; C2 nerves exit between posterior arch of C1 vertebra and lamina of C2 vertebra; C3–C8 spinal nerves through IVF above corresponding cervica vertebra, with the exception of C8 pair which exit via IVF between C7 and T1 vertebra)
- 12 thoracic segments forming 12 pairs of thoracic nerves (exit spinal column through IVF below corresponding vertebra T1–T12)
- 5 lumbar segments forming 5 pairs of lumbar nerves (exit spinal column through IVF, below corresponding vertebra L1–L5)
- 5 sacral segments forming 5 pairs of sacral nerves (exit spinal column through IVF, below corresponding vertebra S1–S5)
- 1 coccygeal segment

Spinal Cord Segments in Some Common Species

Species	Cervical	Thoracic	Lumbar	Sacral	Caudal/Coccygeal	Total
Dog	8	13	7	3	5	36
Cat	8	13	7	3	5	36
Cow	8	13	6	5	5	37
Horse	8	18	6	5	5	42
Pig	8	15/14	6/7	4	5	38
Human	8	12	5	5	1	31

In the fetus, vertebral segments correspond with spinal cord segments. However, because the vertebral column grows longer than the spinal cord, spinal cord segments do not correspond to vertebral segments in the adult, particularly in the lower spinal cord. For example, lumbar and sacral spinal cord segments are found between vertebral levels T9 and L2, and the spinal cord ends around the L1/L2 vertebral level, forming a structure known as the conus medullaris.

Although the spinal cord cell bodies end around the L1/L2 vertebral level, the spinal nerves for each segment exit at the level of the corresponding vertebra. For the nerves of the lower spinal cord, this means that they exit the vertebral column much lower (more caudally) than their roots. As these nerves travel from their respective roots to their point of exit from the vertebral column, the nerves of the lower spinal segments form a bundle called the cauda equina.

There are two regions where the spinal cord enlarges:

- Cervical enlargement – corresponds roughly to the brachial plexus nerves, which innervate the upper limb. It includes spinal cord segments from about C4 to T1. The vertebral levels of the enlargement are roughly the same (C4 to T1).
- Lumbosacral enlargement – corresponds to the lumbosacral plexus nerves, which innervate the lower limb. It comprises the spinal cord segments from L2 to S3 and is found about the vertebral levels of T9 to T12.

Development

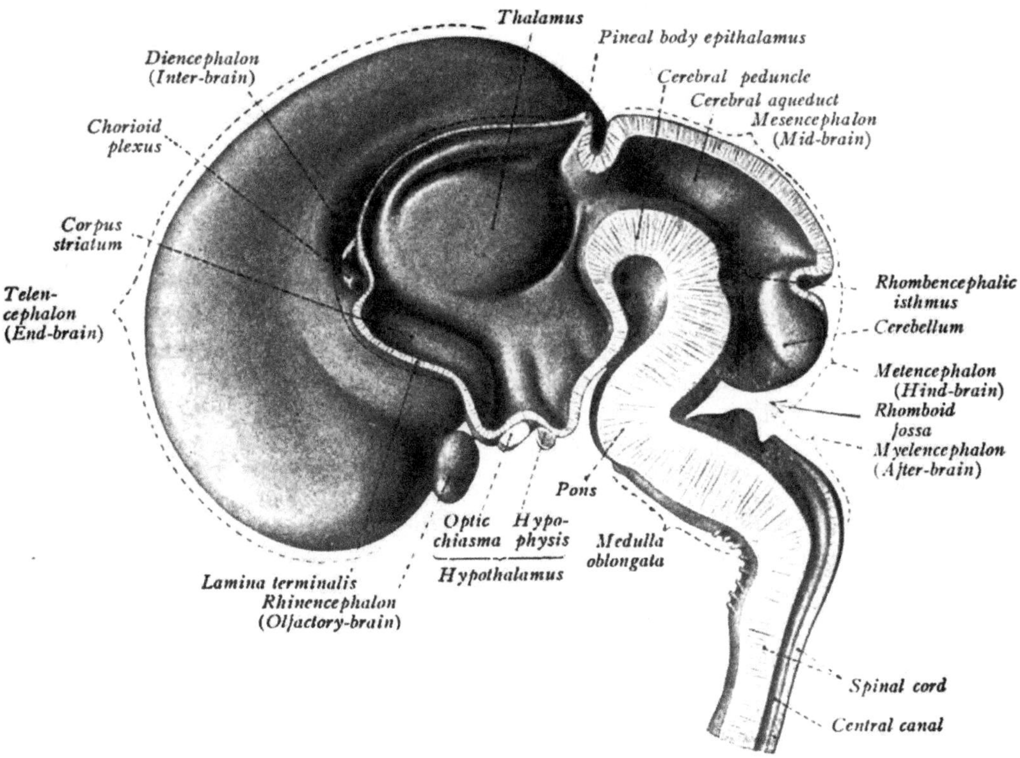

Spinal cord seen in a median section of a five-week-old embryo.

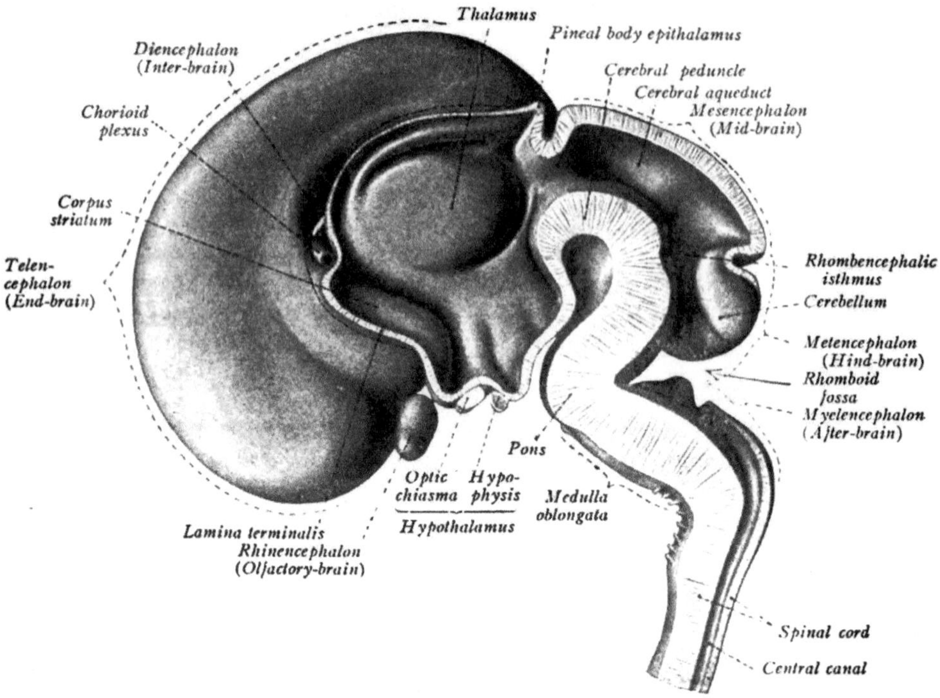

Spinal cord seen in a median section of a 3 month old fetus.

The spinal cord is made from part of the neural tube during development. There are four stages of the spinal cord that arises from the neural tube: The neural plate, neural fold, neural tube, and the spinal cord. Neural differentiation occurs within the spinal cord portion of the tube. As the neural tube begins to develop, the notochord begins to secrete a factor known as Sonic hedgehog or SHH. As a result, the floor plate then also begins to secrete SHH, and this will induce the basal plate to develop motor neurons. During the maturation of the neural tube, its lateral walls thicken and form a longtitudinal groove called the sulcus limitans. This exends the length of the spinal cord into dorsal and ventral portions as well. Meanwhile, the overlying ectoderm secretes bone morphogenetic protein (BMP). This induces the roof plate to begin to secrete BMP, which will induce the alar plate to develop sensory neurons. Dorsal root ganglion neurons differentiate from neural crest progenitors. As the dorsal and ventral column cells proliferate, the lumen of the neural tube narrows to form the small central canal of the spinal cord. The alar plate and the basal plate are separated by the sulcus limitans. Additionally, the floor plate also secretes netrins. The netrins act as chemoattractants to decussation of pain and temperature sensory neurons in the alar plate across the anterior white commissure, where they then ascend towards the thalamus. Following the closure of the caudal neuropore and formation of the brain›s ventricles that contain the choroid plexus tissue, the central canal of the caudal spinal cord is filled with cerebrospinal fluid.

Earlier findings by Viktor Hamburger and Rita Levi-Montalcini in the chick embryo have been confirmed by more recent studies which have demonstrated that the elimination of neuronal cells by programmed cell death (PCD) is necessary for the correct assembly of the nervous system.

Overall, spontaneous embryonic activity has been shown to play a role in neuron and muscle development but is probably not involved in the initial formation of connections between spinal neurons.

Blood Supply

The spinal cord is supplied with blood by three arteries that run along its length starting in the brain, and many arteries that approach it through the sides of the spinal column. The three longitudinal arteries are called the anterior spinal artery, and the right and left posterior spinal arteries. These travel in the subarachnoid space and send branches into the spinal cord. They form anastamoses (connections) via the anterior and posterior segmental medullary arteries, which enter the spinal cord at various points along its length. The actual blood flow caudally through these arteries, derived from the posterior cerebral circulation, is inadequate to maintain the spinal cord beyond the cervical segments.

The major contribution to the arterial blood supply of the spinal cord below the cervical region comes from the radially arranged posterior and anterior radicular arteries, which run into the spinal cord alongside the dorsal and ventral nerve roots, but with one exception do not connect directly with any of the three longitudinal arteries. These intercostal and lumbar radicular arteries arise from the aorta, provide major anastomoses and supplement the blood flow to the spinal cord. In humans the largest of the anterior radicular arteries is known as the artery of Adamkiewicz, or anterior radicularis magna (ARM) artery, which usually arises between L1 and L2, but can arise anywhere from T9 to L5. Impaired blood flow through these critical radicular arteries, especially during surgical procedures that involve abrupt disruption of blood flow through the aorta for example during aortic aneursym repair, can result in spinal cord infarction and paraplegia.

FUNCTION

Somatosensory Organization

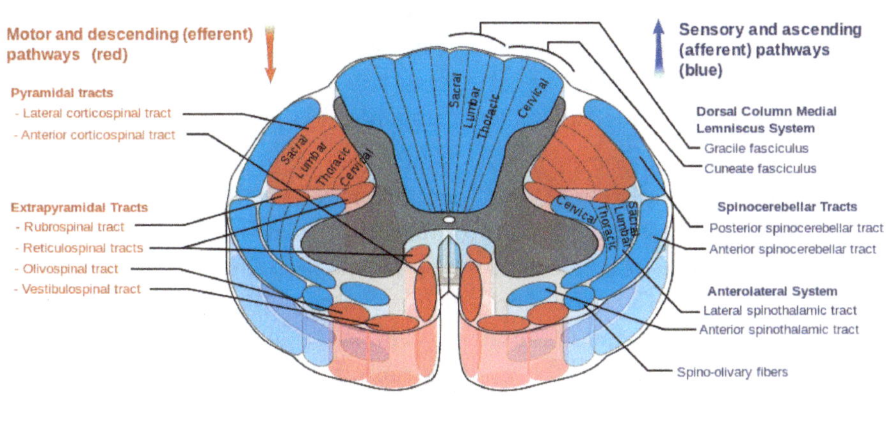

Spinal cord tracts.

Somatosensory organization is divided into the dorsal column-medial lemniscus tract (the touch/proprioception/vibration sensory pathway) and the anterolateral system, or ALS (the pain/temperature sensory pathway). Both sensory pathways use three different neurons to get information from sensory receptors at the periphery to the cerebral cortex. These neurons are designated primary, secondary and tertiary sensory neurons. In both pathways, primary sensory neuron cell bodies are found in the dorsal root ganglia, and their central axons project into the spinal cord.

In the dorsal column-medial leminiscus tract, a primary neuron›s axon enters the spinal cord and then enters the dorsal column. If the primary axon enters below spinal level T6, the axon travels in the fasciculus gracilis, the medial part of the column. If the axon enters above level T6, then it travels in the fasciculus cuneatus, which is lateral to the fasciculus gracilis. Either way, the primary axon ascends to the lower medulla, where it leaves its fasciculus and synapses with a secondary neuron in one of the dorsal column nuclei: either the nucleus gracilis or the nucleus cuneatus, depending on the pathway it took. At this point, the secondary axon leaves its nucleus and passes anteriorly and medially. The collection of secondary axons that do this are known as internal arcuate fibers. The internal arcuate fibers decussate and continue ascending as the contralateral medial lemniscus. Secondary axons from the medial lemniscus finally terminate in the ventral posterolateral nucleus (VPL) of the thalamus, where they synapse with tertiary neurons. From there, tertiary neurons ascend via the posterior limb of the internal capsule and end in the primary sensory cortex.

The proprioception of the lower limbs differs from the upper limbs and upper trunk. There is a four-neuron pathway for lower limb proprioception. This pathway initially follows the dorsal spino-cerebellar pathway. It is arranged as follows: proprioceptive receptors of lower limb -> peripheral process -> dorsal root ganglion -> central process -> Clarke›s column -> 2nd order neuron -> medulla oblogata (Caudate nucleus) -> 3rd order neuron -> VPL of thalamus -> 4th order neuron -> posterior limb of internal capsule -> corona radiata -> sensory area of cerebrum.

The anterolateral system works somewhat differently. Its primary neurons axons enter the spinal cord and then ascend one to two levels before synapsing in the substantia gelatinosa. The tract that ascends before synapsing is known as Lissauer›s tract. After synapsing, secondary axons decussate and ascend in the anterior lateral portion of the spinal cord as the spinothalamic tract. This tract ascends all the way to the VPL, where it synapses on tertiary neurons. Tertiary neuronal axons then travel to the primary sensory cortex via the posterior limb of the internal capsule.

It should be noted that some of the "pain fibers» in the ALS deviate from their pathway towards the VPL. In one such deviation, axons travel towards the reticular formation in the midbrain. The reticular formation then projects to a number of places including the hippocampus (to create memories about the pain), the centromedian nucleus (to cause diffuse, non-specific pain) and various parts of the cortex. Additionally, some ALS axons project to the periaqueductal gray in the pons, and the axons forming the periaqueductal gray then project to the nucleus raphes magnus, which projects back down to where the pain signal is coming from and inhibits it. This helps control the sensation of pain to some degree.

Motor Organization

Actions of the spinal nerves edit	
Level	**Motor Function**
C1–C6	Neck flexors
C1–T1	Neck extensors
C3, C4, C5	Supply diaphragm (mostly C4)
C5, C6	Move shoulder, raise arm (deltoid); flex elbow (biceps)
C6	externally rotate (supinate) the arm
C6, C7	Extend elbow and wrist (triceps and wrist extensors); pronate wrist
C7, C8	Flex wrist; supply small muscles of the hand
T1–T6	Intercostals and trunk above the waist
T7–L1	Abdominal muscles
L1–L4	Flex thigh
L2, L3, L4	Adduct thigh; Extend leg at the knee (quadriceps femoris)
L4, L5, S1	abduct thigh; Flex leg at the knee (hamstrings); Dorsiflexfoot (tibialis anterior); Extend toes
L5, S1, S2	Extend leg at the hip (gluteus maximus); Plantar flex foot and flex toes

The corticospinal tract serves as the motor pathway for upper motor neuronal signals coming from the cerebral cortex and from primitive brainstem motor nuclei.

Cortical upper motor neurons originate from Brodmann areas 1, 2, 3, 4, and 6 and then descend in the posterior limb of the internal capsule, through the crus cerebri, down through the pons, and to the medullary pyramids, where about 90% of the axons cross to the contralateral side at the decussation of the pyramids. They then descend as the lateral corticospinal tract. These axons synapse with lower motor neurons in the ventral horns of all levels of the spinal cord. The remaining 10% of axons descend on the ipsilateral side as the ventral corticospinal tract. These axons also synapse with lower motor neurons in the ventral horns. Most of them will cross to the contralateral side of the cord (via the anterior white commissure) right before synapsing.

The midbrain nuclei include four motor tracts that send upper motor neuronal axons down the spinal cord to lower motor neurons. These are the rubrospinal tract, the vestibulospinal tract, the tectospinal tract and the reticulospinal tract. The rubrospinal tract descends with the lateral corticospinal tract, and the remaining three descend with the anterior corticospinal tract.

The function of lower motor neurons can be divided into two different groups: the lateral corticospinal tract and the anterior cortical spinal tract. The lateral tract contains upper motor neuronal axons which synapse on dorsal lateral (DL) lower motor neurons. The DL neurons are involved in distal limb control. Therefore, these DL neurons are found specifically only in the cervical and lumbosacral enlargements within the spinal cord. There is no decussation in the lateral corticospinal tract after the decussation at the medullary pyramids.

The anterior corticospinal tract descends ipsilaterally in the anterior column, where the axons emerge and either synapse on lower ventromedial (VM) motor neurons in the ventral horn ipsilaterally or descussate at the anterior white commissure where they synapse on VM lower motor neurons contralaterally . The tectospinal, vestibulospinal and reticulospinal descend ipsilaterally in the anterior column but do not synapse across the anterior white commissure. Rather, they only synapse on VM lower motor neurons ipsilaterally. The VM lower motor neurons control the large, postural muscles of the axial skeleton. These lower motor neurons, unlike those of the DL, are located in the ventral horn all the way throughout the spinal cord.

Spinocerebellar Tracts

Proprioceptive information in the body travels up the spinal cord via three tracks. Below L2, the proprioceptive information travels up the spinal cord in the ventral spinocerebellar tract. Also known as the anterior spinocerebellar tract, sensory receptors take in the information and travel into the spinal cord. The cell bodies of these primary neurons are located in the dorsal root ganglia. In the spinal cord, the axons synapse and the secondary neuronal axons decussates and then travel up to the superior cerebellar peduncle where they decussate again. From here, the information is brought to deep nuclei of the cerebellum including the fastigial and interposed nuclei.

From the levels of L2 to T1, proprioceptive information enters the spinal cord and ascends ipsilaterally, where it synapses in Clarke›s nucleus. The secondary neuronal axons continue to ascend ipsilaterally and then pass into the cerebellum via the inferior cerebellar peduncle. This tract is known as the dorsal spinocerebellar tract.

From above T1, proprioceptive primary axons enter the spinal cord and ascend ipsilaterally until reaching the accessory cuneate nucleus, where they synapse. The secondary axons pass into the cerebellum via the inferior cerebellar peduncle where again, these axons synapse on cerebellar deep nuclei. This tract is known as the cuneocerebellar tract.

Motor information travels from the brain down the spinal cord via descending spinal cord tracts. Descending tracts involve two neurons: the upper motor neuron (UMN) and lower motor neuron (LMN). A nerve signal travels down the upper motor neuron until it synapses with the lower motor neuron in the spinal cord. Then, the lower motor neuron conducts the nerve signal to the spinal root where efferent nerve fibers carry the motor signal toward the target muscle. The descending tracts are composed of white matter. There are several descending tracts serving different functions. The corticospinal tracts (lateral and anterior) are responsible for coordinated limb movements.

CLINICAL SIGNIFICANCE

A congenital disorder is diastematomyelia in which part of the spinal cord is split usually at the level of the upper lumbar vertebrae. Sometimes the split can be along the length of the spinal cord.

Injury

Spinal cord injuries can be caused by trauma to the spinal column (stretching, bruising, applying pressure, severing, laceration, etc.). The vertebral bones or intervertebral disks can shatter, causing the spinal cord to be punctured by a sharp fragment of bone. Usually, victims of spinal cord injuries will suffer loss of feeling in certain parts of their body. In milder cases, a victim might only suffer loss of hand or foot function. More severe injuries may result in paraplegia, tetraplegia (also known as quadriplegia), or full body paralysis below the site of injury to the spinal cord.

Damage to upper motor neuron axons in the spinal cord results in a characteristic pattern of ipsilateral deficits. These include hyperreflexia, hypertonia and muscle weakness. Lower motor neuronal damage results in its own characteristic pattern of deficits. Rather than an entire side of deficits, there is a pattern relating to the myotome affected by the damage. Additionally, lower motor neurons are characterized by muscle weakness, hypotonia, hyporeflexia and muscle atrophy.

Spinal shock and neurogenic shock can occur from a spinal injury. Spinal shock is usually temporary, lasting only for 24–48 hours, and is a temporary absence of sensory and motor functions. Neurogenic shock lasts for weeks and can lead to a loss of muscle tone due to disuse of the muscles below the injured site.

The two areas of the spinal cord most commonly injured are the cervical spine (C1-C7) and the lumbar spine (L1-L5). (The notation C1, C7, L1, L5 refer to the location of a specific vertebra in either the cervical, thoracic, or lumbar region of the spine.) Spinal cord injury can also be non-traumatic and caused by disease (transverse myelitis, polio, spina bifida, Friedreich›s ataxia, spinal cord tumor, spinal stenosis etc.)

In the U.S., 10,000-12,000 people become paralyzed annually as a result of various injuries to the spinal cord.

Treatment

Real or suspected spinal cord injuries need immediate immobilisation including that of the head. Scans will be needed to assess the injury. A steroid, methylprednisolone, can be of help as can physical therapy and possibly antioxidants. Treatments need to focus on limiting post-injury cell death, promoting cell regeneration, and replacing lost cells. Regeneration is facilitated by maintaining electric transmission in neural elements. Replacement of lost cells is facilitated by transplants with embryonic stem cells, stem cells from the spinal cord, and spinal cord cells from fetuses.

Lumbar Puncture

The spinal cord ends at the level of vertebrae L1–L2, while the subarachnoid space —the compartment that contains cerebrospinal fluid— extends down to the lower border of S2. Lumbar punctures in adults are usually performed between L3–L5 (cauda equina level) in order to avoid damage to the spinal cord. In the fetus, the spinal cord extends the full length of the spine and regresses as the body grows.

Tumours

Spinal tumours can occur in the spinal cord and these can be either inside (intradural) or outside (extradural) the dura mater.

ADDITIONAL IMAGES

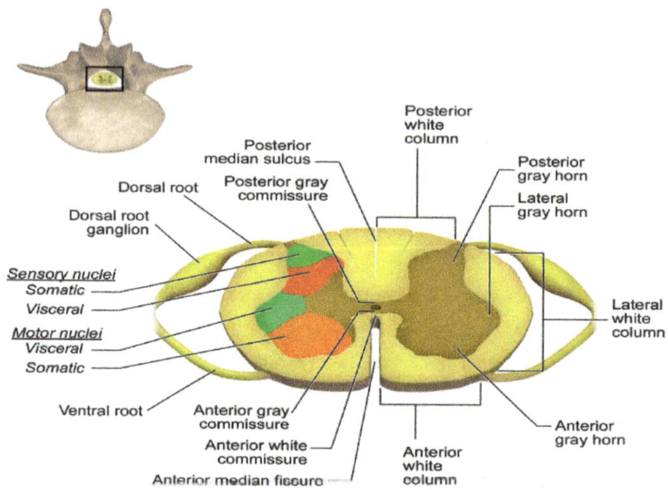

Sectional Organization of the Spinal Cord

Spinal Cord Sectional Anatomy. Animation in the reference.

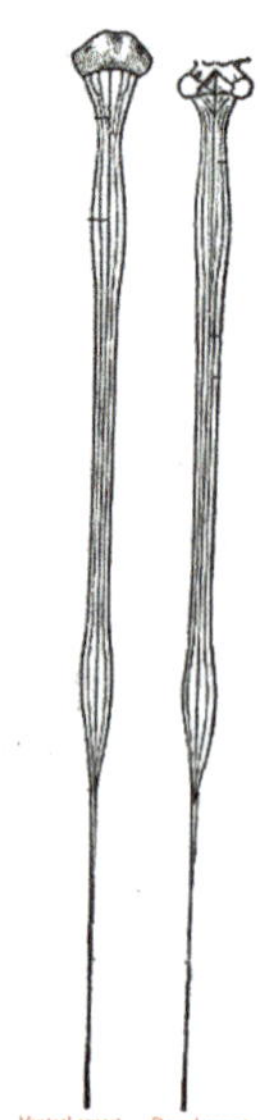

Diagrams of the spinal cord.

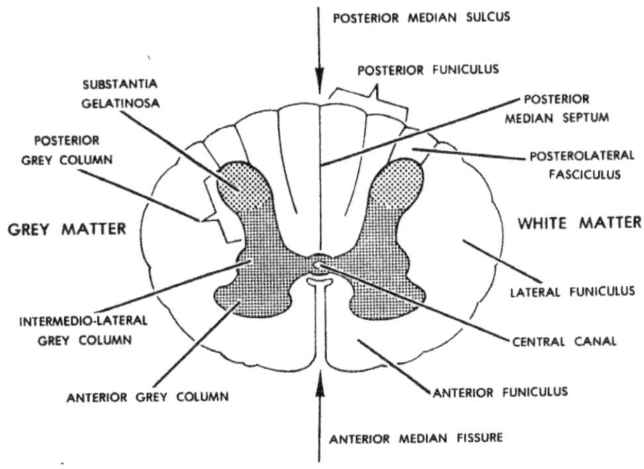

Cross-section through the spinal cord at the mid-thoracic level.

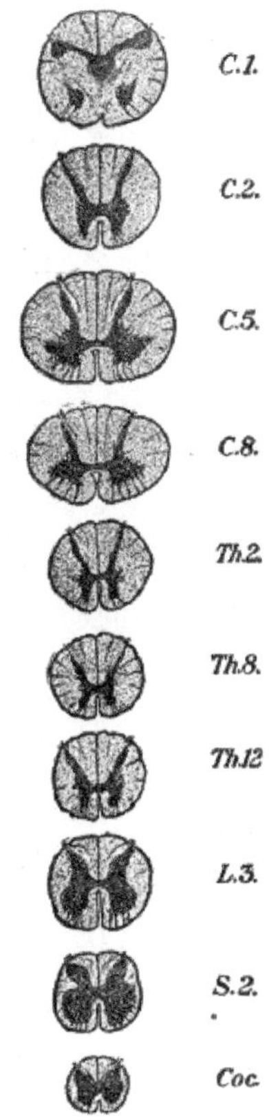

Cross-sections of the spinal cord at varying levels.

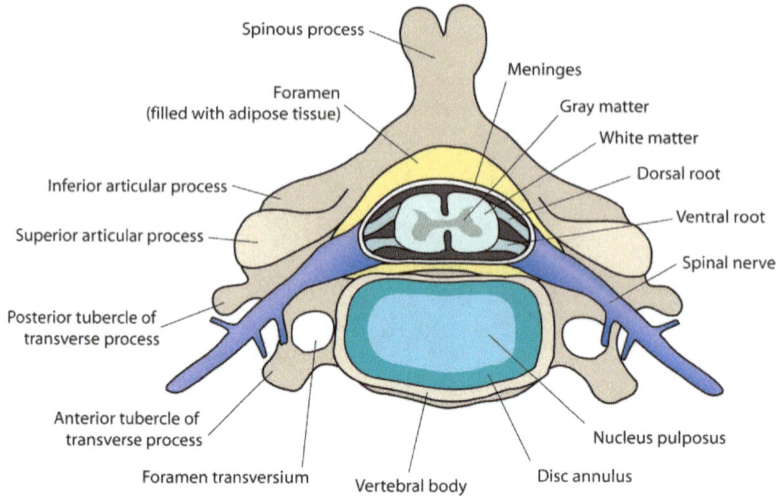

Cervical vertebra

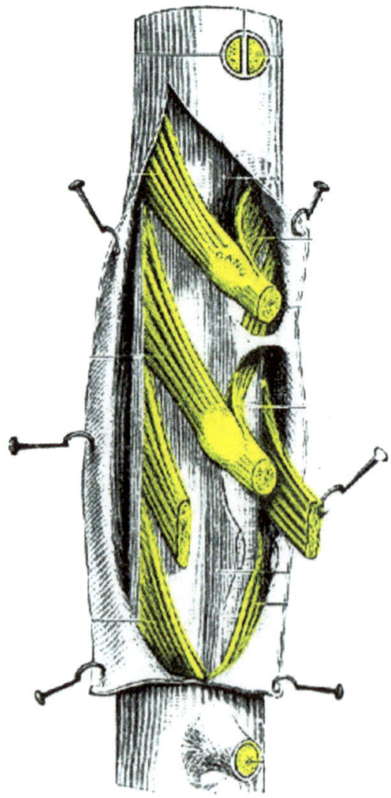

A portion of the spinal cord, showing its right lateral surface. The dura is opened and arranged to show the nerve roots.

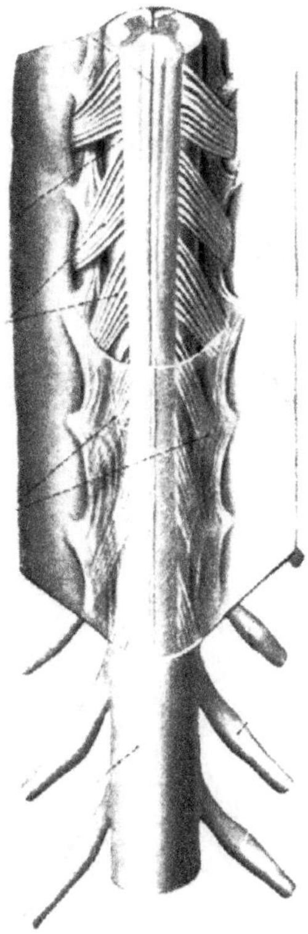

The spinal cord with dura cut open, showing the exits of the spinal nerves.

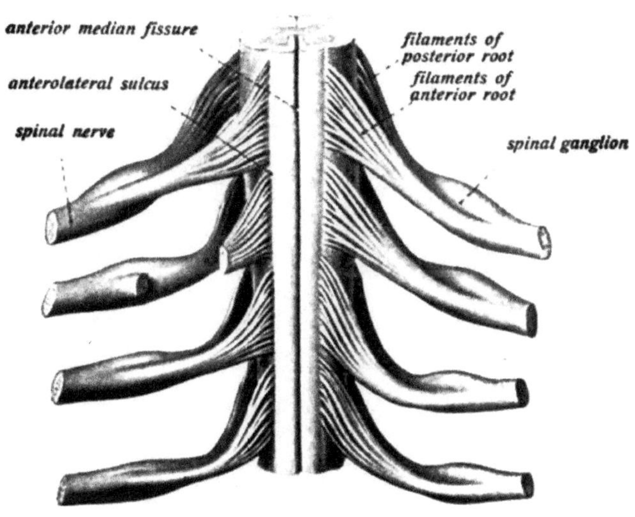

The spinal cord showing how the anterior and posterior roots join in the spinal nerves.

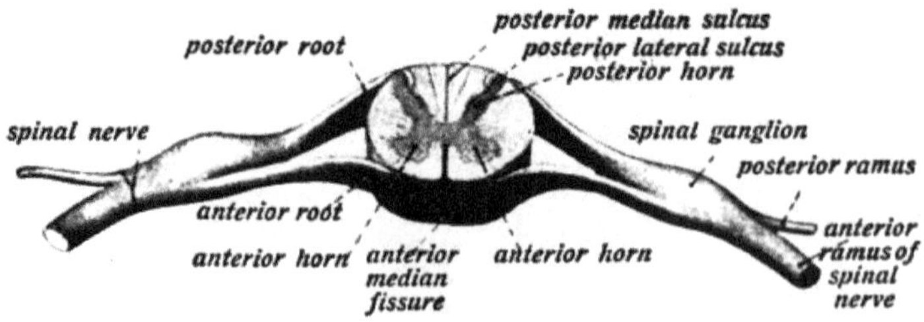

The spinal cord showing how the anterior and posterior roots join in the spinal nerves.

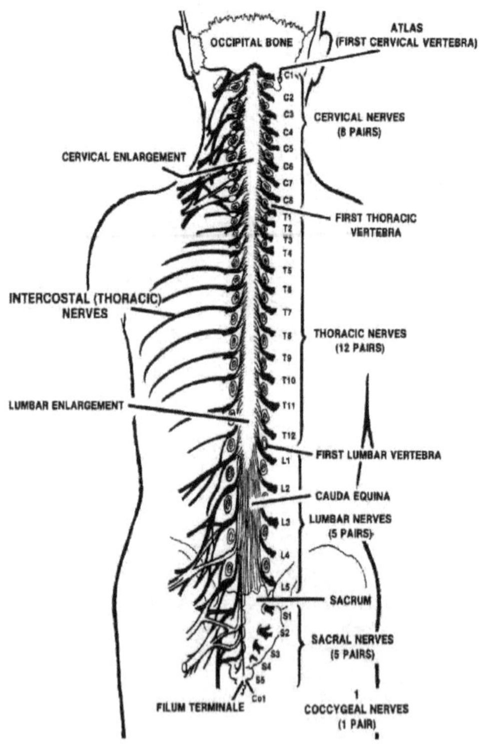

A longer view of the spinal cord.

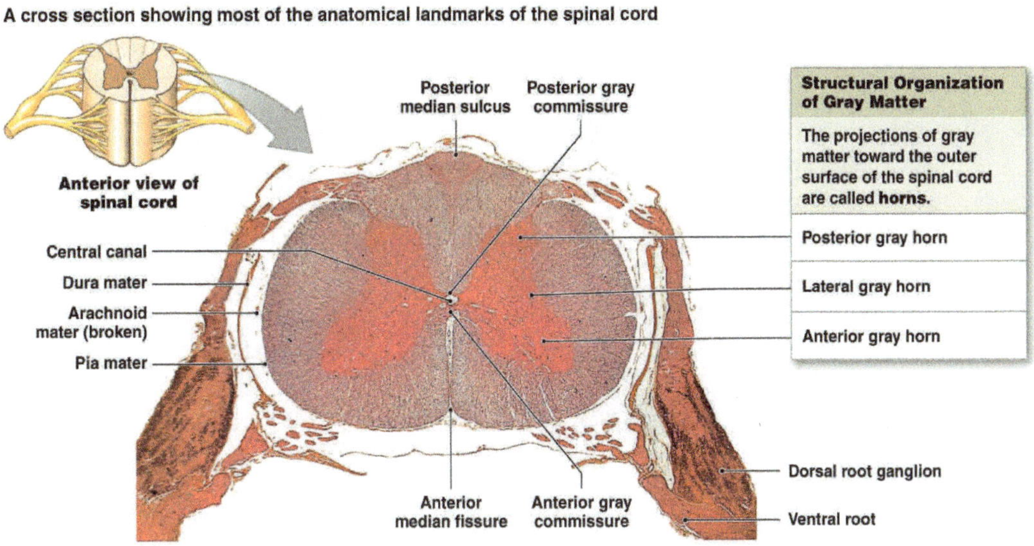

Projections of the spinal cord into the nerves (red motor, blue sensory).

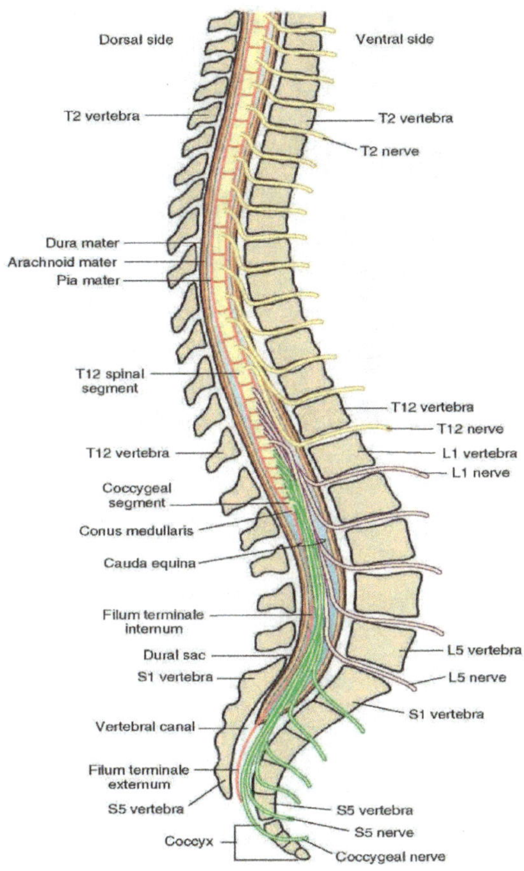

Projections of the spinal cord into the nerves (red motor, blue sensory).

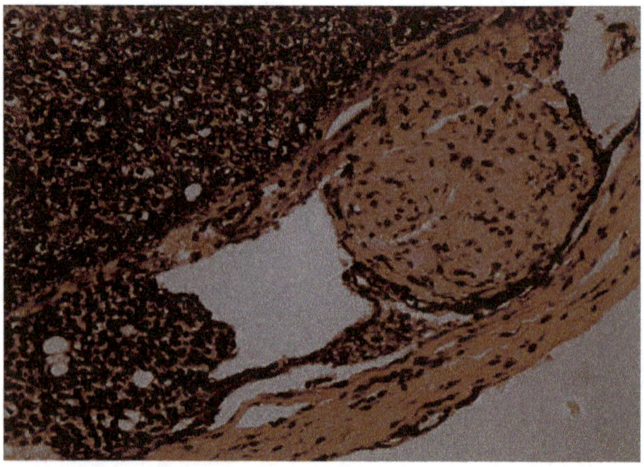

Cross-section of rabbit spinal cord.

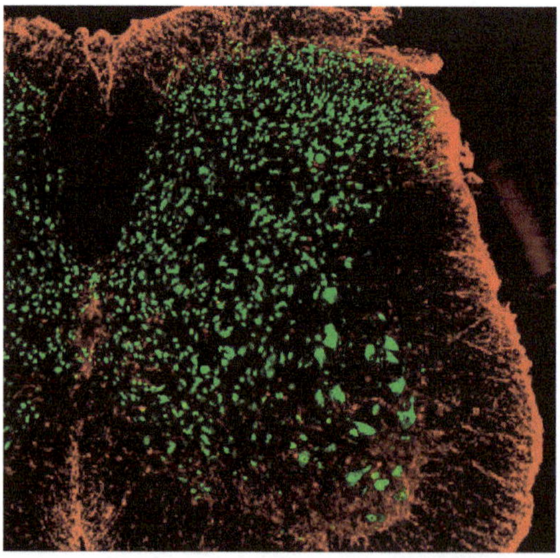

Cross-section of adult mouse spinal cord: astrocytes (red) and neurons (green)

REFERENCES

1. Maton, Anthea; Jean Hopkins; Charles William McLaughlin; Susan Johnson; Maryanna Quon Warner; David LaHart; Jill D. Wright (1993). Human Biology and Health. Englewood Cliffs, New Jersey, United States of America: Prentice Hall. pp. 132–144. ISBN 0-13-981176-1.
2. Myers, Gary. Exploring Psychology. Worth Publishers. p. 41. ISBN 978-1429216357.
3. «Spinal Cord Gross Anatomy». Retrieved December 27, 2015.

4. Kaufman, Bard. "Spinal Cord- Development and Stem Cells». Life Map Discovery Compendium. Retrieved 12 Dec 2015.
5. Kaufman, Bard. "Spinal Cord-Development and Stem Cells». Stem Cell Development Compendium. Retrieved 2 Dec 2015.
6. Saladin. Anatomy & Physiology The Unity of Form and Function. Mc Graw Hill.
7. Moore, Keith; Anne Agur (2007). Essential Clinical Anatomy, Third Edition. Lippincott Williams & Wilkins. p. 298. ISBN 0-7817-6274-X.
8. Biglioli, Paolo; et alia (April 2004). "Upper and lower spinal cord blood supply: the continuity of the anterior spinal artery and the relevance of the lumbar arteries». Journal of Thoracic and Cardiovascular Surgery. **127** *(4): 1188–1192. doi:10.1016/j.jtcvs.2003.11.038. PMID 15052221.*
9. Saladin. Anatomy and Physiology, 5th Ed.
10. Le, Tao (10 January 2014). First Aid for the USMLE Step 1 2014 / Edition 24. McGraw-Hill Professional Publishing. ISBN 9780071831420.

CHAPTER 9

Epigenetics in Stem-Cell Differentiation

Chapter Contents

Stem-cell differentiation is the process by which a more specialised cell is formed from a stem cell, leading to loss of some of the stem cell's developmental potential. Stem-cell differentiation occurs during development of an organism to produce new specialised cells, and also in adults to replenish cells that are lost.

INTRODUCTION

Embryonic stem cells are capable of self-renewing and differentiating to the desired fate depending on its position within the body. Stem cell homeostasis is maintained through epigenetic mechanisms that are highly dynamic in regulating the chromatin structure as well as specific gene transcription programs. Epigenetics has been used to refer to changes in gene expression, which are heritable through modifications not affecting the DNA sequence.

The mammalian epigenome undergoes global remodeling during early stem cell development that requires commitment of cells to be restricted to the desired lineage. There has been multiple evidence suggesting that the maintenance of the lineage commitment of stem cells are controlled by epigenetic mechanisms such as DNA methylation, histone modifications and regulation of ATP-dependent remolding of chromatin structure. Based on the *histone code* hypothesis, distinct covalent histone modifications can lead to functionally distinct chromatin structures that influence the fate of the cell.

This regulation of chromatin through epigenetic modifications is a molecular mechanism that will determine whether the cell will continue to differentiate into the desired fate. A research study performed by *Lee et al.* examined the effects of epigenetic modifications on the chromatin structure and the modulation of these epigenetic markers during stem cell differentiation through in vitro differentiation of murine embryonic stem (ES) cells.

EXPERIMENTAL BACKGROUND

Embryonic stem cells exhibit dramatic and complex alterations to both global and site-specific chromatin structures. *Lee et al.* performed an experiment to determine the importance of deacetylation and acetylation for stem cell differentiation by looking at global acetylation and methylation levels at certain site-specific modification in histone sites *H3K9* and *H3K4*. Gene expression at these histones regulated by epigenetic modifications is critical in restricting the embryonic stem cell to desired cell lineages and developing cellular memory.

For mammalian cells, the maintenance of cytosine methylation is catalyzed by DNA methyltransferases and any disruption to these methyltransferases will cause a lethal phenotype to the embryo. Cytosine methylation is examined at *H3K9*, which is associated with inactive heterochromatin and occurs mainly at CpG dinucleotides while global acetylation is examined at *H3K4*, which is associated with active euchromatin. The mammalian zygotic genome undergoes active and passive global cytosine demethylation following fertilization that reaches a minimal point of 20% CpG methylation at the blastocyst stage to which is then followed by a wave of methylation that reprograms the chromatin structure in order to restore global levels of CpG methylation to 60%. Embryonic stem cells containing reduced or elevation levels of methylation are viable but unable to differentiate and therefore require critical regulation of cytosine methylation for mammalian development.

EFFECTS OF GLOBAL HISTONE MODIFICATIONS DURING EMBRYONIC STEM CELL DIFFERENTIATION

Histones modifications in chromatin were analyzed at various time intervals (along a 6-day period) following the initiation of in vitro embryonic stem cell differentiation. Differentiation was triggered by the removal of Leukemia inhibitory factor (LIF) which inhibits differentiation. Representative data of the histone modifications at the specific sites were assessed using Western blotting. The data confirms that strong deacetylation at the *H3K4* and *H3K9* positions of histone H3 one day after LIF removal, followed by a small increase in acetylation by day two.

The histone *H3K4* methylation also decreased after one day of LIF removal but showed a rebound between days 2–4 of differentiation, finally ending with a decrease in methylation on day five. These results indicate a decrease in the level of active euchromatin epigenetic marks upon initiation of embryonic stem cell differentiation which is then followed immediately by reprogramming of the epigenome.

Histone modifications of *H3K9* position show a decrease in di- and tri-methylation of undifferentiated embryonic stem cells and had a gradual increase in methylation during the six-day time course of in vitro differentiation, which indicated that there is a global increase of inactive heterochromatin levels at this histone mark.

As the embryonic stem cell undergoes differentiation the markers for active euchromatin (histone acetylation and *H3K4* methylation) are decreased after the removal of LIF showing that the cell is indeed becoming more differentiated. The slight rebound in each of these marks allows for further differentiation to occur by allowing another opportunity to decrease the markers once again, bringing the cell closer to its desired fate. Since there is also an increase throughout the six-day period in *H3K9me*, a marker for active heterochromatin, once differentiation occurs it is concluded that the formation of heterochromatin occurs as the cell is differentiated into its desired fate making the cell inactive to prevent further differentiation.

DNA Methylation in Differentiated Versus Undifferentiated Cells

Global levels of cytosine methylation were compared between undifferentiated and differentiated embryonic stem cells. Global 5-methylcytosine levels have been measured prior to differentiation and after in vitro differentiation. The global cytosine methylation pattern appears to be established prior to the reprogramming of the histone code that occurs upon in vitro differentiation of embryonic stem cells.

As the embryonic stem cell undergoes differentiation the level of DNA methylation increases. This is in agreement with findings that show that there is an increase in inactive heterochromatin during differentiation.

Supplemental effects of methylation with DNMTs

In mammals, DNA methylation plays a role in regulating a key component of multipotency—the ability to rapidly self-renew. Khavari et al. discussed the fundamental mechanisms of DNA methylation and the interaction with several pathways regulating differentiation. New approaches studying the genomic status of DNA methylation in various states of differentiation have shown that methylation at CpG sites associated with putative enhancers are important in this process. DNA methylation can modulate the binding affinities of transcription factors by recruiting repressors such as *MeCP2* which display binding specificity for sequences containing methylated CpG dinucleotides. DNA methylation is controlled by certain methyltransferases, *DMNTs*, which perform different functions depending on each one. *DNMT3A* and *DNMT3B* have both been linked to a role in the establishment of DNA methylation pattern in the early development of the stem cell, whereas *DNMT1* is required to methylate a newly synthesized strand of DNA after the cell has undergone replication in order to sustain the epigenetic regulatory state.

Numerous proteins can physically interact with *DNMTs* themselves, which help target *DNMT1* to hemi-methylated DNA.

Several new studies point to the central role of DNA methylation interacting with the regulation of cell cycles and DNA repair pathways in order to maintain the undifferentiated state. In embryonic stem cells, *DNMT1* depletion within the undifferentiated progenitor cell compartment led to cell cycle arrest, premature differentiation and a failure of tissue self-renewal. The loss of *DNMT1* occurred from profound effects associated with activation of differentiation genes and loss of genes promoting cell cycle progression, thus indicating that *DNMT1* and other *DNMTs* do not continuously suppress differentiation and thus maintain the pluripotent state.

These studies point to the important of the interaction of DNMTs in order to maintain stem cell states allowing for further differentiation and formation of heterochromatin to occur.

EPIGENETIC MODIFICATIONS OF REGULATED GENES DURING ESC DIFFERENTIATION

Okamoto et al. previously documented the expression level of the *Oct4* gene decreasing with embryonic stem cell differentiation. *Lee et al* performed a ChIP analysis of the Oct4 promoter, associated with undifferentiated cells, region to examine the epigenetic modifications of regulated genes undergoing development during embryonic stem cell differentiation. This promoter region decreased at *H3K4* methylation and *H3K9* acetylation sites and increased at the *H3K9* methylation site during differentiation. Analysis of a CpG motif of the *Oct4* gene promoter revealed a progressive increase of DNA methylation and was completely methylated at day 10 of differentiation as previously reported in Gidekel and Bergman.

These results indicate that there was a shift from the active eurchromatin to the inactive heterochromatin due to the decrease of acetylation of H3K4 and an increase of H3K9me. This means that the cell is becoming differentiated at the Oct4 gene, which is coincident with the silence of Oct4 gene expression.

Another site specific gene tested for histone modification was a *Brachyury* gene, a marker of mesoderm differentiation and is only slightly expressed in undifferentiated embryonic stem cells. "Brachyury" was induced at day five of differentiation and completely silencing by day 10, corresponding to the last day of differentiation. The ChIP analysis of the "Brachyury" gene promoter revealed increase of expression in mono- and di-methylation of *H3K4* at day 0 and 5 of embryonic stem cell differentiation with a loss of gene expression at day 10. *H3K4* trimethylation coincides with the time of highest Brachyury gene expression since it only had gene expression on day 5. *H3K4* methylations in all forms are absent at day 10 of differentiation, which correlates with the silencing of Brachyury gene expression. Mono-methylation of both histones produced expression at day 0 indication a marker that is not useful for chromatin structure. Acetlyation of H3K9 does not correlate to *Brachyury* gene expression since it was down regulated at the induction of differentiation. Upon examining of DNA methylation expression, there was no formation of intermediate sized bad in the Southern analysis suggesting that CpG motifs upstream of the promoter region are not methylated in the absence of cytosine methylation at this site.

It is demonstrated from these studies that both *H3K9* di-and tri-methylation correlate with the DNA methylation and gene expression while *H3K4* tri-methylation is associated the highest gene expression stage of the *Brachyury* gene. A previous report from Santos-Rosa is in agreement with these data showing that active genes are associated with *H3K4* tri-methylation in yeast.

This data indicated the same results as for the *Oct4* gene, in that heterochromatin is forming as differentiation occurs again coinciding with the silence of *Brachyury* gene expression.

EFFECT OF TSA ON STEM CELL DIFFERENTIATION

Leukemia inhibitory factor (LIF) was removed from all the cell lines. LIF inhibits cell differentiation, and its removal allows the cell lines to go through cell differentiation. The cell lines were treated with Trichostatin A (TSA) - a histone deacetylase inhibitor for 6 days. One group of cell lines was treated with 10nM of TSA. The western analysis showed the lack of initial deacetylation on Day-1 which, was observed in the control for the embryonic stem cell differentiation. The lack of histone deacetylase activity allowed the acetylation of H3K9 and histone H4. Embryonic stem cells were also analyzed morphologically to observe the formation of embryoid body formation as one of the measures of cell differentiation. The 10nM TSA treated cells failed to form the embryoid body by Day-6 as observed in the control cell line. This implies that the ES cells treated with TSA lacked the deacetylation on Day-1 and failed to differentiate after the removal of LIF. Second group,'-TSA Day4' was treated with TSA for 3days. As soon as the TSA treatment was stopped, on day 4 the deacetylation was observed and the acetylation recovered on Day-5. The morphological examination showed the formation of embryoid body formation by Day-6. In addition, "Interestingly" the embryoid body formation was faster than the control cell line. This suggests that the '-TSA Day4' lines were responding to the removal of LIF but, were unable to acquire any differentiation phenotype. They were able to acquire the differentiation phenotype after the cessation of TSA treatment and at rapid rate. The morphological examination of the third group,' 5 nM TSA' showed the intermediate effect between the control and 10nM-TSA group. The lower dose of TSA allowed the formation of some embryoid body formation. This experiment shows that TSA inhibits histone deacetylase and the activity of histone deacetylase is required for the embryonic stem cell differentiation. Without the initial deacetylation on Day-1, the ES cells cannot go through the differentiation.

ALKALINE PHOSPHATASE ACTIVITY

In normal stem cells, the activity of alkaline phosphatase activity is lowered upon differentiation. Trichostatin A causes the cells to maintain the activity of alkaline phosphatase. Significant increase in alkaline phosphatase extinction was observed when Trichostatin A was withdrawn after three days. Alkaline phosphatase activity correlates with the morphology changes. Initial deacetylation of histone is required for embryonic stem cell differentiation.

HDAC1, but not HDAC2 controls differentiation

Dovery et al. (2010) used HDAC knockout mice to demonstrate whether HDAC1 or HDAC2 was important for the embryonic stem cell differentiation. Examination of global histone acetylation in the absence of HDAC 1 showed an increase in acetylation. Global histone acetylation levels were unchanged by the loss of HDAC2. In order to analyze the process of HDAC knockout mouse in detail, the knockout mice embryonic stem cells were used to generate embryoid bodies. It showed that just before or during gastrulation, embryonic stem cells lacking HDAC1 acquired visible developmental defects. The continued culture of HDAC1 knockout embryonic stem cells showed that the embryoid bodies formed became irregular and reduced in size rather than uniformly spherical as in normal mice. Embryonic stem cell proliferation was unaffected by the loss of either HDAC1 or HDAC2 but the differentiation of embryonic stem cells were affected with that lack of HDAC 1. This shows that HDAC1 is required for cell fate determination during differentiation.

THE FUTURE

Any disturbance of a stable epigenetic regulation of gene expression mediated by DNA methylation is associated with a number of human disorders, including cancer as well as congenital diseases such as pseudohypoparathyroidism type IA, Beckwith-Wiedemann, Prader-Willi and Angelman syndromes, which are each caused by altered methylation-based imprinting at specific loci.

Perturbations of both global and gene-specific patterns of cytosine methylation are commonly observed in cancer while histone deacetylation is an important feature of nuclear reprogramming in oocytes during meiosis.

Recent studies have revealed that there is an array of different pathways that cooperates with one another in order to bestow proper epigenetic regulation by DNA methylation. Future studies will be needed to further clarify the certain mechanism pathways such as DNA binding proteins, DNA repair and noncoding RNAs serve in order to regulate DNA methylation to suppress differentiation and sustain self-renewal in somatic stem cells in the epidermis and other tissues. Addressing these questions will help extend insight into these recent findings for a central role in epigenetic regulators of DNA methylation in controlling embryonic stem cell differentiation.

COMPUTATIONAL EPIGENETICS

Computational epigenetics uses bioinformatic methods to complement experimental research in epigenetics. Due to the recent explosion of epigenome datasets, computational methods play an increasing role in all areas of epigenetic research.

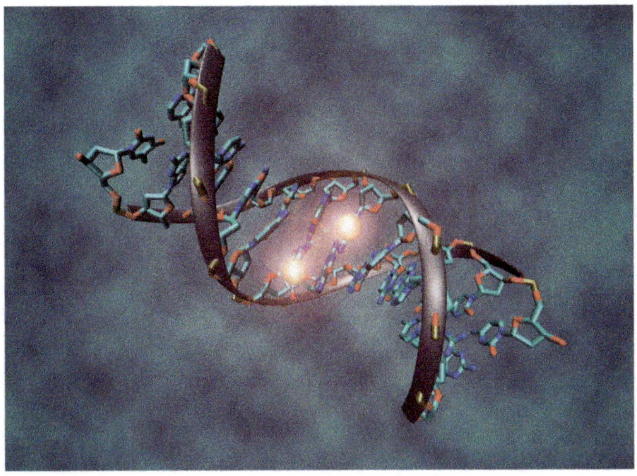

DNA methylation is a epigenetic mechanism that can be studied with bioinformatics

Research in computational epigenetics comprises the development and application of bioinformatics methods for solving epigenetic questions, as well as computational data analysis and theoretical modeling in the context of epigenetics. This includes modelling of the effects of histone and DNA CpG island methylation.

CURRENT RESEARCH AREAS

Epigenetic Data Processing and Analysis

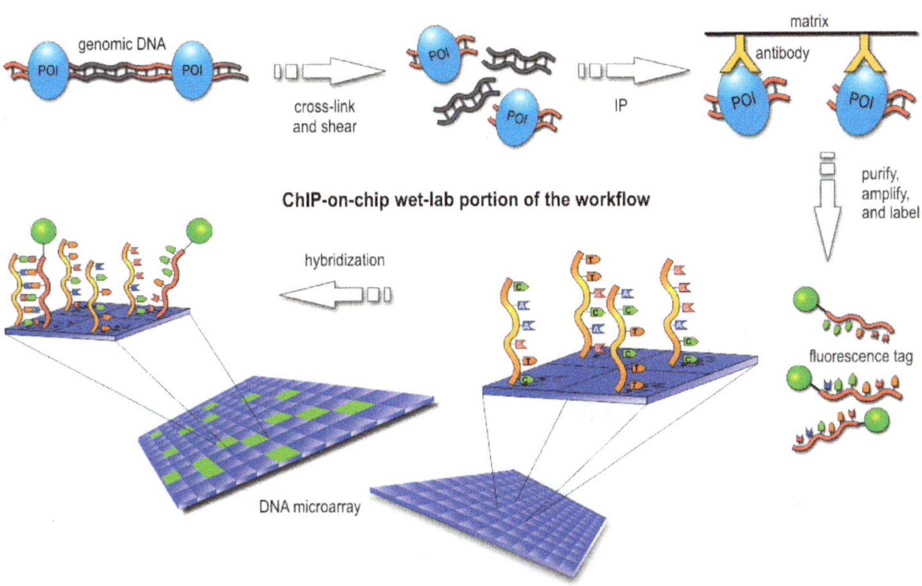

ChIP-on-chip technique.

Various experimental techniques have been developed for genome-wide mapping of epigenetic information, the most widely used being ChIP-on-chip, ChIP-seq and bisulfite sequencing. All of these methods generate large amounts of data and require efficient ways of data processing and quality control by bioinformatic methods.

Epigenome Prediction

A substantial amount of bioinformatic research has been devoted to the prediction of epigenetic information from characteristics of the genome sequence. Such predictions serve a dual purpose. First, accurate epigenome predictions can substitute for experimental data, to some degree, which is particularly relevant for newly discovered epigenetic mechanisms and for species other than human and mouse. Second, prediction algorithms build statistical models of epigenetic information from training data and can therefore act as a first step toward quantitative modeling of an epigenetic mechanism. Successful computational prediction of DNA and lysine methylation and acetylation has been achieved by combinations of various features.

Applications in Cancer Epigenetics

The important role of epigenetic defects for cancer opens up new opportunities for improved diagnosis and therapy. These active areas of research give rise to two questions that are particularly amenable to bioinformatic analysis. First, given a list of genomic regions exhibiting epigenetic differences between tumor cells and controls (or between different disease subtypes), can we detect common patterns or find evidence of a functional relationship of these regions to cancer? Second, can we use bioinformatic methods in order to improve diagnosis and therapy by detecting and classifying important disease subtypes?

Emerging Topics

The first wave of research in the field of computational epigenetics was driven by rapid progress of experimental methods for data generation, which required adequate computational methods for data processing and quality control, prompted epigenome prediction studies as a means of understanding the genomic distribution of epigenetic information, and provided the foundation for initial projects on cancer epigenetics. While these topics will continue to be major areas of research and the mere quantity of epigenetic data arising from epigenome projects poses a significant bioinformatic challenge, several additional topics are currently emerging.

- Epigenetic regulatory circuitry: Reverse engineering the regulatory networks that read, write and execute epigenetic codes.
- Population epigenetics: Distilling regulatory mechanisms from the integration of epigenome data with gene expression profiles and haplotype maps for a large sample from a heterogeneous population.
- Evolutionary epigenetics: Learning about epigenome regulation in human (and its medical consequences) by cross-species comparisons.

- Theoretical modeling: Testing our mechanistic and quantitative understanding of epigenetic mechanisms by in silico simulation.
- Genome browsers: Developing a new blend of web services that enable biologists to perform sophisticated genome and epigenome analysis within an easy-to-use genome browser environment.
- Medical epigenetics: Searching for epigenetic mechanisms that play a role in diseases other than cancer, as there is strong circumstantial evidence for epigenetic regulation being involved in mental disorders, autoimmune diseases and other complex diseases.

Epigenetics Databases

- MethDB Contains information on 19,905 DNA methylation content data and 5,382 methylation patterns for 48 species, 1,511 individuals, 198 tissues and cell lines and 79 phenotypes.
- PubMeth Contains over 5,000 records on methylated genes in various cancer types.
- REBASE Contains over 22,000 DNA methyltransferases genes derived from GenBank.
- MeInfoText Contains gene methylation information across 205 human cancer types.
- MethPrimerDB Contains 259 primer sets from human, mouse and rat for DNA methylation analysis.
- The Histone Database Contains 254 sequences from histone H1, 383 from histone H2, 311 from histone H2B, 1043 from histone H3 and 198 from histone H4, altogether representing at least 857 species.
- ChromDB Contains 9,341 chromatin-associated proteins, including RNAi-associated proteins, for a broad range of organisms.
- CREMOFAC Contains 1725 redundant and 720 non-redundant chromatin-remodeling factor sequences in eukaryotes.
- The Krembil Family Epigenetics Laboratory Contains DNA methylation data of human chromosomes 21, 22, male germ cells and DNA methylation profiles in monozygotic and dizygotic twins.
- MethyLogiX DNA methylation database Contains DNA methylation data of human chromosomes 21 and 22, male germ cells and late-onset Alzheimer's disease.

EPIGENETIC CLOCK

An **epigenetic clock** is a type of **DNA clock** based on measuring natural DNA methylation levels to estimate the biological age of a tissue, cell type or organ. A pre-eminent example for an epigenetic clock is **Horvath›s clock**, which is based on 353 epigenetic markers on the human genome.

The strong effect of age on DNA methylation levels has been known since the late 1960s. A vast literature describes sets of CpGs whose DNA methylation levels correlate with age, e.g. Two publications describe age estimators based on DNA methylation levels in either saliva or blood.

Horvath›s epigenetic clock was developed by Steve Horvath, a professor of human genetics at the David Geffen School of Medicine at UCLA and of biostatistics at the UCLA Fielding School of Public Health. The scientific article was first published on Oct 21, 2013, in Genome Biology. Horvath spent over 4 years collecting publicly available Illumina DNA methylation data and identifying suitable statistical methods. The personal story behind the discovery was featured in Nature. The age estimator was developed using 8,000 samples from 82 Illumina DNA methylation array datasets, encompassing 51 healthy tissues and cell types. The major innovation of Horvath›s epigenetic clock lies in its wide applicability: the same set of 353 CpGs and the same prediction algorithm is used irrespective of the DNA source within the organism, i.e. it does not require any adjustments or offsets. This property allows one to compare the ages of different areas of the human body using the same aging clock.

Relationship to a Cause of Biological Aging

It is not yet known what exactly is measured by DNA methylation age. Horvath hypothesized that DNA methylation age measures the cumulative effect of an epigenetic maintenance system but details are unknown. The fact that DNA methylation age of blood predicts all-cause mortality in later life strongly suggests that it relates to a process that causes aging. However, it is unlikely that the 353 clock CpGs are special or play a direct causal role in the aging process. Rather, the epigenetic clock captures an emergent property of the epigenome.

Motivation for Biological Clocks

In general, biological aging clocks and biomarkers of aging are expected to find many uses in biological research since age is a fundamental characteristic of most organisms. Accurate measures of biological age (**biological aging clocks**) could be useful for

- testing the validity of various theories of biological aging,
- diagnosing various age related diseases and for defining cancer subtypes,
- predicting/prognosticating the onset of various diseases,
- serving as surrogate markers for evaluating therapeutic interventions including rejuvenation approaches,
- studying developmental biology and cell differentiation,
- forensic applications, for example to estimate the age of a suspect based on blood left on a crime scene.

Overall, biological clocks are expected to be useful for studying what causes aging and what can be done against it.

Properties of Horvath's clock

The clock is defined as an age estimation method based on 353 epigenetic markers on the DNA. The 353 markers measure DNA methylation of CpG dinucleotides. Estimated age (predicted age in mathematical usage), also referred to as DNA methylation age, has the following properties: first, it is close to zero for embryonic and induced pluripotent stem cells; second, it correlates with cell passage number; third, it gives rise to a highly heritable measure of age acceleration; and, fourth, it is applicable to chimpanzee tissues (which are used as human analogs for biological testing purposes). Organismal growth (and concomitant cell division) leads to a high ticking rate of the epigenetic clock that slows down to a constant ticking rate (linear dependence) after adulthood (age 20). The fact that DNA methylation age of blood predicts all-cause mortality in later life even after adjusting for known risk factors suggests that it relates to a process that causes aging. Similarly, markers of physical and mental fitness are associated with the epigenetic clock (lower abilities associated with age acceleration).

Salient features of Horvath›s epigenetic clock include its high accuracy and its applicability to a broad spectrum of tissues and cell types. Since it allows one to contrast the ages of different tissues from the same subject, it can be used to identify tissues that show evidence of accelerated age due to disease.

Statistical Approach

The basic approach is to form a weighted average of the 353 clock CpGs, which is then transformed to DNAm age using a calibration function. The calibration function reveals that the epigenetic clock has a high ticking rate until adulthood, after which it slows to a constant ticking rate. Using the training data sets, Horvath used a penalized regression model (Elastic net regularization) to regress a calibrated version of chronological age on 21,369 CpG probes that were present both on the Illumina 450K and 27K platform and had fewer than 10 missing values. DNAm age is defined as estimated ("predicted") age. The elastic net predictor automatically selected 353 CpGs. 193 of the 353 CpGs correlate positively with age while the remaining 160 CpGs correlate negatively with age. R software and a freely available web-based tool can be found at the following webpage.

Accuracy

The median error of estimated age is 3.6 years across a wide spectrum of tissues and cell types . The epigenetic clock performs well in heterogeneous tissues (for example, whole blood, peripheral blood mononuclear cells, cerebellar samples, occipital cortex, buccal epithelium, colon, adipose, kidney, liver, lung, saliva, uterine cervix, epidermis, muscle) as well as in individual cell types such as CD4 T cells, CD14 monocytes, glial cells, neurons, immortalized B cells, mesenchymal stromal cells. However, accuracy depends to some extent on the source of the DNA. In particular, DNAm age is higher than chronological age in female breast tissue that is adjacent to breast cancer tissue. Since normal tissue, which is adjacent to other cancer types, does not exhibit a similar age acceleration effect, this finding suggests that normal female breast tissue ages faster than other parts of the body.

Comparison with other Biological Clocks

The epigenetic clock leads to a chronological age prediction that has a Pearson correlation coefficient of r=0.96 with chronological age (Figure 2 in). Thus the age correlation is close to its maximum possible correlation value of 1. Other biological clocks are based on a) telomere length, b) p16INK4a expression levels (also known as INK4a/ARF locus), and c) microsatellite mutations. The correlation between chronological age and telomere length is r=−0.51 in women and r=−0.55 in men. The correlation between chronological age and expression levels of p16INK4a in T cells is r=0.56. p16INK4aexpression levels only relate to age in T cells, a type of white blood cells. The microsatellite clock measures not chronological age but age in terms of elapsed cell divisions within a tissue.

Applications of Horvath's Clock

By contrasting DNA methylation age (estimated age) with chronological age, one can define measures of age acceleration. Age acceleration can be defined as the difference between DNA methylation age and chronological age. Alternatively, it can be defined as the residual that results from regressing DNAm age on chronological age. The latter measure is attractive because it does not correlate with chronological age. A positive/negative value of epigenetic age acceleration suggests that the underlying tissue ages faster/slower than expected.

Genetic Studies of Epigenetic age Acceleration

The broad sense heritability (defined via Falconer's formula) of age acceleration of blood from older subjects is around 40% but it appears to be much higher in newborns. Similarly, the age acceleration of brain tissue (prefrontal cortex) was found to be 41% in older subjects. Genome-wide association studies of cerebellar age acceleration have identified several SNPs at a genomewide significance level. Gene and SNP sets found by genome-wide association analysis of epigenetic age acceleration exhibit significant overlap with those of Alzheimer's disease, age-related macular degeneration, and Parkinson's disease.

Cancer Tissue

Cancer tissues show both positive and negative age acceleration effects. For most tumor types, no significant relationship can be observed between age acceleration and tumor morphology (grade/stage). On average, cancer tissues with mutated TP53 have a lower age acceleration than those without it. Further, cancer tissues with high age acceleration tend to have fewer somatic mutations than those with low age acceleration. Age acceleration is highly related to various genomic aberrations in cancer tissues. Somatic mutations in estrogen receptors or progesterone receptors are associated with accelerated DNAm age in breast cancer. Colorectal cancer samples with a BRAF (V600E) mutation or promoter hypermethylation of the mismatch repair gene MLH1 are associated with an increased age acceleration. Age acceleration in glioblastoma multiforme samples is highly significantly associated with certain mutations in H3F3A. One study suggests that the epigenetic age of blood tissue may be prognostic of lung cancer incidence.

Obesity

The epigenetic clock was used to study the relationship between high body mass index (BMI) and the DNA methylation ages of human blood, liver, muscle and adipose tissue. A significant correlation (r=0.42) between BMI and epigenetic age acceleration could only be observed for the liver.

Trisomy 21 (Down syndrome)

Down Syndrome (DS) entails an increased risk of many chronic diseases that are typically associated with older age. The clinical manifestations of accelerated aging suggest that trisomy 21 increases the biological age of tissues, but molecular evidence for this hypothesis has been sparse. According to the epigenetic clock, trisomy 21 significantly increases the age of blood and brain tissue (on average by 6.6 years).

Alzheimer›s Disease Related Neuropathology

Epigenetic age acceleration of the human prefrontal cortex was found to be correlated with several neuropathological measurements that play a role in Alzheimer's disease Further, it was found to be associated with a decline in global cognitive functioning, and memory functioning among individuals with Alzheimer's disease. The epigenetic age of **blood** relates to cognitive functioning in the elderly.Overall, these results strongly suggest that the epigenetic clock lends itself for measuring the biological age of the brain.

Cerebellum Ages Slowly

It has been difficult to identify tissues that seem to evade aging due to the lack of biomarkers of tissue age that allow one to contrast compare the ages of different tissues. An application of epigenetic clock to 30 anatomic sites from six centenarians and younger subjects revealed that the cerebellum ages slowly: it is about 15 years younger than expected in a centenarian. This finding might explain why the cerebellum exhibits fewer neuropathological hallmarks of age related dementias compared to other brain regions. In younger subjects (e.g. younger than 70), brain regions and brain cells appear to have roughly the same age. Several SNPs and genes have been identified that relate to the epigenetic age of the cerebellum

Huntington's Disease

Huntington's disease has been found to increase the epigenetic aging rates of several human brain regions.

Centenarians age Slowly

The offspring of semi-supercentenarians (subjects who reached an age of 105–109 years) have a lower epigenetic age than age-matched controls (age difference=5.1 years in blood) and centenarians are younger (8.6 years) than expected based on their chronological age.

HIV Infection

Infection with the Human Immunodeficiency Virus-1 (HIV) is associated with clinical symptoms of accelerated aging, as evidenced by increased incidence and diversity of age-related illnesses at relatively young ages. But it has been difficult to detect an accelerated aging effect on a molecular level. An epigenetic clock analysis of human DNA from HIV+ subjects and controls detected a significant age acceleration effect in brain (7.4 years) and blood (5.2 years) tissue due to HIV-1 infection.

Parkinson's Disease

A large-scale study suggests that the blood of Parkinson's disease subjects exhibits (relatively weak) accelerated aging effects.

Developmental Disorder: Syndrome X

Children with a very rare disorder known as syndrome X maintain the façade of persistent toddler-like features while aging from birth to adulthood. Since the physical development of these children is dramatically delayed, these children appear to be a toddler or at best a preschooler. According to an epigenetic clock analysis, blood tissue from syndrome X cases is not younger than expected.

Menopause Accelerates Epigenetic Aging

The following results strongly suggest that the loss of female hormones resulting from menopause accelerates the epigenetic aging rate of blood and possibly that of other tissues. First, early menopause has been found to be associated with an increased epigenetic age acceleration of blood.Second, surgical menopause (due to bilateral oophorectomy) is associated with epigenetic age acceleration in blood and saliva. Third, menopausal hormone therapy, which mitigates hormonal loss, is associated with a negative age acceleration of buccal cells (but not of blood cells). Fourth, genetic markers that are associated with early menopause are also associated with increased epigenetic age acceleration in blood.

Cellular Senescence Versus Epigenetic aging

A confounding aspect of biological aging is the nature and role of senescent cells. It is unclear whether the three major types of cellular senescence, namely replicative senescence, oncogene-induced senescence and DNA damage-induced senescence are descriptions of the same phenomenon instigated by different sources, or if each of these is distinct, and how they are associated with epigenetic aging. Induction of replicative senescence (RS) and oncogene-induced senescence (OIS) were found to be accompanied by epigenetic aging of primary cells but senescence induced by DNA damage was not, even though RS and OIS activate the cellular DNA damage response pathway. These results highlight the independence of cellular senescence from epigenetic aging. Consistent with this, telomerase-immortalised cells continued to age (according to the epigenetic clock) without having been treated with any senescence inducers or DNA-damaging agents, re-affirming the independence of the process of epigenetic ageing from telomeres, cellular senescence, and the DNA damage response pathway. Although the uncoupling of senescence from cellular aging appears at first sight to be inconsistent with the fact that senescent cells contribute to the physical manifestation of organism ageing, as demonstrated by Baker et al., where removal of senescent cells slowed down aging.However, the epigenetic clock analysis of senescence suggests that cellular senescence is a state that cells are forced into as a result of external pressures such as DNA damage, ectopic oncogene expression and exhaustive proliferation of cells to replenish those eliminated by external/environmental factors. These senescent cells, in sufficient numbers, will probably cause the deterioration of tissues, which is interpreted as organism ageing. However, at the cellular level, aging, as measured by the epigenetic clock, is distinct from senescence. It is an intrinsic mechanism that exists from the birth of the cell and continues. This implies that if cells are not shunted into senescence by the external pressures described above, they would still continue to age. This is consistent with the fact that mice with naturally long telomeres still age and eventually die even though their telomere lengths are far longer than the critical limit, and they age prematurely when their telomeres are forcibly shortened, due to replicative senescence. Therefore, cellular senescence is a route by which cells exit prematurely from the natural course of cellular aging.

Effect of sex and Race/Ethnicity

Men age faster than women according to epigenetic age acceleration in blood, brain, saliva, and many other tissues. The epignetic clock method applies to all examined racial/ethnic groups in the sense that DNAm age is highly correlated with chronological age. But ethnicity can be associated with epigenetic age acceleration. For example, the blood of Hispanics and Tsimane Amerindians ages more slowly than that of other populations which might explain the Hispanic mortality paradox.

Biological Mechanism Behind the Epigenetic Clock

The precise biological mechanism behind the epigenetic clock is currently unknown. However, the following explanations have been proposed in the literature.

Possible explanation 1: Epigenomic maintenance system

Horvath hypothesized that his clock arises from a methylation footprint left by an epigenomic maintenance system.

Possible explanation 2: Unrepaired DNA damages

Endogenous DNA damages occur frequently including about 50 double-strand DNA breaks per cell cycle and about 10,000 oxidative damages per day (see DNA damage (naturally occurring)). During repair of double-strand breaks many epigenetic alterations are introduced, and in a percentage of cases epigenetic alterations remain after repair is completed, including increased methylation of CpG island promoters. Similar, but usually transient epigenetic alterations were recently found during repair of oxidative damages caused by H_2O_2, and it was suggested that occasionally these epigenetic alterations may also remain after repair. These accumulated epigenetic alterations may contribute to the epigenetic clock. Accumulation of epigenetic alterations may parallel the accumulation of un-repaired DNA damages that are proposed to cause aging (see DNA damage theory of aging).

Other age Estimators Based on DNA Methylation Levels

Several other age estimators have been described in the literature.

1) Weidner et al. (2014) describe an age estimator for DNA from blood that uses only three CpG sites of genes hardly affected by aging (cg25809905 in integrin, alpha 2b (ITGA2B); cg02228185 in aspartoacylase (ASPA) and cg17861230 in phosphodiesterase 4C, cAMP specific (PDE4C)). The age estimator by Weidener et al. (2014) applies only to blood. Even in blood this sparse estimator is far less accurate than Horvath's epigenetic clock (Horvath 2014) when applied to data generated by the Illumina 27K or 450K platforms. But the sparse estimator was developed for pyrosequencing data and is highly cost effective.
2) Hannum et al. (2013) report several age estimators: one for each tissue type. Each of these estimators requires covariate information (e.g. gender, body mass index, batch). The authors mention that each tissue led to a clear linear offset (intercept and slope). Therefore, the authors had to adjust the blood-based age estimator for each tissue type using a linear model. When the Hannum estimator is applied to other tissues, it leads to a high error (due to poor calibration) as can be seen from Figure 4A in Hannum et al. (2013). Hannum et al. adjusted their blood-based age estimator (by adjusting the slope and the intercept term) in order to apply it to other tissue types. Since this adjustment step removes differences between tissue, the blood-based estimator from Hannum et al. cannot be used to compare the ages of different tissues/organs. In contrast, a salient characteristic of the epigenetic clock is that one does not have to carry out such a calibration step: it always uses the same CpGs and the same coefficient values. Therefore, Horvath's epigenetic clock can be used to compare the ages of different tissues/cells/organs from the same individual. While the age estimators from Hannum et al. cannot be used to compare the ages of different normal tissues, they can be used to compare the age of a cancerous tissue with that of a corresponding normal (non-

cancerous) tissue. Hannum et al. reported pronounced age acceleration effects in all cancers. In contrast, Horvath's epigenetic clock reveals that some cancer types (e.g. triple negative breast cancers or uterine corpus endometrial carcinoma) exhibit negative age acceleration, i.e. cancer tissue can be much younger than expected. An important difference relates to additional covariates. Hannum's age estimators make use of covariates such as gender, body mass index, diabetes status, ethnicity, and batch. Since new data involve different batches, one cannot apply it directly to new data. However, the authors present coefficient values for their CpGs in Supplementary Tables which can be used to define an aggregate measure that tends to be strongly correlated with chronological age but may be poorly calibrated (i.e. lead to high errors).

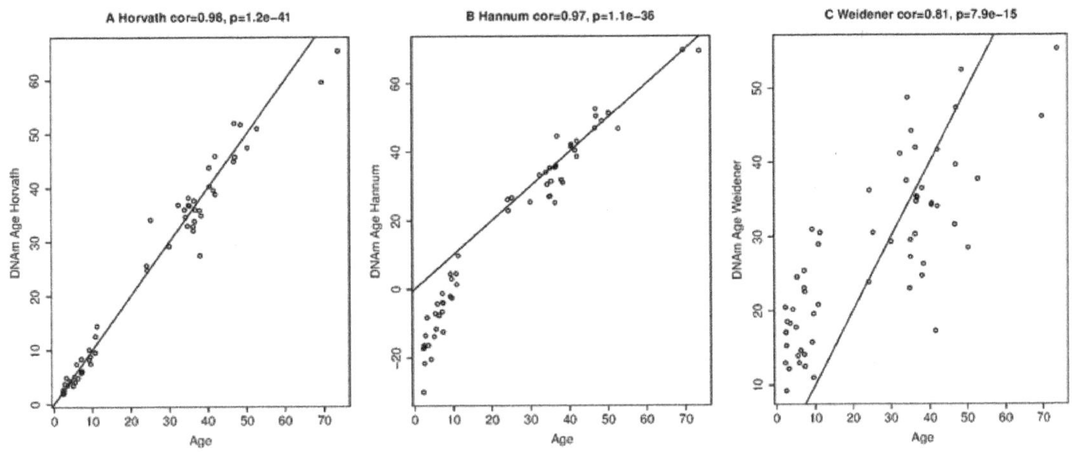

3.) Giuliani et al. identify genomic regions whose DNA methylation level correlates with age in human teeth. They propose the evaluation of DNA methylation at ELOVL2, FHL2, and PENK genes in DNA recovered from both cementum and pulp of the same modern teeth. They wish to apply this method also to historical and relatively ancient human teeth.

In a multicenter benchmarking study 18 research groups from three continents compared all promising methods for analyzing DNA methylation in the clinic and identified the most accurate methods, having concluded that epigenetic tests based on DNA methylation are a mature technology ready for broad clinical use.

EPIGENETIC REGULATION OF NEUROGENESIS

Epigenetics is the study of heritable changes in gene expression which do not result from modifications to the sequence of DNA. Neurogenesis is the mechanism for neuron proliferation and differentiation. It entails many different complex processes which are all time and order dependent. Processes such as neuron proliferation, fate specification, differentiation, maturation, and functional integration of newborn cells into existing neuronal networks are all interconnected. In the past decade many epigenetic regulatory mechanisms have been shown to play a large role in the timing and determination of neural stem cell lineages.

Relevant Mechanisms & Definitions

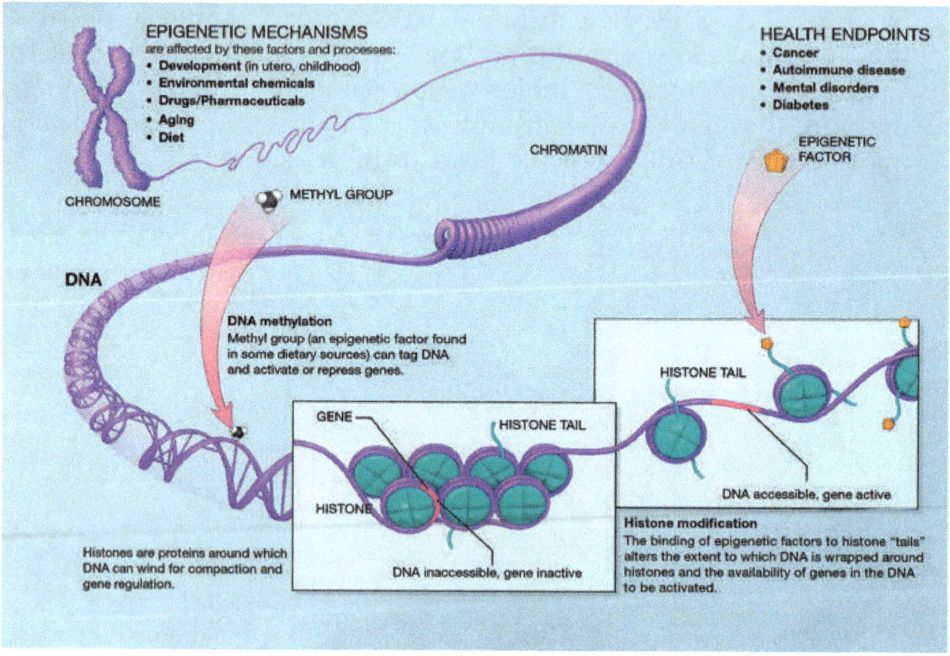

Epigenetic mechanisms.

Three important methods of epigenetic regulation include histone modification, DNA methylation and demethylation, and MicroRNA (miRNA) expression. Histones keep the DNA of the eukaryotic cell tightly packaged through charge interactions between the positive charge on the histone tail and the negative charge of the DNA, as well as between histone tails of nearby nucleosomes.While there are many different types of Histone modifications, in neural epigenetics there are two primary mechanisms which have been explored: histone methylation and histone acetylation. In the former, methyl groups are either added or removed to the histone altering its structure and exposing chromatin and leading to gene activation or deactivation. In the latter, histone acetylation causes the histone to hold the DNA more loosely, allowing for more gene activation. DNA Methylation, in which methyl groups are added to cytosine or adenosine redisdues on the DNA, is a more lasting method of gene inactivation than histone modification, though is still reversible in some cases. MicroRNAs are a small form of non-coding RNA (ncRNA) which often act as “fine-tuning” mechanisms for gene expression by repressing or inducing messenger RNA (mRNA) in neural cells but can also act directly with transcription factors to guide neurogenesis.

Epigenetic Regulation in the Brain

Embryonic Neurogenesis

Histone Modifications

Neural Stem Cells generate the cortex in a precise "inside out" manner with carefully controlled timing mechanisms. Early born neurons form deep layers in the cortex while newer born form the upper layers. This timing program is seen *in vitro* as well as *in vivo*. Histone methylation has been shown to be one of the epigenetic regulatory mechanisms which alters the proportionate production of deep layer and upper layer neurons. Specifically, deletion of Ezh2 encoding histone methyltransferase led to a twofold reduction of BRN2-expressing and SATB2 expressing upper layer neurons without affecting the number of neurons in layer V and VI. Similarly, histone acetylation through histone deacetylase (HDAC) inhibitor Valproic Acid, an epilepsy therapeutic, in mouse embryonic stem cell (ESC) derived neural proginetors not only induces neuronal differentiation, but also selectively enriched the upper layer neuronal population. As such, it has been proposed that HDAC inhibition promotes the progression of neuronal differentiation, leading to a fate-switch from deep-layer producing progenitors into upper-layer progenitors. However, the reasons behind this selective differentiation and timing control as a result of HDAC inhibition are not yet fully understood.

DNA Methylation

DNA methylation's critical nature to corticogenesis has been shown through knockout experiments in mice. When DNMT3b and DNMT1 were ablated separately in mouse embryos they died due to impairment of neural tube development. DNMT3a silencing did not cause embryonic lethality, but did result in a severe detriment in postnatal neurogenesis. This is largely due to the timing in which these epigenetic mechanisms are active. DNMT3b is expressed in early neural progenitor cells and decrease as neural development proceeds and DNMT3a is barely detectable up until embryonic day 10 (E.10). However, at E.10, DNMT3a expression increases significantly from E13.5 and well into adulthood. In the postnatal forebrain, DNMT3a is expressed in the subventricular zone (SVZ) and the hippocampal dentate gyrus, the primary locations for adult neurogenesis. The loss of DNMT3a in post natal neural progenitor cells leads to the down-regulation of neuronic genes such as *Dlx2*, *Neurog2*, and *Sp8*; but upregulation of genes involved in astroglial and oligodendroglial differentiation, indicating a role in the cell-fate switch from neurogenesis to gliogenesis. DNA demethylation, as well as methylation, of certain genes allows for neurogenesis to proceed in a time dependent manner. One such gene is *Hes5*, hypermethylated in E7.5 Embryos but completely demethylated by E9.5, which is one of the target genes in the Notch Signaling pathway. GCM1 and GCM2 demethylate the *Hes5* promoter, allowing it to respond to NOTCH signaling and initiating the generation of neural stem cells. Another example is the *Gfap* gene which is required for astrocyte differentiation. The ability to differentiate into glial cells is repressed in neural stem cells with a neuronal cell fate. This repression is due largely to an irresponsiveness of neural stem cells towards astrocyte-inducing stimulations. The neural stem cells are non-responsive due to hypermethylated DNA in the promoter regions of astrocyte genes such as *Gfap*. The STAT3 binding site in the promoter region of *Gfap* is hypermethylated at E11.5 and barely so at E14.5, at which point it is able to receive astrocyte inducing stimulations and begin cytokine-inducible astrocyte differentiation.

miRNAs

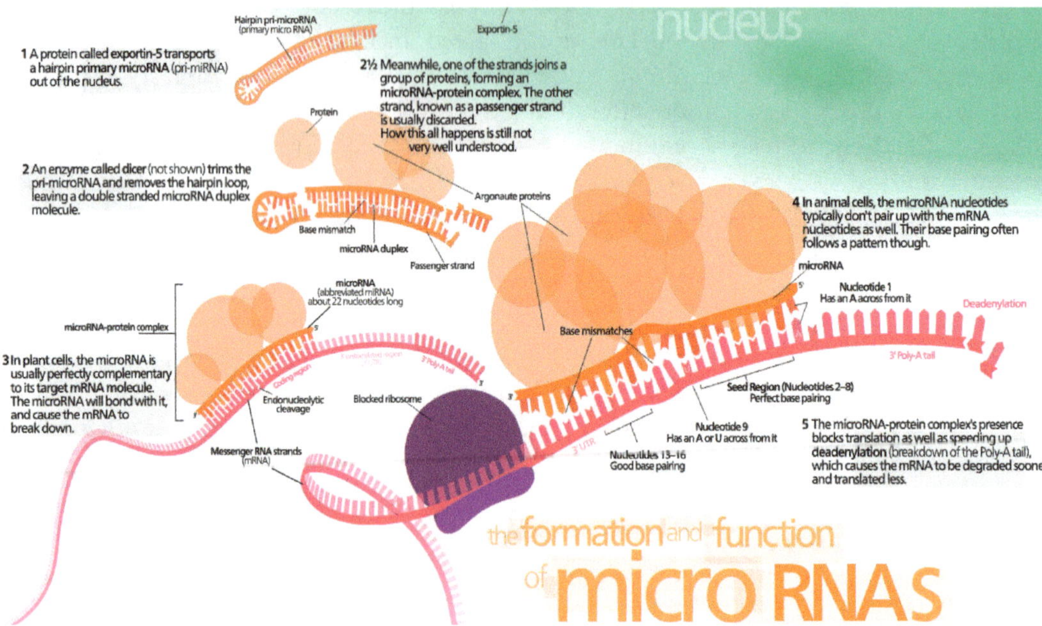

Mechanism of miRNAs.

Studies done by De Pietri Tonelli and Kawase-Koga have shown conditional knockout of Dicer, an enzyme largely used for miRNA synthesis, in mouse neocortex resulted in reduced cortical size, increased neuronal apoptosis, and deficient corticol layering. Neuroepithelial cells and neuroprogenitor cells were not affected until E.14, at which point they also underwent apoptosis. This doesn't show which miRNAs were responsible for the varying factors affected, but it does show that there is a stage-specific requirement for miRNA expression in cortical development. miR-124, the most abundant microRNA in the central nervous system, controls the lineage progression of subventricular zone neural progenitor cells into neuroblasts by suppressing protein production by targeting *Sox9*. Another major microRNA player is miR-9/9*. In embryonic neurogenesis miR-9 has been shown to regulate neuronal differentiation and self-renewal. Ectopic expression of miR-9 in the developing mouse cortex led to premature neuronal differentiation and disrupted the migration of new neurons through targeting *Foxg1*.

Contrary to the idea that microRNAs are only fine-tuning mechanisms, recent studies have shown that miR-9 and miR-124 can act together to guide fibroblasts into neural cells.

Transcription factors and regulatory genes, such as *Neurodl*, *Ascrl*, and *Mytll*, which were previously thought to be responsible for this phenomena did not transform human fibroblasts in the absence of miR-9 and miR-124, but in the presence of the microRNAs and the absence of the transcription factors human fibroblast transformation proceeded, albeit in a less efficient manner.

Adult Neurogenesis

DNA Methylation

Neurogenesis continues after development well through adulthood.Growth arrest and DNA-damage-inducible, beta (GADD45b) is required for the demethylation of promoters of critical genes responsible for new-born neuron development such as brain-derived neurotrophic factor (BDNF) and Basic fibroblast growth factor (FGF2). As such, upregulation of GADD45b leads to increased demethylation, increased BDNF and FGF2, and ultimately more neural progenitor cells.

Histone Modification

Histone deacetylation also plays a large role in the proliferation and self-renewal of post-natal neural stem cells. Neural-expressed HDACs interact with *Tlx*, an essential neural stem cell regulator, to suppress TLX target genes. This includes the cyclin-dependent kinase inhibitor P21 and the tumor suppressor gene *Pten* to promote neural stem cell proliferation. Inhibition of HDACS by the antiepileptic drug valproic acid induces neuronal differentiation as in embryonic neurogenesis, but also inhibits glial cell differentiation of adult neural stem cells. This is likely mediated through upregulation of neuronal specific genes such as the neurogeneic basic helix-loop-helix transcription factors NEUROD, NEUROGENENIN1, and Math1. Conditional loss of HDAC1 and HDAC2 in neural progenitor cells prevented them from differentiating into neurons and their loss in oligodendrytic progenitor cells disrupted oligodendrocyte formations, suggesting that histone deacetlyation plays important but varying roles in different stages of neuronal development.

miRNAs

miR-9 targets the nuclear receptor TLX in adult neurogenesis to promote neural differentiation and inhibit neural stem cell proliferation. It also influences neuronal subtype specification and regulates axonal growth, branching, and targeting in the central nervous system through interactions with HES1, a neural stem cell homeostasis molecule. miR-124 promotes cell cycle exit and neuronal differentiation in adult neurogensis. Mouse studies have shown that ectopic expression of miR-124 showed premature neural progenitor cell differentiation and exhaustion in the subventricular zone.

In Memory

Histone acetylation has a dynamic role in controlling memory formation and synaptic plasticity. HDAC inhibitors exhibited positive effects on mice with cognitive defects such as Alzheimers disease and improved the cognition of wild type mice. HDAC2 has been shown to play a negative role in memory and learning. Sirt1, a histone acetylase, reduces memory formation ability by promoting the expression of miR-134, which targets the critical activity-dependent transcription factor (CREB) essential for learning and memory.

The Growth Arrest and DNA Damage inducible 45 (Gadd45) gene family plays a large role in the hippocampus. Gadd45 facilitates hippocampal long-term potentiation and enhances persisting memory for motor performance, aversive conditioning, and spatial navigation. Additionally, DNA methylation has been shown to be important for activity-dependent modulation of adult neurogenesis in the hippocampus, which is mediated by GADD45b. GADD45b seems to act as a sensor in mature neurons for environmental changes which it expresses through these methylation changes. This was determined by examining the effects of applying an electric stimulus to the hippocampal dentate gyrus (DG) in normal and GADD45b knockout mice. In normal mice application of electrical stimulation to the DG increased neurogenesis by increasing BDNF. However, in GADD45b deficient mice the electrical stimulus had less of an effect. Further examination revealed that around 1.4% of CpG islands in DG neurons are actively methylated and demthylated upon electric shock. This shows that the post-mitotic methylation states of neurons are not static and given that electric shock equipment such as that used in the study has been shown to have therapeutic effects to human patients with depression and other psychiatric disorders, the possibility remains that epigenetic mechanisms may play an important role in the pathophysiology of neuropsychiatric disorders. DNMT1 and DNMT3a are both required in conjunction for learning, memory, and synaptic plasticity.

Epigenetic Misregulation & Neurological Disorders

Alterations on epigenomic machinery cause DNA methylation and Histone acetylation processes to go rogue, leading to alterations on the transcriptional level of genes involved in the pathogenesis of neural degenerative diseases such as Parkinsons Disease, Alzheimer›s Disease, Schizophrenia, and Bipolar Disease.

Alzheimer's Disease

MicroRNA expression is critical for neurogenesis. In patients with Alzheimer's disease miR-9 and miR-128 is upregulated, while miR-15a is downregulated. Alzheimer's patients also show decreases in brain-derived neurotrophic factor, which has been shown to be repressed through DNA methylation.Although what has been argued as the most evidence for epigenetic influence in Alzheimer's is the gene which controls the protein responsible for amyloid plaque formation, *App*. This gene has very high GC content in its promoter region, meaning that it is highly susceptible to DNA methylation. This promoter site has been shown to naturally reduce methylation with aging, exemplifying the parallels between aging and Alzheimer's already well known. Heavy metals also seem to interfere with epigenetic mechanisms. Specifically in the case of APP, lead exposure earlier in life has been shown to cause a marked over-expression of the APP protein, leading to more amalyoid plaque later in life in the aging brain.

DNA methylation's age relation has been further investigated in the promoter regions of several Alzheimer's related genes in the brains of postmortem late-onset Alzheimer's disease patients. The older patients seem to have more abnormal epigenetic machinery than the younger patients, despite the fact that both had died from Alzheimers. Though this in of itself is not conclusive evidence of anything, it has led to an age-related epigenetic drift theory where abnormalities in epigenetic machinery and exposure to certain environmental factors which occur earlier in life lead to aberrant DNA methylation patterns far later, contributing to sporadic Alzheimer's Disease predisposition.

Histone modifications may also have an impact in Alzheimer›s disease, but the differences between HDAC effects in rodent brains compared to human brains have researchers puzzled. As the focus for neurodegenerative diseases begins to shift towards epigenetic pharmacology, it can be expected that the interactions of histone modifications with respect to neurogenesis will become more clear.

REFERENCES

1. Horvath, S (2013). DNA methylation age of human tissues and cell types. Genome Biology. 2013 (14): R115. doi:10.1186/gb-2013-14-10-r115. PMC 4015143. PMID 24138928.
2. Horvath, S (2015). Erratum to: DNA methylation age of human tissues and cell types. Genome Biology. 16 (1): 96. doi:10.1186/s13059-015-0649-6. PMID 25968125.
3. University of California, Los Angeles (UCLA), Health Sciences (20 October 2013). Scientist uncovers internal clock able to measure age of most human tissues; Women›s breast tissue ages faster than rest of body. ScienceDaily. Retrieved 22 October 2013.
4. University of California, Los Angeles (UCLA), Health Sciences (21 October 2013). Scientists discover new biological clock with age-measuring potential. Forbes. Retrieved 21 October 2013.
5. Berdyshev, G; Korotaev, G; Boiarskikh, G; Vaniushin, B (1967). Nucleotide composition of DNA and RNA from somatic tissues of humpback and its changes during spawning. Biokhimiia. 31: 88–993.
6. Rakyan, VK; Down, TA; Maslau, S; Andrew, T; Yang, TP; Beyan, H; Whittaker, P; McCann, OT; Finer, S; Valdes, AM; Leslie, RD; Deloukas, P; Spector, TD (2010). Human aging-associated DNA hypermethylation occurs preferentially at bivalent chromatin domains. Genome Res. 20: 434–439. doi:10.1101/gr.103101.109.
7. Teschendorff, AE; Menon, U; Gentry-Maharaj, A; Ramus, SJ; Weisenberger, DJ; Shen, H; Campan, M; Noushmehr, H; Bell, CG; Maxwell, AP; Savage, DA; Mueller-Holzner, E; Marth, C; Kocjan, G; Gayther, SA; Jones, A; Beck, S; Wagner, W; Laird, PW; Jacobs, IJ; Widschwendter, M (2010). Age-dependent DNA methylation of genes that are suppressed in stem cells is a hallmark of cancer. Genome Res. 20: 440–446. doi:10.1101/gr.103606.109.

8. Koch, CM; Wagner, W (Oct 2011). Epigenetic-aging-signature to determine age in different tissues. Aging. 3 (10): 1018–27.

9. Horvath, S; Zhang, Y; Langfelder, P; Kahn, R; Boks, M; van Eijk, K; van den Berg, L; Ophoff, RA (2012). Aging effects on DNA methylation modules in human brain and blood tissue. Genome Biol. 13 (10): R97. doi:10.1186/gb-2012-13-10-r97. PMID 23034122.

10. Bell, JT; Tsai, PC; Yang, TP; Pidsley, R; Nisbet, J; Glass, D; Mangino, M; Zhai, G; Zhang, F; Valdes, A; Shin, SY; Dempster, EL; Murray, RM; Grundberg, E; Hedman, AK; Nica, A; Small, KS; Dermitzakis, ET; McCarthy, MI; Mill, J; Spector, TD; Deloukas, P (2012). Epigenome-wide scans identify differentially methylated regions for age and age-related phenotypes in a healthy ageing population. PLoS Genet. 8: e1002629. doi:10.1371/journal.pgen.1002629.

11. Bocklandt, S; Lin, W; Sehl, ME; Sánchez, FJ; Sinsheimer, JS; Horvath, S; Vilain, E (2011). Epigenetic Predictor of Age. PLoS ONE. 6 (6): e14821. doi:10.1371/journal.pone.0014821. PMC 3120753. PMID 21731603.

12. ^ Jump up to:[a] [b] Hannum, G; Guinney, J; Zhao, L; Zhang, L; Hughes, G; Sadda, S; Klotzle, B; Bibikova, M; Fan, JB; Gao, Y; Deconde, R; Chen, M; Rajapakse, I; Friend, S; Ideker, T; Zhang, K (2013). Genome-wide methylation profiles reveal quantitative views of human aging rates. Mol Cell. 49: 359–367. doi:10.1016/j.molcel.2012.10.016. PMID 23177740.

13. Biome on 21st October 2013 Novel epigenetic clock predicts tissue age

14. Gibbs, WT (2014). Biomarkers and ageing: The clock-watcher. Nature. 508: 168–170. doi:10.1038/508168a.

15. Chen, B; Marioni, ME (2016). "DNA methylation-based measures of biological age: meta-analysis predicting time to death.". Aging (US Albany). 8 (9): 1844–1865. doi:10.18632/aging.101020. PMC 5076441. PMID 27690265.

16. Marioni, R; Shah, S; McRae, A; Chen, B; Colicino, E; Harris, S; Gibson, J; Henders, A; Redmond, P; Cox, S; Pattie, A; Corley, J; Murphy, L; Martin, N; Montgomery, G; Feinberg, A; Fallin, M; Multhaup, M; Jaffe, A; Joehanes, R; Schwartz, J; Just, A; Lunetta, K; Murabito, JM; Starr, J; Horvath, S; Baccarelli, A; Levy, D; Visscher, P; Wray, N; Deary, I (2015). DNA methylation age of blood predicts all-cause mortality in later life. Genome Biology. 16 (1): 25. doi:10.1186/s13059-015-0584-6.

17. Christiansen, L (2015). DNA methylation age is associated with mortality in a longitudinal Danish twin study. Aging Cell. 15 (1): 149–154. doi:10.1111/acel.12421. PMC 4717264. PMID 26594032.

18. Horvath, S (2015). Decreased epigenetic age of PBMCs from Italian semi-supercentenarians and their offspring.. Aging (Albany NY) (Dec).

19. Marioni, R; Shah, S; McRae, A; Ritchie, S; Muniz-Terrera, GH; SE; Gibson, J; Redmond, P; SR, C; Pattie, A; Corley, J; Taylor, A; Murphy, L; Starr, J; Horvath, S; Visscher, P; Wray, N; Deary, I (2015). The epigenetic clock is correlated with physical and cognitive fitness in the Lothian Birth Cohort 1936. Int J of Epidemiology. 44: 1388–1396. doi:10.1093/ije/dyu277. PMID 25617346.

20. DNA methylation age software
21. Collado, M; Blasco, MA; Serrano, M (Jul 2007). Cellular senescence in cancer and aging. Cell. 130 (2): 223–33. doi:10.1016/j.cell.2007.07.003.
22. Forster P, Hohoff C, Dunkelmann B, Schürenkamp M, Pfeiffer H, Neuhuber F, Brinkmann B. (2015) Elevated germline mutation rate in teenage fathers. Proc Biol Sci 282:20142898
23. Nordfjäll, K; Svenson, U; Norrback, KF; Adolfsson, R; Roos, G (Mar 2010). Large-scale parent-child comparison confirms a strong paternal influence on telomere length. Eur J Hum Genet. 18 (3): 385–9. doi:10.1038/ejhg.2009.178. PMID 19826452.
24. Wang, Y; Zang, X; Wang, Y; Chen, P (2012). High expression of p16INK4a and low expression of Bmi1 are associated with endothelial cellular senescence in the human cornea (PDF). Molecular Vision. 18: 803–815.
25. Levine, M (2015). "Epigenetic age of the pre-frontal cortex is associated with neuritic plaques, amyloid load, and Alzheimer's disease related cognitive functioning". Aging (Albany NY). 7 (Dec): 1198–211. PMC 4712342. PMID 26684672.
26. Lu, A (2016). Genetic variants near MLST8 and DHX57 affect the epigenetic age of the cerebellum.. Nature Communications. 7: 10561. doi:10.1038/ncomms10561.
27. Levine, M (2015). DNA methylation age of blood predicts future onset of lung cancer in the women›s health initiative.. Aging (Albany NY). 7: 690–700. doi:10.18632/aging.100809. PMC 4600626. PMID 26411804.
28. Horvath, S; Erhart, W; Brosch, M; Ammerpohl, O; von Schoenfels, W; Ahrens, M; Heits, N; Bell, JT; Tsai, PC; Spector, TD; Deloukas, P; Siebert, R; Sipos, B; Becker, T; Roecken, C; Schafmayer, C; Hampe, J (2014). Obesity accelerates epigenetic aging of human liver. Proc Natl Acad Sci U S A. 111: 15538–43. doi:10.1073/pnas.1412759111. PMID 25313081.
29. Horvath, S; Garagnani, P; Bacalini, MG; Pirazzini, C; Salvioli, S; Gentilini, D; Di Blasio, AM; Giuliani, C; Tung, S; Vinters, HV; Franceschi, C (Feb 2015). Accelerated epigenetic aging in Down syndrome. Aging Cell. 14: 491–5. doi:10.1111/acel.12325. PMID 25678027.
30. Horvath, S; Mah, V; Lu, AT; Woo, JS; Choi, OW; Jasinska, AJ; Riancho, JA; Tung, S; Coles, NS; Braun, J; Vinters, HV; Coles, LS (2015). "The cerebellum ages slowly according to the epigenetic clock" (PDF). Aging (Albany NY). 7 (5): 294–306. doi:10.18632/aging.100742. PMID 26000617.
31. Horvath, S (2016). Huntington›s disease accelerates epigenetic aging of human brain and disrupts DNA methylation levels. Aging (Albany NY). 8 (7): 1485–512. doi:10.18632/aging.101005. PMC 4993344. PMID 27479945.
32. Horvath, S; Levine, AJ (2015). HIV-1 infection accelerates age according to the epigenetic clock. J Infect Dis. 212: 1563–73. doi:10.1093/infdis/jiv277. PMID 25969563.

33. Horvath, S (2015). Increased epigenetic age and granulocyte counts in the blood of Parkinson›s disease patients.. Aging (Albany NY). 7: 1130–42. doi:10.18632/aging.100859. PMC 4712337. PMID 26655927.
34. Walker, RF; Liu, JS; Peters, BA; Ritz, BR; Wu, T; Ophoff, RA; Horvath, S (2015). Epigenetic age analysis of children who seem to evade aging. Aging (Albany NY). 7 (5): 334–9. PMID 25991677.
35. Levine, M (2016). Menopause accelerates biological aging. Proc Natl Acad Sci USA. 113: 201604558. doi:10.1073/pnas.1604558113. PMID 27457926.
36. Lowe, D (2016). "Epigenetic clock analyses of cellular senescence and ageing.". Oncotarget. 7 (8): 8524–8531. doi:10.18632/oncotarget.7383. PMID 26885756.
37. Baker, DJ (2011). Clearance of p16Ink4a-positive senescent cells delays ageing-associated disorders.. Nature. 479 (7372): 232–6. doi:10.1038/nature10600. PMC 3468323. PMID 22048312.
38. ^ Jump up to:[a] [b] [c] Horvath S, Gurven M, Levine ME, Trumble BC, Kaplan H, Allayee H, Ritz BR, Chen B, Lu AT, Rickabaugh TM, Jamieson BD, Sun D, Li S, Chen W, Quintana-Murci L, Fagny M, Kobor MS, Tsao PS, Reiner AP, Edlefsen KL, Absher D, Assimes TL (2016). An epigenetic clock analysis of race/ethnicity, sex, and coronary heart disease.. Genome Biol. 17 (1): 171. doi:10.1186/s13059-016-1030-0. PMC 4980791. PMID 27511193.
39. Vilenchik MM, Knudson AG (2003). Endogenous DNA double-strand breaks: production, fidelity of repair, and induction of cancer. Proc. Natl. Acad. Sci. U.S.A. 100 (22): 12871–6. doi:10.1073/pnas.2135498100. PMC 240711. PMID 14566050.
40. Cuozzo C, Porcellini A, Angrisano T, Morano A, Lee B, Di Pardo A, Messina S, Iuliano R, Fusco A, Santillo MR, Muller MT, Chiariotti L, Gottesman ME, Avvedimento EV (2007). DNA damage, homology-directed repair, and DNA methylation. PLoS Genet. 3 (7): e110. doi:10.1371/journal.pgen.0030110. PMC 1913100. PMID 17616978.
41. O›Hagan HM, Mohammad HP, Baylin SB (2008). Double strand breaks can initiate gene silencing and SIRT1-dependent onset of DNA methylation in an exogenous promoter CpG island. PLoS Genet. 4 (8): e1000155. doi:10.1371/journal.pgen.1000155. PMC 2491723. PMID 18704159.
42. Morano A, Angrisano T, Russo G, Landi R, Pezone A, Bartollino S, Zuchegna C, Babbio F, Bonapace IM, Allen B, Muller MT, Chiariotti L, Gottesman ME, Porcellini A, Avvedimento EV (2014). Targeted DNA methylation by homology-directed repair in mammalian cells. Transcription reshapes methylation on the repaired gene. Nucleic Acids Res. 42 (2): 804–21. doi:10.1093/nar/gkt920. PMC 3902918. PMID 24137009.
43. Ding N, Bonham EM, Hannon BE, Amick TR, Baylin SB, O›Hagan HM (2016). Mismatch repair proteins recruit DNA methyltransferase 1 to sites of oxidative DNA damage. J Mol Cell Biol. 8 (3): 244–54. doi:10.1093/jmcb/mjv050. PMID 26186941. free version at http://jmcb.oxfordjournals.org/content/early/2015/08/06/jmcb.mjv050

44. Weidner, C. I.; Lin, Q.; Koch, C. M.; Eisele, L.; Beier, F.; Ziegler, P.; Wagner, W. (2014). Aging of blood can be tracked by DNA methylation changes at just three CpG sites. Genome Biology. 15 (2): R24. doi:10.1186/gb-2014-15-2-r24. PMID 24490752.

45. Horvath S (2014-02-18 16:34) Comparison with the epigenetic clock (2014). Reader Comment.

46. Wagner W (2014) Response to comment comparison with the epigenetic clock by Horvath 2013

47. Horvath S (2013-11-04 11:00) Erratum in cancer tissues Reader Comment

48. Genome-wide methylation profiles reveal quantitative views of human aging rates.. Mol Cell. 49: 359–67. Jan 2013. doi:10.1016/j.molcel.2012.10.016. PMID 23177740.

49. Aging of blood can be tracked by DNA methylation changes at just three CpG sites.. Genome Biol. 15: R24. 2014. doi:10.1186/gb-2014-15-2-r24. PMID 24490752.

50. Giuliani, C.; Cilli, E.; Bacalini, M. G.; Pirazzini, C.; Sazzini, M.; Gruppioni, G.; Franceschi, C.; Garagnani, P.; Luiselli, D. (2016). Inferring chronological age from DNA methylation patterns of human teeth. Am. J. Phys. Anthropol. 159: 585–595. doi:10.1002/ajpa.22921.

51. Christoph Bock et al. (2016). Quantitative comparison of DNA methylation assays for biomarker development and clinical applications. Nature Biotechnology, doi:10.1038/nbt.3605

Index